VisualDx: Essential Pediatric Dermatology

VisualDx: Essential Pediatric Dermatology

SENIOR EDITORS:

Craig N. Burkhart, MD

Assistant Professor of Dermatology
Department of Dermatology
University of North Carolina-Chapel Hill
Chapel Hill, North Carolina

Dean S. Morrell, MD

Associate Professor of Dermatology
Department of Dermatology
University of North Carolina-Chapel Hill
Chapel Hill, North Carolina

ASSOCIATE EDITORS:

Lowell A. Goldsmith, MD, MPH

Dean Emeritus
University of Rochester School of Medicine and Dentistry
Rochester, New York
Professor of Dermatology
University of North Carolina-Chapel Hill
Chapel Hill, North Carolina

Art Papier, MD

Associate Professor of Dermatology
University of Rochester School of Medicine and Dentistry

ASSISTANT EDITORS:

Brian Green, DO, MS

Resident in Dermatology
University of North Carolina-Chapel Hill
Chapel Hill, North Carolina

David Dasher, MD

Resident in Dermatology
University of North Carolina-Chapel Hill
Chapel Hill, North Carolina

Sethuraman Gomathy, MD, MNAMS

Associate Professor
Department of Dermatology
All India Institute of Medical Sciences, New Delhi, India

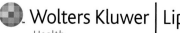 **Wolters Kluwer** | **Lippincott Williams & Wilkins**
Health

Philadelphia • Baltimore • New York • London
Buenos Aires • Hong Kong • Sydney • Tokyo

Acquisitions Editor: Sonya Seigafuse
Product Managers: Kerry Barrett/Nicole Walz
Vendor Manager: Alicia Jackson
Senior Manufacturing Manager: Benjamin Rivera
Marketing Manager: Kimberly Schonberger
Design Coordinator: Terry Mallon
Production Service: SPi Technologies

Printed in China.

ISBN-13: 978-1-6054-7770-1
ISBN-10: 1-60547-770-2
Cataloging-in-Publication Data available upon request

Care has been taken to confirm the accuracy of the information presented and to describe generally accepted practices. However, the authors, editors, and publisher are not responsible for errors or omissions or for any consequences from application of the information in this book and make no warranty, expressed or implied, with respect to the currency, completeness, or accuracy of the contents of the publication. Application of the information in a particular situation remains the professional responsibility of the practitioner.

The authors, editors, and publisher have exerted every effort to ensure that drug selection and dosage set forth in this text are in accordance with current recommendations and practice at the time of publication. However, in view of ongoing research, changes in government regulations, and the constant flow of information relating to drug therapy and drug reactions, the reader is urged to check the package insert for each drug for any change in indications and dosage and for added warnings and precautions. This is particularly important when the recommended agent is a new or infrequently employed drug.

Some drugs and medical devices presented in the publication have Food and Drug Administration (FDA) clearance for limited use in restricted research settings. It is the responsibility of the health care provider to ascertain the FDA status of each drug or device planned for use in their clinical practice.

To purchase additional copies of this book, call our customer service department at (800) 638-3030 or fax orders to (301) 223-2320. International customers should call (301) 223-2300.

Visit Lippincott Williams & Wilkins on the Internet: at LWW.com. Lippincott Williams & Wilkins customer service representatives are available from 8:30 am to 6 pm, EST.

10 9 8 7 6 5 4 3 2 1

Dr. Green's work as author was performed outside the scope of his employment as a US government employee. This work represents his personal and professional views and not necessarily those of the US government.

Dedication

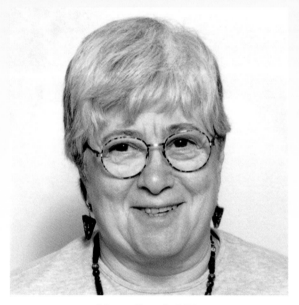

Nancy Esterly, MD

This book is dedicated to Nancy Esterly, MD, a true doyen of pediatric dermatology. She was one of a handful of physicians who specialized in this ever-enlarging and very important subspecialty of dermatology. In addition to her own scientific and clinical contributions, her role as a trainer of a cohort of academic pediatric dermatologists has been an important contribution to both dermatology and pediatrics.

Board certified in both dermatology and pediatrics, Dr. Esterly established the first pediatric dermatology fellowship in the United States at Children's Memorial Hospital in Chicago, Illinois. She has received numerous awards from the American Academy of Pediatrics, the Dermatology Foundation, the Society for Pediatric Dermatology, and the Society for Investigative Dermatology. She is a widely published author—her works include such respected textbooks as the *Textbook of Neonatal Dermatology* and the *Handbook of Genetic Skin Disorders*—and was the founding editor of the journal *Pediatric Dermatology*.

Dr. Esterly is a meticulous photographer who donated her clinical images to Logical Images, where they are the basis of pediatric and neonatal disease sections in VisualDx. In this book, her clinical photographs are an essential part of the illustrative materials.

We are highly indebted to Dr. Esterly for the images used in this book and for her considerable contributions to medical knowledge, patient care, and the careers of those in pediatric dermatology.

Table of Contents

Foreword

The authors of this text show they love books and that books have a central place in skin care and skin education, even with all the new ways to access information available today. Every book has a history, and this book has a long pedigree. *Dermatologic Differential Diagnosis* (Year Book Medical Publishers, 1962) by Thomas B. Fitzpatrick and Sheldon A. Walker contained tables of morphological characteristics organized into diagnostic lists using the classical dermatologic terms fashioned in the 18th and 19th centuries. That "field guide," as described by its authors, was well-known to us (Jerry Lazarus and Lowell Goldsmith, the series editor) during our residency training. The "field guide" approach led to our book, *Diagnosis of Skin Disease* in 1980 and then *Adult and Pediatric Dermatology: A Color Guide to Diagnosis and Treatment* when we were joined by Michael Tharp in 1997. The *essential* books are the next logical step in the evolution of skin disease diagnosis and treatment.

VisualDx: Essential Pediatric Dermatology has outstanding color pictures illustrating the pediatric diseases critical for any diagnostic text. Having separate essential books for pediatric and adult diseases is an excellent strategy because the practitioners for these age groups are often different. Lowell and his colleagues followed changes in computer and imaging technology, and VisualDx, an online clinical decision support system allowing diagnosis and education, was developed. The VisualDx system builds upon the morphologic-driven differential diagnosis lists of *Fitzpatrick's Dermatology in General Medicine* and allows simultaneous online searching across multiple morphologic and patient characteristics. The VisualDx system displays the full spectrum of disease variation, complementing the *essential* textbooks. The VisualDx system has been created and refined by a medical informatics team led by dermatologist Art Papier, trained in Rochester, and a technical team led by Bill Haake at Logical Images.

This current book, *VisualDx: Essential Pediatric Dermatology*, connects learning and using the dermatology fundamentals with a highly crafted text that seamlessly interfaces with a Web-based system. This project provides the best of both the printed page and the online medical-information world and is a model for similar publications. The Lippincott Williams & Wilkins team headed by Kerry Barrett helped the authors produce a book like none other for the 21st century.

Gerald S. Lazarus, MD
Professor of Dermatology
Johns Hopkins University School of Medicine
Dean and CEO Emeritus
University of California, Davis Medical Center

Harzell Professor Emeritus and Chair—
Emeritus of Dermatology
University of Pennsylvania

James L. Callaway Professor Emeritus and
Chief Division of Dermatology
Duke University Medical Center

Preface

VisualDx: *Essential Pediatric Dermatology* is a foundation textbook for diagnosing and managing common and serious pediatric skin diseases. The authors of this text are practicing pediatric dermatologists who have seen thousands of children with common, rare, and very unusual skin diseases at the University of North Carolina, Northwestern University, and the Medical College of Wisconsin. In addition to knowledge that can be referenced, it is the combined experience of the editors that brings special value to this book for practicing clinicians, those who see children with skin disease either very frequently or infrequently, and especially those who see patients with severe and challenging skin diseases. The chapters emphasize important details that are not often discussed in many other texts: approach to the patient, office-based diagnostic and biopsy procedures, and details of therapy, the latter of which is summarized in a special therapy chapter. Special diagnostic issues that may be present in the skin of heavily pigmented patients or immunosuppressed patients are also clearly addressed. This is a modern textbook that is in touch with newer ways of learning and using information.

Visualdx: Essential Pediatric Dermatology has a complementary intrinsic diagnostic system and online decision support resource, and more than 500 images in the book are further served by thousands of online images and extensive references for each condition. This differentiates this text and series from those with images and text online. In addition to functionality that allows searching for a differential diagnosis and therapeutic information by diagnosis, online point-of-care tools are also organized by problems and symptoms. Material can be printed from the online source to distribute to the parents of the pediatric patients. Further, the online system has training modules that allow the user to be a better user of the book and the online data.

As educators and clinicians, we aim to be at the forefront of developments combining the best features of all media for education and patient care. Lippincott Williams & Wilkins is an enthusiastic partner with us in these endeavors.

Art Papier, MD
Lowell A. Goldsmith, MD, MPH
Craig N. Burkhart, MD
Dean S. Morrell, MD

Acknowledgments

The majority of the photographs in this book are part of a collection of pediatric dermatology conditions taken by Dr. Nancy Esterly during her outstanding career as a clinician and educator that have been contributed to Logical Images. Other photographs are from institutions that have donated clinician photographs to Logical Images, which include the slide collections of the Departments of Dermatology at New York University and the School of Medicine and Dentistry of the University of Rochester and their editors and authors. Additional image contributors include Karen Wiss, MD; Charles Crutchfield III, MD; Tor Shwayder, MD, FAAP, FAAD; Victor D. Newcomer, MD; Elaine Siegfried, MD; Stephen Estes, MD; Robert Chalmers, MD, MRCP, FRCP; Noah Craft, MD, PhD, DTM&H; and David Elpern, MD. Additional contributions to the content were made by Cynthia Christy, MD; Sheila Galbraith, MD; Lynn Garfunkel, MD; Karen McKoy, MD; Sarah Stein, MD; and Karen Wiss, MD.

All the authors and editors are grateful for the meticulous care that Frances Reed gave to the preparation and redaction of the text and the precision and professional skill with which Heidi Halton prepared the large number of clinical photographs for this text. Kerry Barrett from Lippincott Williams & Wilkins helped make this complex project a reality.

Introduction to the VisualDx Essential Dermatology Series

Welcome to the VisualDx Essential Dermatology Series. The goal of the series is to assist you in making the diagnosis and planning for the treatment of the most common skin disorders you will encounter in your daily clinical practice.

With *VisualDx: Essential Pediatric Dermatology*, you have two stand-alone and complementary products:

1. Book: The book contains an approach to pediatric patients, techniques of diagnosis and laboratory testing, a special approach leading you to the correct diagnosis and differential diagnosis, and four-color figures showing the clinical variation of the condition. The book is designed for quick use while the patient is still in your office.

   Each disease or set of related diseases has special sections of text on the diagnostic criteria, skin characteristics, best laboratory tests, differential diagnosis, and special characteristics of the condition in immunocompromised patients and those with darker skin colors and treatments.

2. Website access includes:
   - Online searching of more than 20 morphological characteristics of the skin lesion, the general health of the patient, onset of the disease, disease distribution, and signs and symptoms in other organ systems.
   - A module which allows for a rapid, accurate diagnosis of rashes.
   - Clickable printouts of patient information sheets.
   - An exhaustive image bank for study of a disorder that can be downloaded for presentations.

We certainly hope that this product will be useful to you and the patients you care for.

Please look for other titles in the VisualDx: Essential Dermatology Series.

Introduction: VisualDx: Essential Pediatric Dermatology Online

To use the chapter, go to www.essentialdermatology.com and register using the code found in the front of this book.

VisualDx is a diagnostic clinical decision support system that integrates search, imagery, and text in an easy-to-use Web browser-based system. VisualDx allows you to simultaneously "look up" information by multiple parameters rather than by a single index term, as found in print-based resources. It is important to know that online VisualDx is note based on a simple search of this textbook or a search of text in an online database. Our authors and editors have reviewed the medical literature and created a search technology that allows you, the user, to search by patient findings. Through organization by patient characteristics such as symptoms, signs, visual clues, laboratory, etc., you will receive highly relevant information results. This distinction is important: When using a search engine such as Google or Yahoo, one is searching millions of pages of text; in decision support systems such as VisualDx, you do not experience the randomness of millions of pages of search and results; you are searching purposefully designed medical relationships derived from the medical literature. The search results are more accurate, easier to read, and more comprehensive from the point of view of clinical differential diagnosis. And the process takes much less time than it took to read this paragraph! Investigate this distinction and prove it for yourself:

1. Open an Internet search engine or a medical electronic resource.
2. Type the following search terms into the search box: neonate, toxic, pustules, and widespread.
3. View the results.

Now log in to VisualDx via www.essentialdermatology.com:

1. Once registered and logged in to VisualDx, follow the choice/path for building a differential diagnosis. Enter by age and the other characteristics of a widespread location/distribution (Fig. 1) and lesion morphology of pustule (Fig. 2).

Compare the results of the information display optimized for medical diagnosis (Fig. 3) with those from a generic search engine or medical reference system organized by diagnosis, and you will immediately recognize the difference between search engines that search text and a clinical decision support system designed to search structured relationships between findings and diagnoses.

In addition to a structured search of medical findings-to-diagnosis relationships, the VisualDx interface is optimized to display images prominently. The information task our engineers are addressing is best summarized by the question, "What am I looking at?" To address this universal information need for the health care professional, we have designed the VisualDx interface around pictures, diagrams, and graphics. This allows the search by findings to result in a visual differential diagnosis. The near-limitless ability to electronically access pictures means that our authors can go beyond displaying the "classic" examples of disease. Online VisualDx presents the typical *and* the common—and even very unusual—variants (Figs. 4–6). The computer interface has a

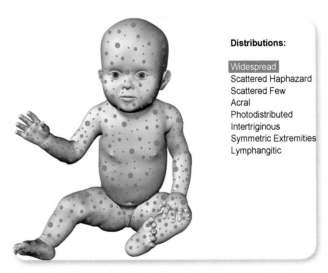

Distributions:

Widespread
Scattered Haphazard
Scattered Few
Acral
Photodistributed
Intertriginous
Symmetric Extremities
Lymphangitic

Figure 1 A widespread distribution selected for neonate/infant.

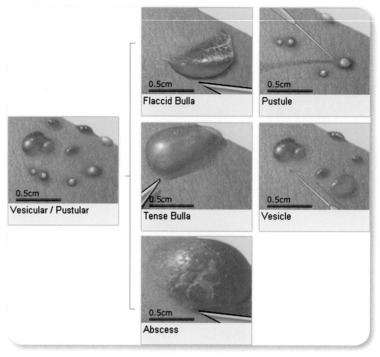

Figure 2 Vesicular/pustular lesion morphology and its subtypes, including pustule.

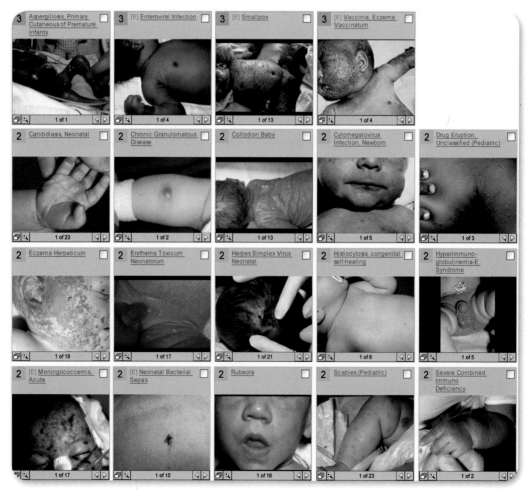

Figure 3 As findings are entered, VisualDx returns a visual differential diagnosis organized by the diagnoses with most matched findings.

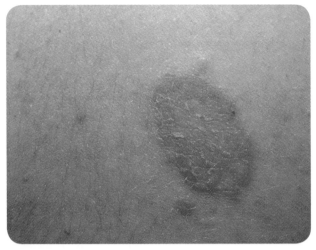

Figure 4 Variation in pityriasis rosea. In light skin, a "classic" oval erythematous, scaly herald plaque.

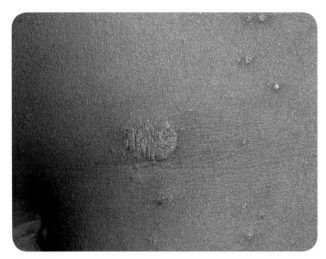

Figure 5 Variation in pityriasis rosea. In dark skin, small papules are common as well as the more typical scaly plaques.

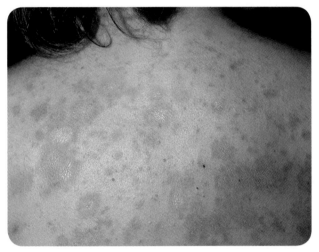

Figure 6 Variation in pityriasis rosea. In light skin, classic morphology with thin, scaly, salmon-colored plaques; however, this child does not have a "Christmas tree" pattern to the lesions, which is often cited as a clue to this diagnosis.

unique "stacking" of each diagnosis thumbnail that is dependent on the entered morphology search term; the picture variants resort within the stacks to match the morphology you search. This means that, in addition to the differential diagnosis created by your patient factors, VisualDx will also display extra relevant image examples. Moreover, while this textbook is typically limited to four images per disease, VisualDx has thousands of pictures. The images are organized by your search entry and displayed in uniform color and standard size.

Use VisualDx at www.essentialdermatology.com to

- Develop a differential diagnosis using the data from the actual patients being examined. This process fulfills practice-based learning goals and allows more comprehensive and relevant differential diagnoses as you work.
- If you have an exam room computer, log in and bookmark VisualDx so that you can quickly search for images to use them for patient education and reassurance. There is nothing like a picture to reassure a parent of a patient that a rash is common and there is no worry.
- Use the LearnDerm link for interactive training in dermatology exam, morphology, and disease variation.
- Review many more diagnoses and pictures.

CHAPTER 1

Approach to the Pediatric Dermatology Patient

History

What does the approach to the patient have to do with the prevention, diagnosis, and treatment of skin diseases? Everything. Before the care provider, physician, nurse, or physician's assistant enters the patient's room, both the provider and the patient are being influenced by social changes that are the challenge of our generation of physicians (with the word *physician* being the placeholder for the constellation of health care workers involved in patient care). In all of medicine, including dermatology, the traditional roles of the patient and the physician are rapidly changing and are being challenged at many levels: the legal system, including malpractice; the public's interest in autonomy in decision making; medical advertising by physicians and pharmaceutical companies directed at the public; and the availability of large amounts of undigested medical information via the Internet.

Before seeing the doctor, patients have a personal version of their skin condition—when and how it began, what helped it, what did not help it, and what the condition means to themselves and their family. Children, and those not able to care for themselves, have their personal views on their condition, as does their caretaker. Thus, in addition to the purely medical history of the condition, these other—sometimes conflicting—versions of the disease exist. Today, all of this detail is embellished with information from both respected medical sites and marketing sites on the Internet.

History taking in dermatology serves more than one purpose: the process gathers information that is focused and deeper than the notes the patient may bring, it supplements the often incomplete and unreadable notes from other physicians, and it is the substrate for the relationship between the physician and the patient. This first interaction portends the relationship between the patient and the physician. The most useful histories are supplemented by information from the physical examination, and, in a follow-up, information from laboratory tests and biopsies. Information that may seem extraneous for the patient is still very valuable, as it suggests the mindset of the patient and his or her approach to following therapeutic plans. The best histories are taken when the physician is considering a variety of conditions and asking insightful questions.

Obtaining a history may be especially challenging when the patient's native language is not one the physician can speak, or the patient communicates with sign language, or when ethnic or religious reasons prevent full frankness of discussion. Social and occupational histories, focused family history, and a noncutaneous medical history are more than niceties; they establish the full and rich substrate for the physician–patient relations. This may seem an archaic approach for the time-challenged physician but remains an essential part of exemplary patient care. At the end of the history, through thoughtful questions, the physician should have established in the patient's mind that the medical encounter is proceeding successfully, that he or she is a very competent professional, and that the patient will be part of the short- and long-term solutions to the matters at hand.

The patient has thought extensively about the history and there may be some questions the physician asked that the patient had not considered, but the physical exam is where the special skills of the physician come to the fore. Thoroughness establishes the physician as the consummate professional and expert. Looking in the mouth and between the toes, carefully parting the hair to examine the scalp, and inspecting all of the nails may not have been performed by previous examiners, and the patient will be positively impressed by the assiduous search for disease and etiology. Talking with the patient and explaining what you are observing makes the patient part of the process, and ultimately enlists him or her in the diagnostic, prevention, or treatment plans. Explaining the need for photographs, with the reassurance of confidentiality, is logically done at this stage. The physical examination is an intense and demanding process for the physician, who is both gathering and integrating historical and physical information and considering the need for further information. *Cognitive bias* is a term that is frequently used today to describe that the physicians see what they think should be rather than being a critical observer of what actually exists on the patient being examined. This bias can affect the student and even the sophisticated physician who is misled by a false "clue" from the history, a recent patient, or an article that was read just before seeing the patient. Lesions and diseases may be at a stage of their evolution where a diagnosis is not possible either histologically or clinically; this unsettling fact must be communicated to the patient with compassion and knowledge.

Biopsies and Laboratory Testing

Biopsy and laboratory tests are most useful when purposely performed to establish an important diagnosis. In many parts of the world, these tests may cost the patients, their insurers, or their governments more than visits to the physician. Significant judgment goes into the decision to do tests, especially when genetic testing is contemplated. If one individual with an autosomal dominant disease, such as epidermolytic hyperkeratosis, has a proven genomic K1 mutation, there is little or no justification in testing another affected individual in the same family. Similarly, in a patient with stable systemic lupus erythematosus, periodic antinuclear antibody titers serve no useful purpose. Classical psoriasis with multiple plaques covering 10% of the body or classical acanthosis nigricans in an obese adolescent is not an indication for a biopsy. The physician should discuss with the patient why a biopsy or any laboratory test will be performed.

Communication

Communication of biopsy and laboratory tests is important for continued patient rapport. This can be performed over the phone, but additional communication by letter or e-mail is useful, even if the patient is seen again. This completes the communication loop and is appreciated by the patient.

Communication of the physician's considerations of what is happening in the patient's skin, the diagnosis (e.g., will the condition be acute or chronic?), the prognosis, and what can be done for the disease in the patient (i.e., treatment) is what the patient carries away from the visit.

Patients and their parents would like certainty of diagnosis and treatment. The uncertainty that is intrinsic to many portions of medicine is more unsettling to the patient than the doctor. Clear communication of the diagnostic and therapeutic processes may allay some of the anxiety; any anxiety by the physician is readily perceived and can be magnified manyfold by the patient or parent. A physician's handling and communicating of his or her own anxiety is a learned skill.

Topical medicines with their multiple strengths and chemical entities, even among corticosteroids, are often confusing, and we can compare the various steroids to the strengths of a bicycle, a Honda, a Mercedes, and—when occlusion is used—a supercharged Mercedes. Patients remember this therapeutic ladder more than chemical names.

Children as Patients

In the skin care of children, there are special medical and social circumstances that must be addressed at all times for successful patient encounters. Several common skin diseases of children are rarely seen in adults, and even when the same disorder affects adults and children, it may have a very different distribution, intensity, and/or prognosis. After a diagnosis is made, the approach to therapy may be complicated by different therapeutic options, doses, and regimens. Lastly, the patient–doctor relationship is altered by the nearly universal presence of a parent during the provision of medical care. This creates the need to communicate and develop a relationship with both the child patient and the adult caregiver during the encounter.

Broad communication techniques for interacting with children and their families have recently and exhaustively been reviewed; the following three tables are derived from the useful article by Levetown and American Academy of Pediatrics Commitee on Bioethics.[1]

Strategies for Interacting with a Child

- Speak *with* the child, not *at* the child.
- Communicate in a private setting.
- Determine whom the child would like to be present during the interview.
- Begin with nonthreatening topics.
- Actively listen.
- Watch body language and pay attention to tone of voice.
- Utilize drawings, games, or other creative communication tools.
- Elicit fears and concerns by referencing one's self or a third party.

Strategies for Disclosing Bad News to Parents

- Avoid disclosing bad news over the telephone.
- For possibly very upsetting information, avoid telling a lone parent without a support person present.
- Hold or touch the affected child with obvious care.
- Recognize that parents have primary responsibility for their child.
- Show a caring and compassionate sense of connection with the patient and family.
- Pace the discussion to the emotional state of the parents.
- Avoid jargon.
- Ensure that parents do not blame themselves or others for the problem.
- Write out the name of the illness for the parents.
- Confirm effective transmission of information by asking the parents to use their own words to explain what you discussed.
- Address the implications to the future of the child.
- Acknowledge the parents' emotions and be prepared for tears and the need for time.

- Avoid being aloof or detached.
- Give parents time to integrate the information and formulate additional questions.
- Be able to recommend community-based resources, where appropriate.
- Arrange a follow-up plan and appointment for continued conversation.

Strategies for Approaching Diagnostic and Surgical Procedures

- Discuss in a private setting with both the family and the child.
- Use words and language the child and family can understand.
- Use visual aids.
- Provide information in a logical sequence.
- Be prepared to repeat information.
- Acknowledge emotional distress.
- Discuss indications, risks, benefits, and alternatives.
- Personalize the information.
- Avoid last-minute surprises.
- Ask parents and children to repeat what they understand and clarify as needed.

Sexual Abuse

Physical and sexual abuse can occur at any age and must be considered in disorders affecting the genitals and when the physical signs suggest an external etiology of the lesions.

Approach to Dealing with Potential Sexual Abuse[2,3]

- If there is any suspicion of sexual abuse, report it to the appropriate local child protective services agency.
- In general, the identification of any sexually transmissible agent in children beyond the neonatal period is suspicious for abuse.
- A positive test for *Chlamydia trachomatis*, gonorrhea, *Trichomonas vaginalis*, HIV, syphilis, or herpes is highly suspicious for sexual abuse.
- A full physical examination looking for signs of abuse should be performed on all children in whom sexual abuse is suspected.
- In children with symptoms suggestive of a sexually transmissible infection (STI), test for other common STIs before initiating treatment that may interfere with their diagnosis.
- If unsure whether to report, discuss the case with local child abuse consultants and/or a local child protective services agency.

References

1. Levetown M, American Academy of Pediatrics Committee on Bioethics. Communicating with children and families: From everyday interactions to skill in conveying distressing information. *Pediatrics.* 2008;121(5): e1441–e1460.

2. Workowski KA, Berman SM, Centers for Disease Control and Prevention. Sexually transmitted diseases treatment guidelines, 2006. *MMWR Recomm Rep.* 2006;55(RR-11):83–86.

3. Kellogg N, American Academy of Pediatrics Committee on Child Abuse and Neglect. The evaluation of sexual abuse in children. *Pediatrics.* 2005;116(2):506–512.

CHAPTER 2

Examination of the Skin

Examining the Skin

The Patient

It is best to first interact with the patient and then quickly acknowledge and identify the patient's support team. We prefer to have the adults identify their own relationship to the patient, as complications may ensue when you assume who the parents, grandparents, and other family members are. In addition to dealing with a potentially apprehensive child with unpredictable preparation/expectations, adult family members also have pre-existing expectations, concerns, and/or fears.

It is best to examine younger infants on a well-supported surface (examination table) with a parent at their side. For infants with good head control through approximately 2 years of age—approved by the parent—many physical examinations are successful on the lap of a parent with a seated clinician. If children are resistant to any type of examination, providing them with a choice can foster a successful and nontraumatic interaction. A statement such as, "We can look at your skin on the table or on your mother's lap" will often be more successful than an open-ended question such as, "Where should we look at you?"

Once the parent and child are prepared for the examination, it is more acceptable and less invasive to start with the fingers and nails. The children feel a soft touch to a safe zone. After establishing comfort and observing for nail-related findings, the examiner can work his or her way to the rest of the body, verbalizing where he or she is going in advance and what is being seen. Verbalizing your findings will allow the parent input, reassurance, and confidence in the clinical interaction and distracts the patient from potential fear.

The patient should completely undress for a comprehensive skin examination. Often, patients or parents ask the physician to examine a particular lesion or area of involved skin, and the physician focuses on the patient complaint without looking elsewhere. Looking at an isolated lesion without examining the patient completely, however, may lead to misdiagnosis or nondiagnosis of potentially serious lesions. Encourage your patient to disrobe completely and wear a gown by explaining how other clues or problems might be hidden on the back.

When performing a skin examination, the entire skin surface should be examined, including the scalp, oral cavity, genitals, and nails. Gloves are worn for examination of the genitals, intraoral palpation, and palpation of potentially infectious lesions that are moist, hemorrhagic, or crusted. Wearing gloves for the complete examination may cause the patient further embarrassment or self-consciousness. Gloves are not necessary unless there is a concern about infection.

Lighting

Good lighting, either artificial or natural, is essential for a good skin examination. Fixed or standing lighting frees both hands for examination or manipulation of lesions.

Oblique illumination (side lighting) of a slightly elevated papule confirms its raised character by the shadow it casts. This should be done in a dimly-lit or dark room (Fig. 2-1).

Intense light (e.g., the head of an ophthalmologic penlight) is used to transilluminate cystic lesions and reveal the homogeneity of the structure. Focused, intense light should not be used for the complete examination because it can wash out important details.

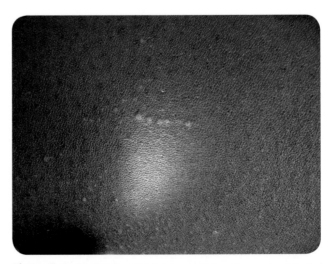

Figure 2-1 Side lighting. Faint degrees of elevation can be detected by side lighting, as seen in this side lighting of the tiny linear papules of lichen nitidus.

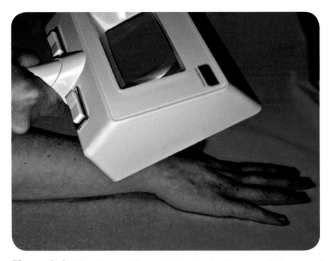

Figure 2-2 Wood lamp. After adapting to the dark, small degrees of decreased or increased pigmentation can be seen with the Wood lamp.

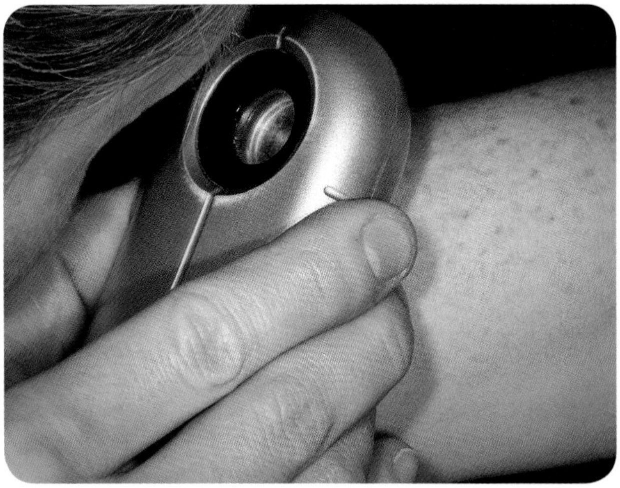

Figure 2-3 Episcope. Using bright optics and polarization, especially pigmented and vascular lesions can be examined in more detail.

Wood Light

The Wood lamp ("black light") produces long-wave ultraviolet rays (365 nm peak UVA [ultraviolet A] range) with relatively low energy. No special precautions are required for its routine use, except that the room should be as dark as possible (Fig. 2-2). Melanin absorbs strongly at 365 nm, so minor losses of melanin are accentuated. Hypopigmented areas are paler than normal skin, and depigmented areas are stark or milk white under Wood light. The Wood lamp is especially useful in the diagnosis of vitiligo or the hypopigmentation of tinea versicolor in their early stages. Certain conditions have characteristic fluorescent patterns (Table 2-1). The lamp is also useful for checking urine specimens for uroporphyrins (pink fluorescence), characteristic of porphyria cutanea tarda. Multiple exogenous substances, including markers, lint, dyes, and lipstick, can fluoresce on the skin.

Magnification

Magnifying lenses (5× to 10×) should be strong enough to allow the physician to observe lesions easily. Lenses are especially useful for detecting altered skin markings and

contours in tumors, and especially melanoma. Lenses are also used to observe nail fold telangiectasia in connective tissue diseases or to detect the subtle surface changes (Wickham striae) in lichen planus. When mineral oil or immersion oil is placed on the skin, the stratum corneum becomes more transparent, revealing deeper structures in more detail. This technique allows easier visualization of telangiectases, Wickham striae, and similar findings. Episcopes or dermatoscopes allow the examination of skin lesions under magnification with excellent illumination and permit resolution of fine detail and size (Fig. 2-3). They are especially useful for viewing complex pigmented lesions and melanomas.

Compression

Observing the changes in a skin lesion with compression (diascopy) is often useful in the diagnosis of skin diseases. Compression may be performed with a magnifying glass, microscope slide, or clear plastic plate. These instruments are all considered *diascopes*. Blue to red lesions that blanch when compressed are vascular lesions, and their gradual refilling is observed by seeing the red color return. Purpuric lesions do not blanch completely with pressure; raised, purpuric, nonblanchable lesions indicate vasculitis. Compression of brown to yellow-brown papules may reveal the apple jelly nodules of granulomatosis.

Palpation of Skin Lesions

Palpation reveals the lesion's depth, extension, texture, firmness, and fixation to underlying structures of skin. Light pressure can reveal a thrill in a vascular lesion, implying an arteriovenous malformation. Lateral compression of dermatofibromas causes them to become depressed and to indent the overlying skin (Fitzpatrick sign). Firm stroking of apparently normal skin can induce histamine release, redness, and edema; this phenomenon, known as dermographism, is accentuated in urticaria (Fig. 2-4). Stroking of individual

TABLE 2-1 Fluorescent Characteristics of Certain Conditions	
Characteristics	**Conditions**
Yellow-green fluorescence of hair	*Microsporum canis infection*
Yellow-green fluorescence of skin	*Pseudomonas* infection
Pink fluorescence of urine	Uroporphyrins of porphyria cutanea tarda
Coral fluorescence of toes, axillae, and groin	Erythrasma infection

Figure 2-4 Dermographism. Histamine release is accentuated in patients with reactive vasculature in hypersensitivity reactions.

Figure 2-5 Darier sign. Gentle stroking can cause erythema more persistent than that in dermographism and can form blisters as well. Diagnostic for cutaneous mast cell proliferation (urticaria pigmentosum).

papules leading to local erythema and edema (and, rarely, vesiculation) is diagnostic of urticaria pigmentosa. This phenomenon is named Darier sign (Fig. 2-5). Stroking the skin of atopic patients produces a white line without a red phase (white dermographism). In nevus anemicus, firm rubbing makes the surrounding normal skin bright red but does not induce erythema in the hypopigmented skin.

In blistering diseases, rubbing apparently normal skin may induce new blisters; this occurs in patients with pemphigus vulgaris and toxic epidermal necrolysis (Nikolsky sign). Extension of an intact blister by applying pressure to the lesion (Asboe–Hansen sign) indicates an intraepidermal blister.

Special Diagnostic Procedures

Organism Detection and Presumptive Identification

Organism identification is essential for the rational treatment of skin infections and infestations. Procedures important for dermatology are outlined in this section; standard infectious disease and microbiology texts should be consulted for further details. Superficial crusts, exudate, and medications should be swabbed with alcohol to remove saprophytes and secondary contaminating bacteria.

Potassium Hydroxide Preparation for Fungus

1. With an alcohol swab, cleanse the skin of any ointment.
2. With the edge of a microscope slide or scalpel, vigorously scrape the skin onto a second microscope slide. The best areas for scraping are the following:
   - Inner surface of a blister roof or the blister base
   - Moist, macerated areas, such as between toes
   - Rim of lesion
   - Under nail or under paronychial fold
   - Base of a plucked hair

3. Place a drop of 10% KOH on the scale-covered slide and apply a coverslip.
4. Warm gently. Avoid actual boiling, as this causes the KOH to crystallize (Fig. 2-6).
5. Examine with a microscope with 10× and 40× objective at low illumination. This is achieved by setting a low level of light and racking the condenser down (Fig. 2-7).

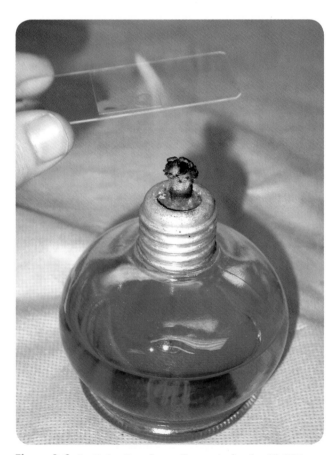

Figure 2-6 Gentle heating of a small amount of scale with KOH over an alcohol lamp is the key for a useful fungal preparation.

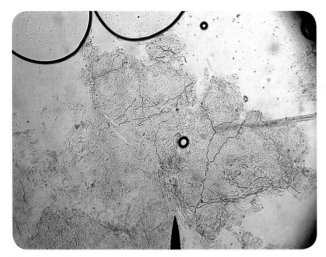

Figure 2-7 Identification of hyphal elements with a 10× objective and low illumination allows hyphae to show up as dark objects against the background. Using a 40× objective confirms the diagnosis.

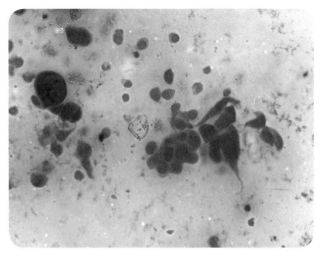

Figure 2-8 Multinucleated cells or giant nuclei characterize herpes simplex or herpes zoster infections of the skin.

Small amounts of scrapings on a slide frequently yield the best results because the coverslip rests on the slide, producing the best optical properties. KOH hydrolyses the epidermal proteins but not the fungal elements. The cell envelopes of the stratum corneum remain and should not be confused with fungi.

Tzanck Smear for Giant Cells

A Tzanck smear is very important for the rapid diagnosis of patients with vesicles and does not require special techniques such as PCR or fluorescent microscopy. The demonstration of multinucleated giant cells indicates that the causative agent is either herpes simplex virus or varicella–zoster virus. The procedure is as follows:

1. Select a fresh umbilicated vesicle.
2. Unroof the vesicle with a scalpel blade.
3. Gently scrape the base of the vesicle with the scalpel and smear scrapings onto a microscope slide.

4. Fix with 95% alcohol.
5. Stain with Wright or Giemsa stain, using the technique that is used for routine white cell differential counts.
6. Examine under the microscope using the 10× or 40× objective. A positive preparation demonstrates very large multinucleated giant cells with a high nuclear–cytoplasmic ratio. Examination with the oil immersion objective is often required in equivocal cases (Fig. 2-8).

Examination for Lice

Nits (eggs of lice) on pubic, axillary, scalp, or other hairs may be directly examined with the microscope. Organisms or empty, highly refractile egg cases are easily observed with 10× objective (Fig. 2-9). Adult lice can be seen with the naked eye and are dramatic under the lower objective (Fig. 2-10)

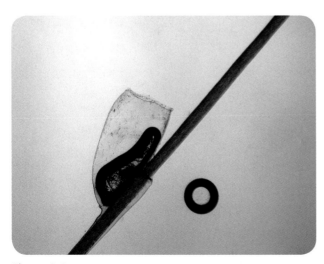

Figure 2-9 Hair with a louse egg case (nit). 10× objective.

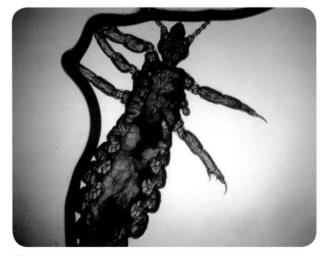

Figure 2-10 Adult louse from scalp. 10× objective.

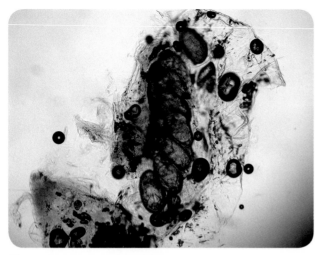

Figure 2-11 Scraping from burrow with an adult *Sarcoptes* mite, in lower-left corner, and a string of eggs containing organisms.

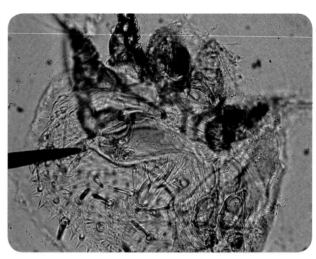

Figure 2-12 Close-up of adult *Sarcoptes* mite, the cause of scabies.

Examination for Scabies

Scabetic mites may be removed from burrows with a scalpel after applying 10% KOH or mineral oil to the suspected burrow. The oil optically clears the stratum corneum, enhancing visualization of the mite. Application of a tetracycline solution (500 mg tetracycline in 20 mL glycerin and 80 mL absolute ethanol), followed 1 min later by shining a Wood lamp on the skin, accentuates the burrow. Burrows fluoresce a brilliant green, allowing easy removal of a suspected organism. A small drop of ink placed on the opening of the burrow and then rapidly removed with a tissue may also reveal tracks (Figs. 2-11–2-13).

Gram Stain for Bacteria and Candida

1. Air-dry the slide.
2. Cover with 1% crystal violet for 15 s. Wash with water.
3. Cover with Gram iodine for 15 s. Wash with water.
4. Decolorize for 15 s with acetone alcohol. Wash with water.
5. Cover with 2.5% safranin for 15 s. Wash with water and air-dry.
6. Examine with 10×, 40×, and oil immersion lenses.

Special Techniques Usually Not Performed in the Primary Care Office

Patch Testing

Patch testing is done to determine delayed hypersensitivity to exogenous substances. The materials are specially prepared or may be available in the form of kits (e.g., T.R.U.E. TEST). The patches are applied for 48 h under occlusion and then examined for a delayed hypersensitivity that may vary from mild edema to actual vesiculation (Fig. 2-14). False negative tests are frequent, and many positives (e.g., to nickel) may not be clinically relevant to the condition at hand.

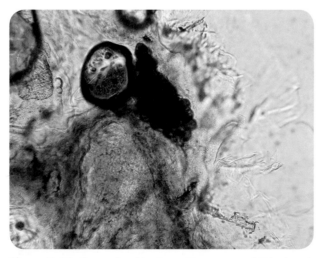

Figure 2-13 Clump of scabies feces. The presence of this alone is diagnostic of scabies.

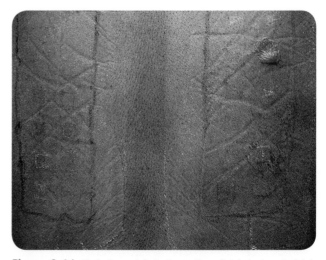

Figure 2-14 Vesicular patch test reaction. Patch test material is often applied on a small disc under occlusion.

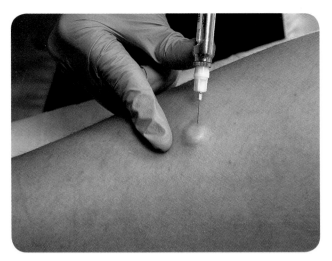

Figure 2-15 Biopsy. Intradermal injection of local anesthetic using a 30-gauge needle.

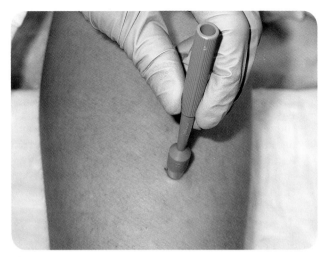

Figure 2-16 Biopsy. Firm pressure is applied to the cutaneous surface while rotating the punch biopsy instrument between the thumb and forefinger.

Culture Techniques

Sabouraud medium is useful for the isolation of most fungi. It is available commercially, stored cool, and then incubated with specimens at room temperature. Sabouraud medium with cycloheximide (actidone) and chloramphenicol suppresses bacterial and saprophytic fungi. It is very important not to use this medium if *Cryptococcus* is suspected because cycloheximide suppresses the growth of *Cryptococcus*.

India Ink Stain for *Cryptococcus*

A smear of an exudate is mixed with one small drop of commercial India ink, and a coverslip is applied. If the preparation is too dark, water may be added to dilute the ink. The large, translucent capsules of the *Cryptococcus*, with a small central nucleus that may contain a nucleolus, are seen. The buds have a narrow base; *Blastomyces* and other fungi have a broad base.

Acid-fast Stain

In suspected lepromatous leprosy and orificial tuberculosis, direct stains may be positive. In other forms of cutaneous leprosy and cutaneous tuberculosis, the chance of a positive smear is so small that a direct smear is not indicated. *Nocardia* in mycetomas will also stain with the acid-fast stain.

Punch Biopsy

The punch biopsy is the most common biopsy used by pediatric dermatologists. When properly performed, the procedure can be done rapidly with a very low incidence of adverse events or significant scarring.

1. Prepare a punch biopsy tray: Alcohol pads, local anesthetic, gloves, punch instrument, forceps, scissors, gauze, needle driver, and suture.
2. Prepare the patient: Explain the procedure to the child and parent step by step in a gentle, reassuring manner using child-appropriate words. If parts of the procedure are likely to be painful, do not lie to the child about impending discomfort.

3. Anesthetize the patient: Use topical lidocaine or EMLA under occlusion to reduce the discomfort caused by needle sticks. Once the cutaneous surface is appropriately anesthetized with topical anesthetic, wipe the area clean with an alcohol pad and use a syringe with a 30-gauge needle to inject local anesthetic into the deep dermis (Fig. 2-15).
4. Distract the patient: While the procedure is being performed, music, books, conversation, squeezing the child's hand, or other activities should be used to distract the patient. With drapes and positioning, hide the surgical site, surgical trays, and blood-soaked material from the child's view.
5. Punch biopsy: The punch biopsy is performed by applying slight downward pressure on the skin while rotating the punch instrument clockwise and counterclockwise (Fig. 2-16). One will feel a pop as the instrument penetrates the dermis into the subcutaneous tissue.

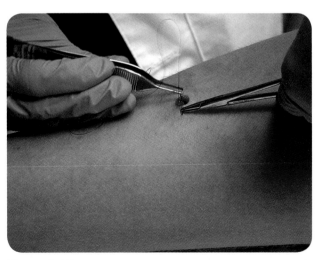

Figure 2-17 Biopsy. Wound edges are approximated with simple interrupted sutures.

6. Remove the biopsy tissue: Gently grasp the sample with forceps, lift until resistance is felt, and cut the tissue free at the subcutaneous level.
7. Close the defect with 1 to 3 simple interrupted sutures (Fig. 2-17): Choose the appropriate suture based on the patient's age, anatomic site, and size of the biopsy. In general, nonabsorbable (nylon or polypropylene) 4-0 suture is appropriate for superficial suturing of lesions on the trunk and extremities, and 5-0 suture is preferred for the face and genitalia. 6-0 absorbable sutures (polyglactin, polyglycolic acid, or surgical gut) can be used in children who are apprehensive about suture removal.
8. Dress the wound: Apply a thin layer of white petrolatum or antibiotic ointment covered with a nonadherent pad (e.g., Telfa [Kendall, Mansfield, MA]) and secured by adhesive tape.
9. Provide the patient's parents with written postoperative instructions explaining proper wound care, activity restrictions, and a number to call should adverse events occur.
10. Remove sutures: The patient should return in 5 to 7 days for removal of facial sutures and 10 to 14 days for removal of sutures on the torso and extremities.

CHAPTER 3

Morphology and Distribution

Learning to describe skin findings is the fundamental and essential skill of dermatologic diagnosis. Learn to describe what you see with the words defined in this chapter and online at www.essentialdermatology.com. In this chapter, there are precise definitions of the key morphologic terms with illustrative case examples. Online, there are additional images, an interactive self-assessment, and further training in configurations, distributions, and a lesson in variants of disease presentation. Master these definitions in this chapter and online.

Morphology

The ability to use the standard morphologic descriptive terminology of dermatology has been the key to developing accurate skin-based differential diagnoses for over a century. The characterization of visual skin findings requires both careful observation and the use of universally accepted terminology. Once you know these terms, you will be able to use the differential diagnosis index in Chapter 4 and use the online differential diagnosis engine of VisualDx more effectively. In this section, as in VisualDx, the primary morphologic terms are grouped into logical categories. For example, vesicles, bullae, and pustules are grouped because these are terms that represent fluid-filled lesions. The grouping is purposeful. As you examine the patient, ask yourself questions such as, Are these lesions raised? Are these lesions solid or fluid filled? Do these lesions blanch, or are they nonblanching as in the purpuras? The categories match the skin exam method. In addition to the main categories, further describe papules and plaques by checking for surface change such as scale or crust. Visit www.essentialdermatology.com for access to the LearnDerm interactive tutorial. The tutorial includes more images, image descriptions, and an interactive self-study test with virtual examination tools.

Group	Lesion Type	Definition
FLAT 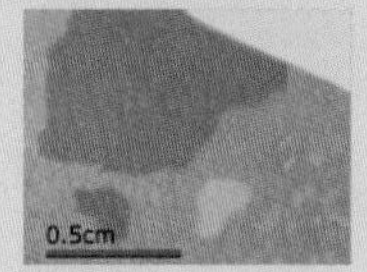	Macule 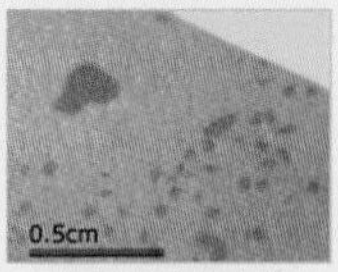	A flat, generally <0.5 cm area of skin or mucous membranes with different color from surrounding tissue. Macules may have nonpalpable, fine scale (see Fig. 3-1).
	Patch* 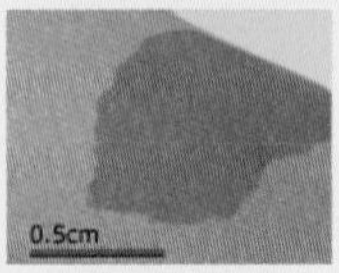	A flat, generally >0.5 cm area of skin or mucous membranes with different color from surrounding tissue. Patches may have nonpalpable, fine scale. *When used to describe an early clinical stage of cutaneous T-cell lymphoma (mycosis fungoides), the term patch may include fine textural change such as "cigarette paper" thinning, poikilodermatous atrophy, or slickness secondary to follicular loss (see Fig. 3-2).
RAISED AND SMOOTH 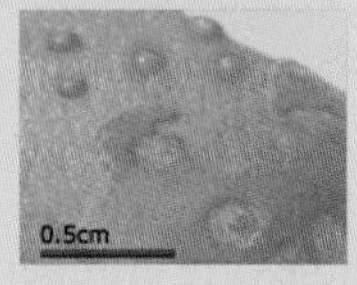	Papule 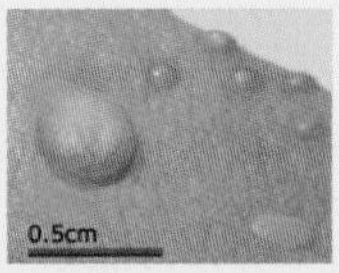	A discrete, solid, elevated body usually <0.5 cm in diameter. Papules are further classified by shape, size, color, and surface change (see Fig. 3-3).
	Plaque 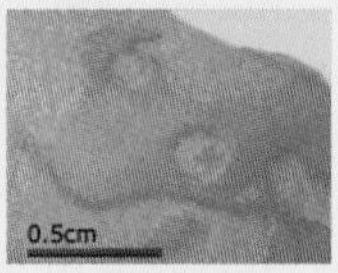	A discrete, solid, elevated body usually broader than it is thick measuring more than 0.5 cm in diameter. Plaques may be further classified by shape, size, color, and surface change (see Fig. 3-4).
	Nodule 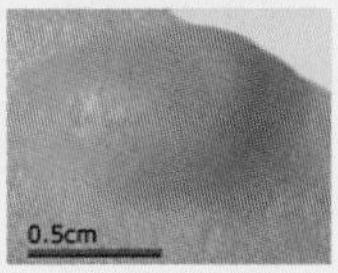	A dermal or subcutaneous firm, well-defined lesion usually >0.5 cm in diameter (see Fig. 3-5).
	Cyst 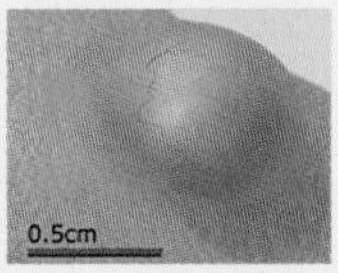	A closed cavity or sac containing fluid or semisolid material. A cyst may have an epithelial, endothelial, or membranous lining (see Fig. 3-6).
SURFACE CHANGE 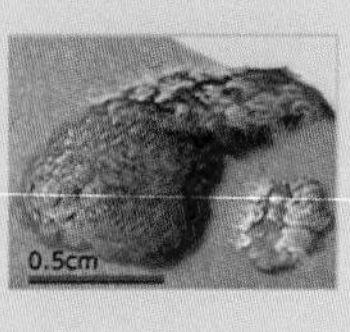	Crust 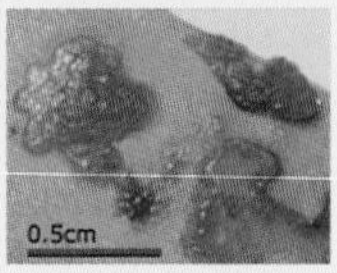	A hardened layer that results when serum, blood, or purulent exudate dries on the skin surface. Crusts may be thin or thick and can have varying color. Crusts are yellow-brown when formed from dried serum, green or yellow-green when formed from purulent exudate, or red-black when formed by blood (see Fig. 3-7).
	Scale 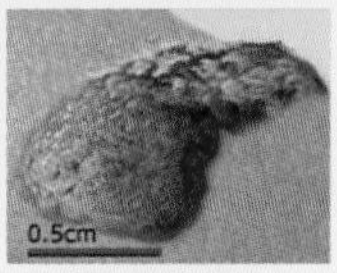	Excess stratum corneum accumulated in flakes or plates. Scale usually has a white or gray color (see Fig. 3-8).

(Continued)

(*Continued*)

Group	Lesion Type	Definition
FLUID-FILLED 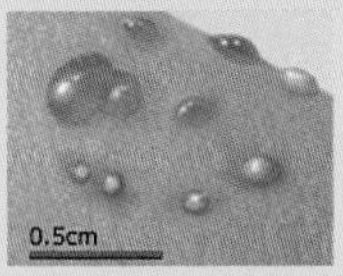	Abscess 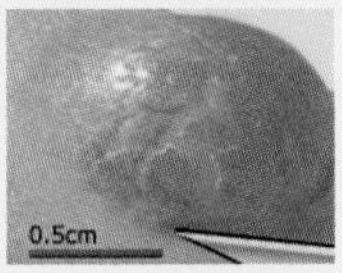	A localized accumulation of pus in the dermis or subcutaneous tissue. Frequently red, warm, and tender (see Fig. 3-9).
	Bulla 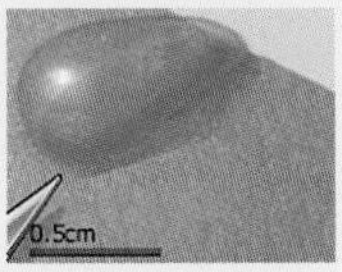	A fluid-filled blister >0.5 cm in diameter. Fluid can be clear, serous, hemorrhagic, or pus filled (see Fig. 3-10).
	Pustule 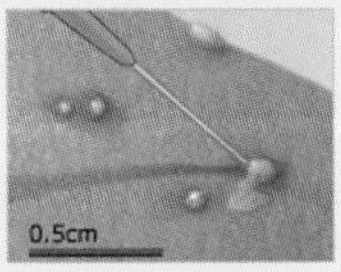	A circumscribed elevation that contains pus. Pustules are usually <0.5 cm in diameter (see Fig. 3-11).
	Vesicle 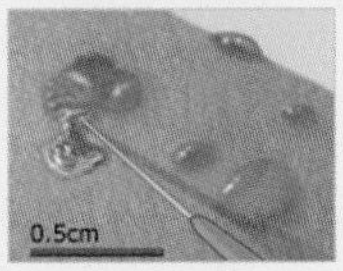	Fluid-filled cavity or elevation <0.5 cm in diameter. Fluid may be clear, serous, hemorrhagic, or pus filled (see Fig. 3-12).
RED BLANCHABLE 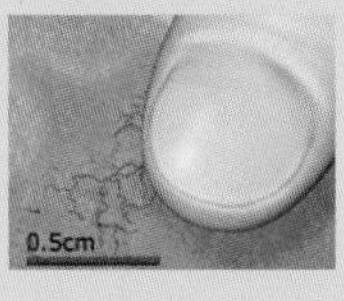	Erythema 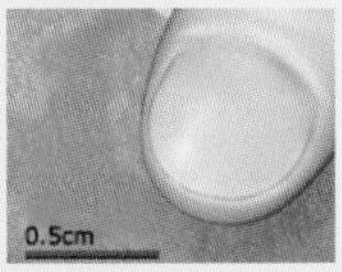	Localized, blanchable redness of the skin or mucous membranes (see Fig. 3-13).
	Erythroderma 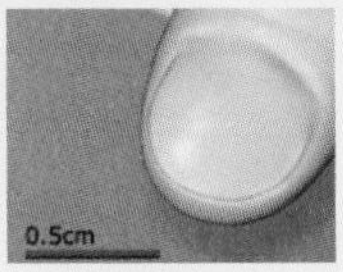	Generalized, blanchable redness of the skin that may be associated with desquamation (see Fig. 3-14).
	Telangiectasia 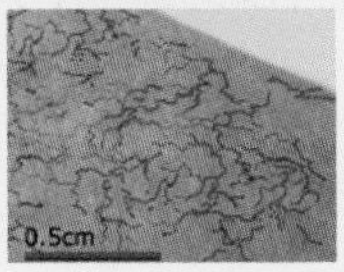	Visible, persistent dilation of small, superficial cutaneous blood vessels. Telangiectases will blanch (see Fig. 3-15).

(*Continued*)

(Continued)

Group	Lesion Type	Definition
PURPURIC 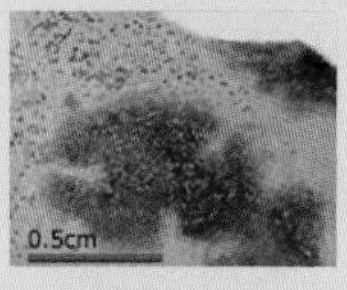 	Ecchymosis 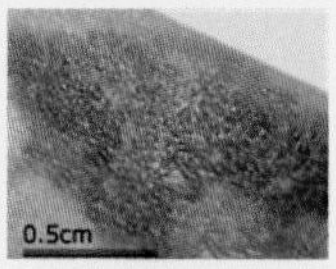 	Extravasation of blood into the skin or mucous membranes. Area of flat color change may progress over time from blue-black to brown-yellow or green (see Fig. 3-16).
	Petechiae 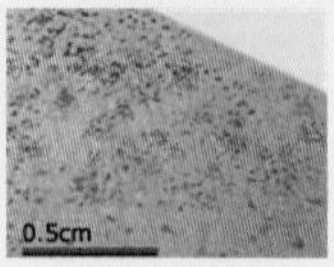 	Tiny 1–2 mm, initially purpuric, nonblanchable macules resulting from tiny hemorrhages (see Fig. 3-17).
	Palpable Purpura 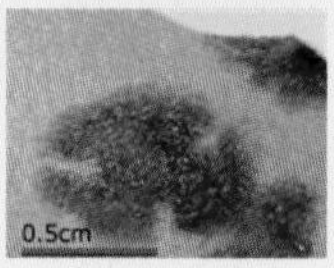 	Raised and palpable, nonblanchable, red or violaceous discoloration of skin or mucous membranes due to vascular inflammation in the skin and extravasation of red blood cells (see Fig. 3-18).
SUNKEN 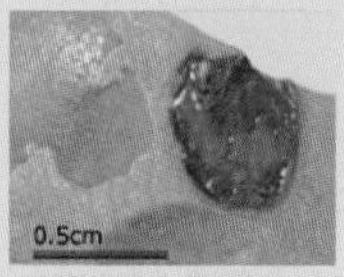 	Atrophy 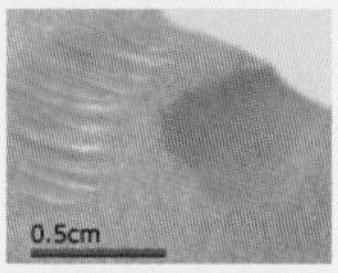 	A thinning of tissue defined by its location, such as epidermal atrophy, dermal atrophy, or subcutaneous atrophy (see Fig. 3-19).
	Erosion 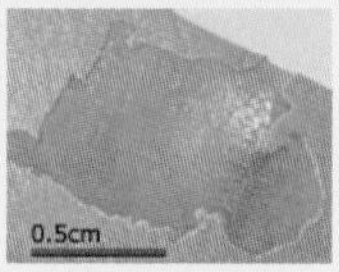 	A localized loss of the epidermal or mucosal epithelium (see Fig. 3-20).
	Ulcer 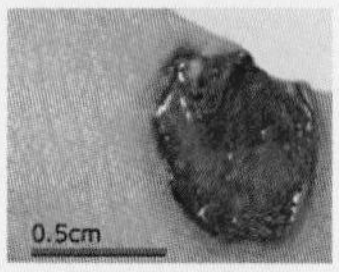 	A circumscribed loss of the epidermis and at least upper dermis. Ulcers are further classified by their depth, border/shape, edge, and tissue at its base (see Fig. 3-21).
GANGRENE	Gangrene 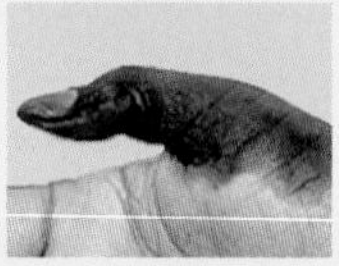 	Necrotic, usually black tissue due to obstruction, diminution, or loss of blood supply. Gangrene may be wet or dry (see Fig. 3-22).
ESCHAR	Eschar 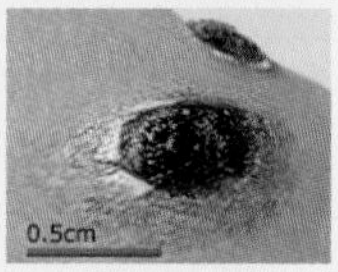 	An adherent thick, dry, black crust (see Fig. 3-23).

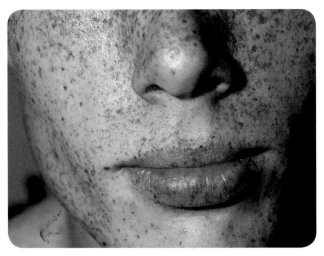

Figure 3-1 Numerous small, hyperpigmented macules of Peutz–Jeghers syndrome.

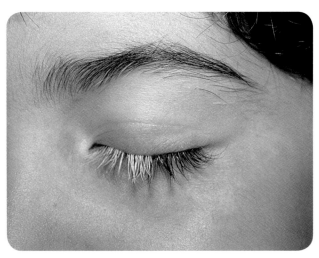

Figure 3-2 Hypopigmented patch of vitiligo involving the superior eyelid and eyelashes.

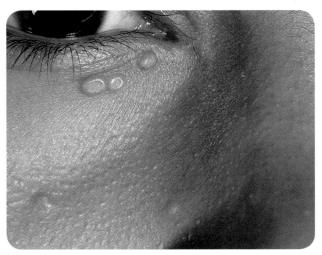

Figure 3-3 Smooth, umbilicated (central indentation) papules of molluscum contagiosum.

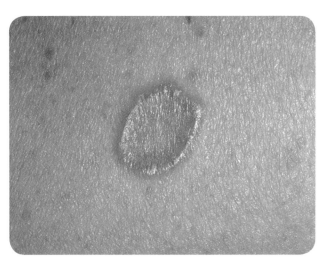

Figure 3-4 Annular (ring-shaped) plaque of granuloma annulare.

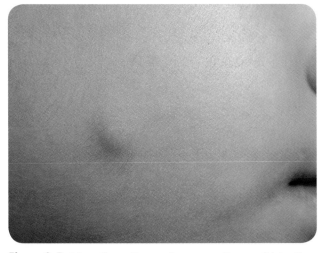

Figure 3-5 A juvenile xanthogranuloma presenting as a faint yellow-orange nodule on the cheek.

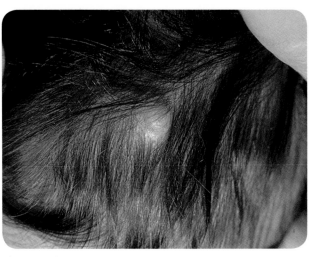

Figure 3-6 An infant with a dermoid cyst located in the scalp.

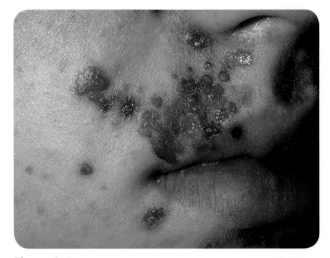

Figure 3-7 Nonbullous impetigo frequently presents with honey-colored crusts.

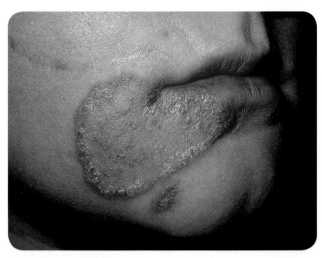

Figure 3-8 A child with a typical peripheral scaling plaque of tinea faciale (dermatophyte infection of the face).

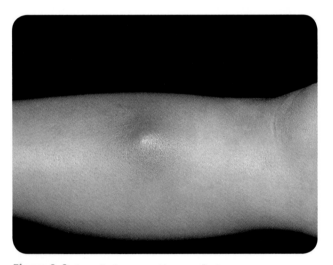

Figure 3-9 A small abscess on the arm of a teenager.

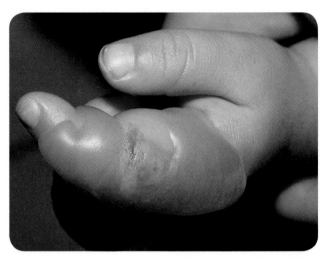

Figure 3-10 A giant bulla involving the digit of a child with bullous impetigo.

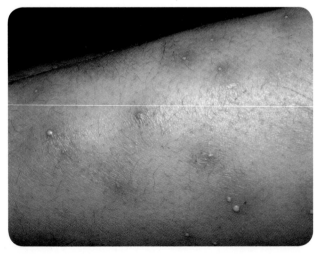

Figure 3-11 Small pustules are localized to the follicle in this child with bacterial folliculitis.

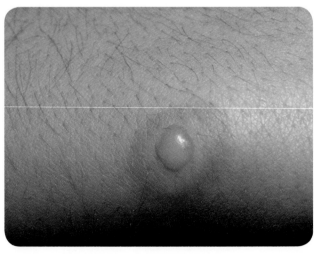

Figure 3-12 A tense, clear, fluid-filled vesicle caused by an insect bite.

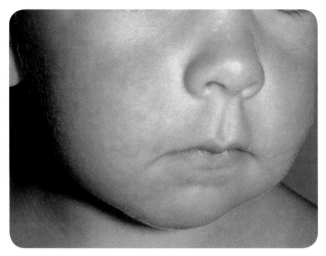

Figure 3-13 Erythematous patches involving the cheeks is the typical presentation of erythema infectiosum (fifth disease).

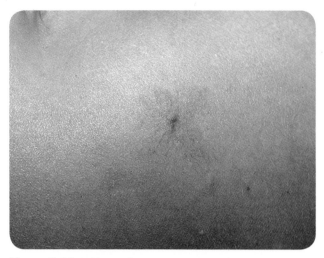

Figure 3-15 Spider angiomas are common telangiectases on the face of children.

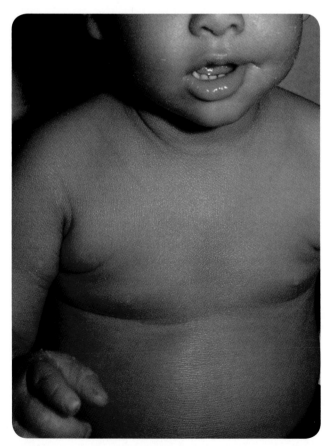

Figure 3-14 Erythroderma of the total body in an infant with generalized psoriasis.

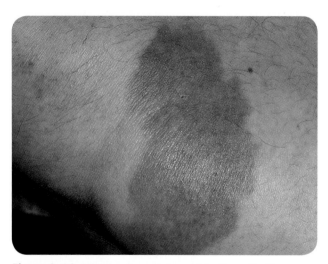

Figure 3-16 A large ecchymosis in a child with capillaritis.

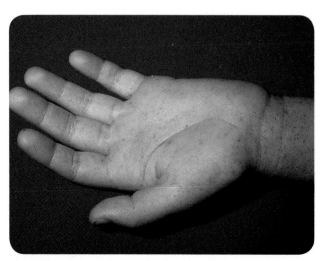

Figure 3-17 Hand petechiae in a child with Rocky Mountain spotted fever.

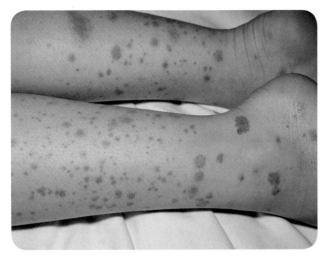

Figure 3-18 Symmetric palpable purpura due to vasculitis in a child with Henoch–Schönlein purpura.

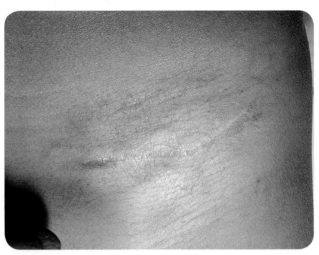

Figure 3-19 Topical steroid-induced atrophy is apparent with skin thinning and transparency.

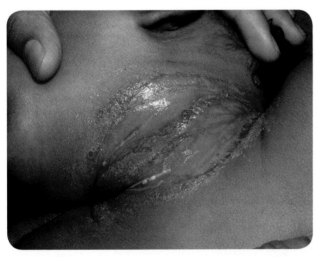

Figure 3-20 A large erosion at the neck of an infant with intertrigo.

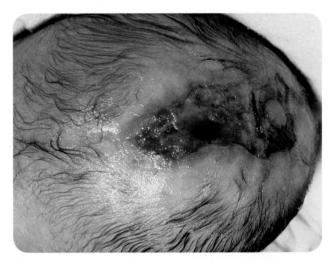

Figure 3-21 An ulcer of the scalp in aplasia cutis congenita.

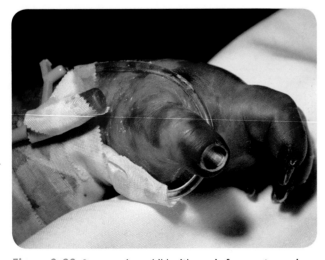

Figure 3-22 Gangrene in a child with sepsis from acute meningococcemia.

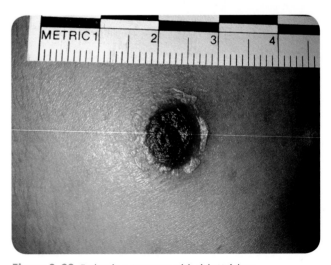

Figure 3-23 Eschar in a teenager with rickettsialpox.

Distributions

Skin lesions can occur at a discrete body location or form a distribution pattern by involving multiple body surfaces. Distribution refers to the pattern in which multiple lesions are arranged. Both location and distribution can be powerful clues in the process of developing a differential diagnosis. Learn the most important distributions in this section and visit www.essentialdermatology.com for additional definitions and an interactive self-study quiz.

Distribution	Definition
Acral	An acral pattern of skin lesions involves the distal aspects of the head (ears and nose) and the extremities (hands, fingers, feet, and toes).
Dermatomal	Dermatomal distribution includes an area of skin following the sensory skin innervation of a particular nerve root. Dermatomal distributions do not cross the midline of the body.
Intertriginous	Intertriginous distribution involves skin creases and folds. An intertriginous pattern includes involvement of the axillae, crural fold, gluteal crease, and possibly the inframammary fold.
Lymphangitic	A lymphangitic pattern of skin lesions or subcutaneous lesions appears along the path of the lymph channels of the leg or arm. Sporotrichosis, a deep fungal infection, typically presents with a lymphangitic pattern.

(Continued)

(Continued)

Distribution	Definition
Photodistributed	A photodistributed pattern follows the sun-exposed skin. Typical areas of involvement are the forehead, chest, upper back, upper ears, nose, cheeks, upper lip, neck, forearms, and dorsa of the hands.
Scattered	Skin lesions occurring across many body locations can appear to be distributed randomly or haphazardly. A severe case of poison ivy dermatitis could appear widely scattered.
Symmetric	Skin lesions that are found symmetrically on the extremities can be indicative of diagnoses of many etiologies, including infectious, metabolic, genetic, and inflammatory causes.
Widespread	A widespread distribution involves the entire—or almost the entire—body.

Essential Pediatric Skin Diseases

This chapter contains 112 diseases organized according to their common presentations. These presentations are divided and are in the order as shown in Morphology Index 4-1 and 4-2 for multiple lesions; Morphology Index 4-3 for lesions that are often present as solitary growths; and Morphology Index 4-4 for lesions on the scalp, nails, perineum, or in the mouth.

Alphabetical Index 4-5 contains all of the discrete diseases in an alphabetical list with the appropriate page number for the disorder.

Disorders that are often of acute onset (i.e., hours to a few days) are in italic.

MORPHOLOGY INDEX 4-1   Multiple Lesions or Rash in the Well Child

Erythemas
Asymmetric Periflexural Exanthem of Childhood
Cold Panniculitis
Cutis Marmorata
Erythema Infectiosum (*Fifth Disease*)
Erythema Multiforme Minor
Erythema Toxicum Neonatorum
Lyme Disease
Urticaria

Flat Pigmentary
Capillaritis
Dermal Melanocytosis (Mongolian Spot)
Drug-induced Pigmentation
Fixed Drug Eruption
Vitiligo

Smooth Papules and Plaques
Acne Vulgaris
Acne, Neonatal (Benign Cephalic Pustulosis)
Bite or Sting, Arthropod
Erythema Nodosum
Folliculitis
Granuloma Annulare
Histiocytosis, Langerhans Cell
Juvenile Xanthogranuloma
Keratosis Pilaris
Milia
Miliaria Rubra
Molluscum Contagiosum
Morphea
Neurofibromatosis
Trichoepithelioma
Tuberous Sclerosis
Wart, Flat

Scaly Papules and Plaques
Acanthosis Nigricans
Acne Excoriée
Candidiasis, Diaper Dermatitis
Dermatitis, Atopic (Eczema)
Dermatitis, Contact
Dermatitis, Diaper Irritant
Dermatitis, Dyshidrotic
Dermatitis, Nummular
Dermatitis, Seborrheic—Child
Dermatitis, Seborrheic—Neonate/Infant
Epidermal Nevus
Ichthyosis Vulgaris
Ichthyosis, X-linked
Juvenile Plantar Dermatosis
Lichen Planus
Lichen Striatus
Lupus Erythematosus, Neonatal
Pityriasis Lichenoides et Varioliformis Acuta
Pityriasis Rosea
Psoriasis
Psoriasis, Guttate
Psoriasis, Infantile
Scabies
Tinea Corporis
Tinea Pedis (*Athlete's Foot*)
Tinea Versicolor
Wart, Common
Wart, Plantar

Fluid-Filled (Vesicles, Pustules, and Bullae)
Acropustulosis of Infancy (Infantile Acropustulosis)
Candidiasis, Neonatal
Dermatitis, Poison Ivy–Oak–Sumac
Epidermolysis Bullosa Simplex
Herpes Simplex Virus, Orofacial
Impetigo, Bullous
Miliaria Crystallina
Neonatal Pustular Dermatosis, Transient
Varicella (*Chickenpox*)
Varicella, Neonatal
Zoster (*Shingles*)

Atrophy/Erosions/Ulcer
Intertrigo
Keratolysis, Pitted
Striae

MORPHOLOGY INDEX 4-2 Multiple Lesions or Rash in the Febrile, Ill, or Toxic-appearing Child

Cellulitis
Drug Eruptions
Drug Hypersensitivity Syndrome (DRESS Syndrome)
Gianotti–Crosti Syndrome
Hand-Foot-and-Mouth Disease
Henoch–Schönlein Purpura
Kawasaki Disease

Lupus Erythematosus, Systemic
Meningococcemia, Acute
Staphylococcal Scalded Skin Syndrome
Stevens–Johnson Syndrome
Toxic Epidermal Necrolysis (Lyell Disease)
Toxic Shock Syndrome
Viral Exanthem

MORPHOLOGY INDEX 4-3 Single Lesion or Growth

Lumps and Bumps
Abscess
Cyst, Epidermoid (Sebaceous Cyst)
Granuloma, Pyogenic
Hemangioma, Infantile
Keloid
Lipoma
Pilomatricoma
Spider Angioma

Pigmented Lesions
Congenital Nevus Including Giant Congenital Nevus
Lentigo Simplex
Melanoma
Nevus, Atypical

MORPHOLOGY INDEX 4-4 Special Locations

Scalp
Aplasia Cutis Congenita
Alopecia Areata
Nevus Sebaceus
Pediculosis Capitis (Head Lice)
Tinea Capitis

Perineum
Balanitis, Nonspecific
Candidiasis, Male Genital
Condyloma Acuminatum (Genital Wart)
Herpes Simplex Virus, Genital
Lichen Sclerosus
Perineal Streptococcal Infection

Nails
Onychomycosis
Paronychia, Candidal

Mouth
Ulcer, Aphthous

ALPHABETICAL INDEX 4-5 Alphabetical List of all of the Essential Skin Disease

(Continued)

ALPHABETICAL INDEX 4-5   *(Continued)*

■■ Diagnosis Synopsis

Asymmetric periflexural exanthem of childhood (APEC), also known as unilateral laterothoracic exanthem of childhood, is a self-limited inflammatory condition of infancy and early childhood. It is typically a mildly pruritic exanthem that usually follows a mild URI (upper respiratory) or GI (gastrointestinal) illness. APEC occurs primarily in late winter and early spring and shows a 2:1 female-to-male predominance. Most patients are 2 to 3 years of age, although it has been described in children from 8 months to 10 years.

Fever is found in 40% of cases. Pruritus is noted in two third of patients: mild intensity in one fourth, moderate in nearly one half, and severe in another one third. Very rarely, children have an associated enanthem. Children may have low-grade or more significant fever. Lesions spontaneously resolve in 2 to 6 weeks.

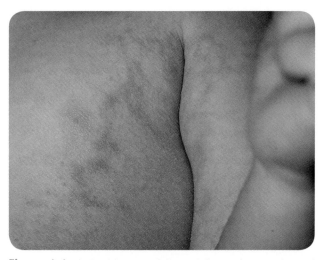

Figure 4-1 APEC with rows of linear inflammatory papules and eczematous plaques on the chest and arm.

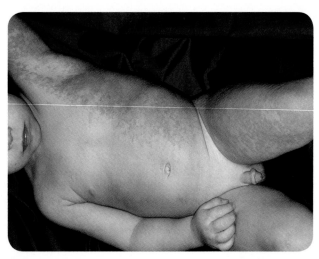

Figure 4-2 APEC with unilateral zone of confluent papules extending from arm to chest to thigh.

◉ Look For

Discrete 1 mm erythematous papules with occasional purpuric areas that coalesce into plaques. The lesions begin unilaterally, on the trunk or near large flexural areas (most often the axilla followed by inguinal), and spread centrifugally (Figs. 4-1–4-4). New lesions appear on the adjacent trunk

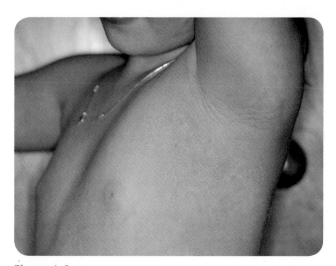

Figure 4-3 APEC with unilateral erythema on upper arm, axilla, and chest.

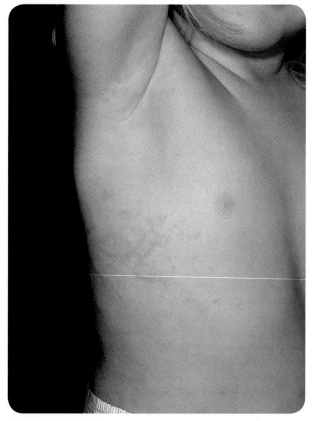

Figure 4-4 APEC with grouped plaques on chest and axilla. Pityriasis rosea is an important differential diagnosis.

and extremity, with normal skin in between. A second stage involving the contralateral side occurs in most cases (65% to 70%) over 2 to 4 weeks, but the exanthem remains more prominent on one side. Lesions disappear with moderate desquamation within another 2 to 4 weeks.

Diagnostic Pearls

- The asymmetry of the eruption extending from a flexural area in combination with young age suggests the diagnosis.
- Patients may have had an antecedent febrile viral illness.
- When patients or their parents show the eruption, it is through a "Statue of Liberty" (one arm extended upward) or "touchdown" (both arms extended upward) motion/position.

?? Differential Diagnosis and Pitfalls

- Seborrheic dermatitis can present with a flexural distribution.
- Gianotti–Crosti syndrome is a more diffuse papular exanthem that is not limited to one side and occurs more prominently over the knees and elbows as well as extensor surfaces.
- Other eruptive disorders of childhood, either infectious or systemic, may mimic APEC. APEC may be confused with more chronic dermatitis, especially atopic dermatitis,

because of the associated pruritus and distribution of lesions during the final stage of eruption. The asymmetry, pruritus, and erythema suggest contact dermatitis in some children.

✓ Best Tests

This is a clinical diagnosis.

▲▲ Management Pearls

APEC is a self-limited illness.

Therapy

Oral antihistamines, antipruritic agents (e.g., pramoxine), and topical steroids may help pruritus.

Suggested Readings

Coustou D, Léauté-Labrèze C, Bioulac-Sage P, et al. Asymmetric periflexural exanthem of childhood: A clinical, pathologic, and epidemiologic prospective study. *Arch Dermatol.* 1999;135(7):799–803.

McCuaig CC, Russo P, Powell J, et al. Unilateral laterothoracic exanthem. A clinicopathologic study of forty-eight patients. *J Am Acad Dermatol.* 1996;34(6):979–984.

Taïeb A, Mégraud F, Legrain V, et al. Asymmetric periflexural exanthem of childhood. *J Am Acad Dermatol.* 1993;29(3):391–393.

Cold Panniculitis

Diagnosis Synopsis

Cold panniculitis is the crystallization of subcutaneous fat with subsequent inflammation in response to cold injury. The typical scenario is an infant or young child that has had prolonged cold exposure to the cheeks or limbs from low ambient temperatures, local therapeutic application of cold (e.g., during cardiac surgery), or other cold exposure (e.g., from a popsicle).

Look For

Painful, firm, red-to-violaceous, ill-defined, 1 to 3 cm, indurated nodules form 1 to 3 days after cold exposure. The cheeks are the most common site of involvement (Fig. 4-5). The buttocks and other fatty areas, however, also may be affected (Fig. 4-6). The infant is otherwise well.

Diagnostic Pearls

- The development of lesions 12 to 72 h after cold exposure is highly important in making the diagnosis.
- Exposure of the face to subfreezing temperatures results in symmetric involvement of the cheeks, whereas local exposure to ice (e.g., a popsicle) will result in unilateral cheek involvement.

?? Differential Diagnosis and Pitfalls

- Infectious cellulitis or panniculitis may appear very similar to cold panniculitis. However, infants with infections

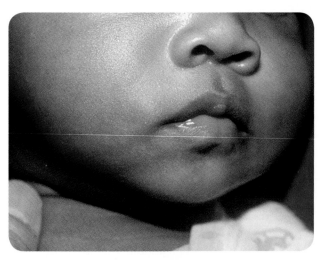

Figure 4-5 Cold panniculitis is often due to cold from metal or a popsicle and is less well defined than typical dermatitis.

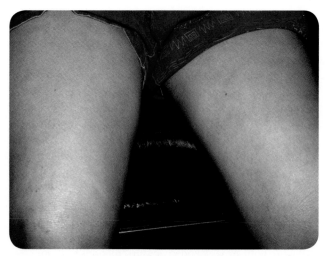

Figure 4-6 Cold panniculitis due to cold exposure during snow sledding.

are febrile, appear toxic, and have lesions that are warm to touch.
- Identical appearing nodules may form 1 to 2 weeks after abrupt cessation of systemic steroids; however, they usually affect more extensive areas of the body (face, trunk, and extremities).
- In newborns, especially those with unusually large plaques (i.e., those >3 cm) or affected by perinatal complications (asphyxia, hypothermia, seizures, pre-eclampsia, or meconium aspiration), subcutaneous fat necrosis of the newborn should be highly considered.
- Traumatic panniculitis (blunt trauma or injection) should be distinguished by history.
- Sclerema neonatorum is characterized by diffuse bound down hardening of the skin that is cold rather than warm on palpation.
- Metastatic neuroblastomas are firm bluish nodules rather than ill defined and erythematous.

✓ Best Tests

There are no definitive laboratory studies. A skin biopsy may demonstrate necrotic fat cells, cystic spaces, and a polymorphous infiltrate or only a nonspecific lobular panniculitis.

▲▲ Management Pearls

Parents should be reassured that cold panniculitis is self-limited, not associated with any systemic disease, and is nonscarring.

Therapy

No therapy is recommended. Cold panniculitis resolves spontaneously, often leaving temporary residual discoloration that may last for months.

Suggested Readings

Cohen BA. Disorders of the subcutaneous tissue. In: Eichenfield LF, Frieden IJ, Esterly NB, eds. *Neonatal Dermatology*. 2nd Ed. Philadelphia, PA: WB Saunders; 2008:447–460.

Epstein EH Jr, Oren ME. Popsicle panniculitis. *N Engl J Med*. 1970;282(17): 966–967.

⬛ Diagnosis Synopsis

Cutis marmorata refers to the netlike, violaceous pattern seen in newborns as a result of transient shifts in cutaneous blood flow. This is a common condition, occurring more frequently in premature infants and may persist to the fourth week of life. Trisomy 18, Down syndrome, Cornelia de Lange syndrome, and hypothyroidism have been associated with cutis marmorata that persists beyond early infancy.

◉ Look For

A symmetric, blanchable, reticular (netlike), violaceous pattern that preferentially affects the extremities over the trunk (Figs. 4-7–4-10). The pattern is more exaggerated with cooling of the skin and it lessens with warming.

●● Diagnostic Pearls

It may be associated with cold-induced acrocyanosis, which is a bluish discoloration secondary to peripheral vasoconstriction of hands and feet.

?? Differential Diagnosis and Pitfalls

- Unlike cutis marmorata, cutis marmorata telangiectatica congenita (CMTC) is persistent on warming, asymmetric, well localized and often associated with cutaneous and/or underlying limb atrophy.
- Cardiac and pulmonary disease is associated with central cyanosis (cyanosis of the lips, face, and trunk) rather than cutis marmorata.

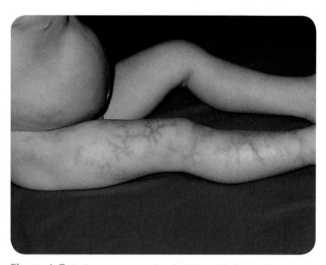

Figure 4-7 Cutis marmorata telangiectasia with deep lesions.

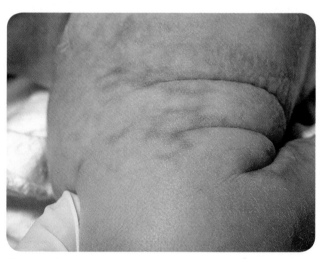

Figure 4-8 Cutis marmorata with a subtle netlike vascular pattern is common with cold exposure in childhood.

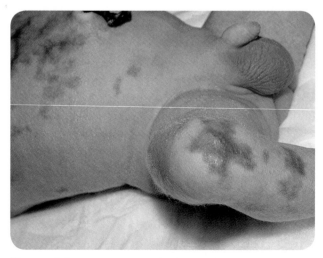

Figure 4-9 CMTC with irregular linear and reticulate atrophy accentuated over joints.

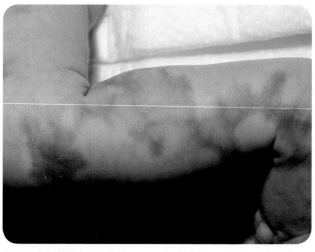

Figure 4-10 CMTC with more obvious reticular pattern, also accentuated over joints.

Best Tests

This is a clinical diagnosis. Lesions should be blanchable and improve on warming of the infant.

Management Pearls

Consider an evaluation for systemic disease (hypothyroidism) in infants with cutis marmorata that does not respond to rewarming or that lasts beyond 6 months of age.

Therapy

Maintain a warm environment for the infant.

Suggested Readings

Lucky AW. Transient benign cutaneous lesions in the newborn. In: Eichenfield LF, Frieden IJ, Esterly NB, eds. *Neonatal Dermatology*. Philadelphia, PA: WB Saunders; 2008:85–98.

Paller AS, Mancini AJ. Cutaneous disorders of the newborn. In: Paller AS, Mancini AJ, eds. *Hurwitz Clinical Pediatric Dermatology. A Textbook of Skin Disorders of Childhood and Adolescence*. 3rd Ed. Philadelphia, PA: Elsevier Saunders; 2006:17–47.

Erythema Infectiosum (Fifth Disease)

▪▪ Diagnosis Synopsis

Erythema infectiosum, or fifth disease, is a common illness in young children due to infection with parvovirus B19. Infection can result in a mild exanthem, no exanthem, or the typical "slapped cheeks" rash.

Children may have a prodromal headache with associated low-grade fever and rhinorrhea beginning 2 days before the onset of the rash. Children recover spontaneously without therapy.

◉ Look For

Erythema of the cheeks. Classically, the rash in children with erythema infectiosum goes through three phases. After several days of a nonspecific flulike illness, an exanthem abruptly

begins with the appearance of asymptomatic, macular, diffuse erythema involving the bilateral cheeks (slapped cheek appearance) (Figs. 4-11 and 4-12). One to four days later, a lacy reticulated eruption consisting of discrete erythematous macules and papules appears on the proximal extremities (Fig. 4-13). The trunk later becomes involved (Fig. 4-14). The third stage is marked by a recurrence of a milder form of the eruption after exposure to heat, friction, or sunlight, or in response to crying or exercise. Roughly 7% of children with erythema infectiosum develop mild arthralgias that resolve within several weeks.

●● Diagnostic Pearls

Bright redness of the cheeks, most intense beneath the eyes, is the classic initial sign with sparing of eyelids, chin, and perioral area.

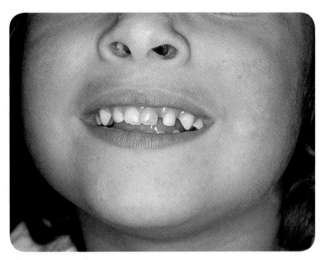

Figure 4-11 Erythema infectiosum (fifth disease) with the characteristic red slapped cheeks and circumoral pallor.

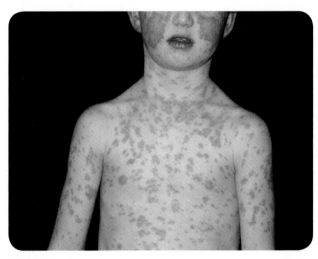

Figure 4-12 Erythema infectiosum (fifth disease) with slapped cheeks and disseminated macular and papular eruption.

Figure 4-13 Erythema infectiosum (fifth disease) with reticulate erythema of proximal extremities.

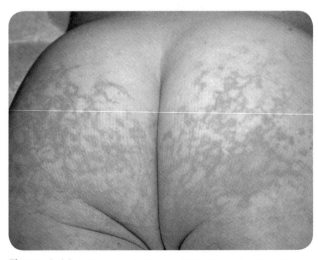

Figure 4-14 Erythema infectiosum (fifth disease) with reticulate erythema on buttocks.

?? Differential Diagnosis and Pitfalls

- Scarlet fever: Typically begins on the neck and trunk, then later involves the extremities. Patients also display signs and symptoms of streptococcal pharyngitis.
- Rubella: Starts on the face and progresses caudad, covering the entire body in one day and resolving by the third day. Red macules or petechiae may be seen on the soft palate and uvula (Forchheimer sign).
- Roseola infantum: Three days of high fever followed by the appearance of a morbilliform erythema upon defervescence consisting of rose-colored macules on the neck, trunk, and buttocks. Mucous membranes are spared.
- Erysipelas of the face: An acute β-hemolytic group A streptococcal infection of the skin involving the superficial dermal lymphatics. Skin lesions have a distinctive raised sharply demarcated advancing edge.
- Rubeola (measles): Is marked by the appearance of morbilliform lesions on the scalp and behind the ears that spread to involve the trunk and extremities over 2 to 3 days. Koplik spots are pathognomonic and appear during the prodromal phase.
- A careful history should help distinguish from a potential drug eruption.

✓ Best Tests

This is usually a clinical diagnosis; however, serologic testing in patients with acute exanthems will reveal elevated specific IgM and IgG antibodies. IgM antibodies persist for 2 to 3 months after acute infection. Specific IgG will also be elevated in patients with previous infections.

▲▲ Management Pearls

- Reassure the parents that the eruption can persist and be exacerbated by warmth and sunlight over a period of weeks to months.
- Patients are infectious from 7 days before the onset of the rash and not infectious once the exanthem appears.
- Pregnant women up to 21 weeks of pregnancy, immunocompromised patients, and patients with hemoglobinopathies are at elevated risk for complications.
- Those with elevated risk who have shared a room for greater than 15 min or had face-to-face contact with a laboratory-confirmed case should be evaluated by their physician, and laboratory evaluation (serologies or viral titers) should be considered to rule out infection.

Therapy

No therapy is necessary, as the condition is self-limited.

Suggested Readings

Crowcroft NS, Roth CE, Cohen BJ, et al. Guidance for control of parvovirus B19 infection in healthcare settings and the community. *J Public Health Med.* 1999;21(4):439–446.

Young NS, Brown KE. Parvovirus B19. *N Engl J Med.* 2004;350(6):586–597.

Diagnosis Synopsis

Erythema multiforme (EM) is a self-limited hypersensitivity reaction of the skin and mucous membranes characterized by the acute onset of fixed lesions of concentric color change (target lesions). Typically, all cutaneous lesions appear within 24 to 72h and persist for 1 to 4 weeks before fading. The eruption recurs on repeated exposure to the inciting agent. In children, herpes simplex virus (HSV) is the most common etiology, although several viruses and histoplasmosis have been associated as triggers.

Look For

A symmetric eruption that may affect any cutaneous surface but favors the extremities, including the palms and soles (Figs. 4-15–4-18). The early lesion consists of a well-defined, fixed erythematous macule or papule that rapidly develops a dusky, grayish central discoloration. The central color change may be preceded by a vesicle that involutes, leaving behind a sharply marginated, central dusky hue (the target lesion). Alternatively, a well-defined wheal with a dusky or vesicular center develops within the erythematous macule that flattens, leaving behind concentric circles consisting of a

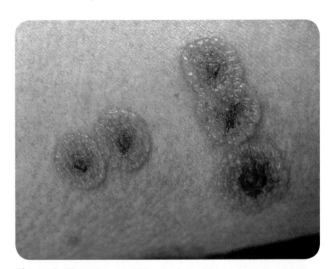

Figure 4.17 Erythema multiforme minor with prominent target lesions.

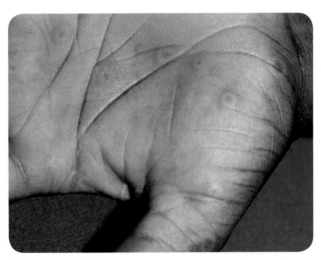

Figure 4.15 Erythema multiforme minor with three target lesions on the palms.

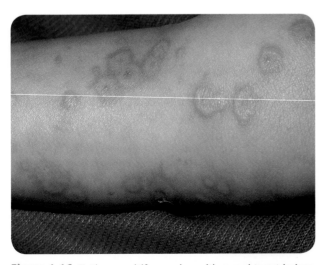

Figure 4.16 Erythema multiforme minor with several target lesions.

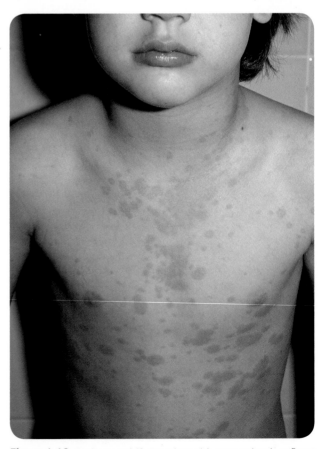

Figure 4.18 Erythema multiforme minor with scattered and confluent truncal lesions.

well-circumscribed erythematous border, pale middle zone, and a dusky center (also called the target lesion). Individual lesions persist for 1 to 4 weeks. Occasionally, mucosal involvement is limited to the mouth and consists of erosions, swelling, and crusting of the lips, tongue, and buccal mucosa.

Patients are otherwise well with, at most, mild systemic symptoms consisting of low-grade fever, malaise, arthralgias, or myalgias.

Diagnostic Pearls

- The gingival surface is rarely involved by lesions of EM; thus, gingival involvement suggests oral HSV infection as the precipitating factor.
- If the resolved lesions of EM are hyperpigmented and sparse, consider the diagnosis of a fixed drug eruption.

?? Differential Diagnosis and Pitfalls

Hypersensitivity Reactions

- Urticaria
- Kawasaki disease
- Fixed drug eruption
- Id reaction
- Acute hemorrhagic edema of infancy

Autoimmune Diseases

- Linear IgA bullous dermatosis
- Bullous pemphigoid
- Neonatal lupus
- Urticarial vasculitis
- Henoch–Schönlein purpura

Annular Erythemas

- Erythema annulare centrifugum
- Erythema migrans (Lyme disease)

Infections and Infestations

- Viral exanthem
- Insect bites
- Disseminated bacterial or fungal infection
- Scabies
- Molluscum contagiosum
- Syphilis

Malignancies

- Lymphoma
- Leukemia
- Lymphomatoid papulosis

Best Tests

This is usually a clinical diagnosis; however, a skin biopsy will show focal keratinocyte necrosis, exostosis, and interface change. If present, a culture, viral PCR, or direct fluorescent antibody test should be obtained from oral lesions to rule out HSV infection.

Management Pearls

A thorough history should be obtained, searching for inciting factors (infections, drugs, and vaccinations) that the child has been exposed to within 3 to 4 weeks of onset of the eruption. HSV infections usually occur 3 to 14 days prior to the onset of EM.

Therapy

As EM is typically a self-limiting and mild illness, symptomatic therapy is sufficient once the underlying etiology has been eliminated. Systemic antihistamines (hydroxyzine 1 mg/kg at night and 0.5 mg/kg daily) and acetaminophen (15 mg/kg every 4 to 6 h) usually control any pruritus or discomfort the child might have.

Children experiencing recurring episodes often have associated HSV infection and can be treated with suppressive doses of acyclovir (20 mg/kg/day for 6 to 12 months).

Special Considerations in Infants

EM is extremely rare in infants, and Kawasaki disease and urticaria should be strongly considered alternative diagnoses. Infants with Kawasaki disease will appear ill and have a high fever. Urticarial lesions resolve and recur in different sites within 24 h, whereas individual lesions of EM are static. Urticaria and Kawasaki disease may be associated with edema of the hands and feet, whereas EM is not.

Suggested Readings

Ayangco L, Rogers RS III. Oral manifestations of erythema multiforme. *Dermatol Clin.* 2003;21:195–205.

Schofield JK, Tatnall FM, Leigh IM. Recurrent erythema multiforme: Clinical features and treatment in a large series of patients. *Br J Dermatol.* 1993;128(5):542–545.

Weston WL, Morelli JG. Herpes simplex virus-associated erythema multiforme in prepubertal children. *Arch Pediatr Adolesc Med.* 1997;151(10):1014–1016.

■■ Diagnosis Synopsis

Erythema toxicum neonatorum is a common benign skin eruption of the newborn of uncertain cause. It is seen in term infants and is rare in the premature infants. The rash develops in most infants between the second and fourth day of life and resolves within hours to days.

◉ Look For

The characteristic lesion is a 1 to 2 mm pale-to-yellow papule or pustule within a large (over 1 cm) inflammatory wheal (Figs. 4-19–4-22). Early on, however, the rash may only consist of blotchy, irregular erythematous macules. Any skin surface may be involved, usually sparing the palms and soles.

●● Diagnostic Pearls

Erythema toxicum very rarely presents at birth or affects the palms and soles, distinguishing it from congenital candidiasis and transient neonatal pustular melanosis, in which this is characteristic.

?? Differential Diagnosis and Pitfalls

Vesiculopustular rashes in the neonate may be divided into infectious, transient, or persistent dermatoses.

Infectious Vesiculopustular Dermatoses

- Congenital cutaneous candidiasis
- Superficial staphylococcal infection

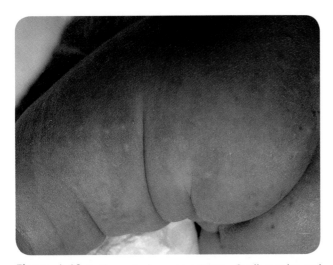

Figure 4-19 Erythema toxicum neonatorum. Small papules and vesicles with a wide rim of erythema.

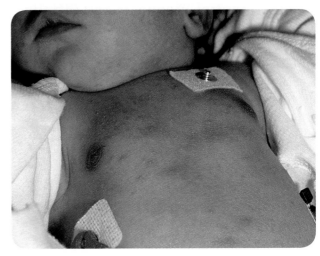

Figure 4-20 Erythema toxicum neonatorum. Tiny wheals and vesicles with extensive erythema.

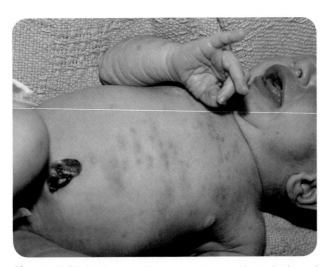

Figure 4-21 Erythema toxicum neonatorum. Tiny wheals and papules, many with significant surrounding erythema.

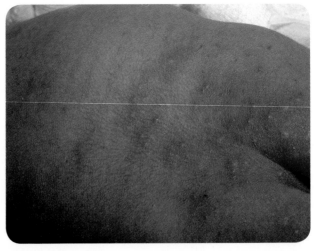

Figure 4-22 Erythema toxicum neonatorum with mainly vesicles and erythema.

- *Listeria monocytogenes*
- *Haemophilus influenza*
- Group A streptococcal infection
- *Pseudomonas*
- *Cytomegalovirus*
- *Aspergillus*
- Herpes simplex
- Neonatal varicella
- Scabies

Transient Noninfectious Vesiculopustular Dermatoses

- Neonatal pustular melanosis
- Miliaria crystallina and rubra
- Neonatal acne
- Acropustulosis of infancy
- Pustular eruption in Down syndrome

Persistent Noninfectious Vesiculopustular Dermatoses

- Incontinentia pigmenti
- Eosinophilic pustular folliculitis
- Langerhans cell histiocytosis
- Hyperimmunoglobulin E syndrome
- Pustular psoriasis

 Best Tests

Wright stain of vesicular fluid will reveal numerous eosinophils.

 Management Pearls

Reassure the parent that this is a transient and benign common rash.

Therapy

None. The condition is self-limiting.

Suggested Readings

Berg FJ, Solomon LM. Erythema neonatorum toxicum. *Arch Dis Child.* 1987;62(4):327–328.

Chang MW, Jiang SB, Orlow SJ. Atypical erythema toxicum neonatorum of delayed onset in a term infant. *Pediatr Dermatol.* 1999;16(2):137–141.

Van Praag MC, Van Rooij RW, Folkers E, et al. Diagnosis and treatment of pustular disorders in the neonate. *Pediatr Dermatol.* 1997;14(2):131–143.

Wagner A. Distinguishing vesicular and pustular disorders in the neonate. *Curr Opin Pediatr.* 1997;9(4):396–405.

Diagnosis Synopsis

Lyme disease is a complex of symptoms and signs related to infection by the tick-borne spirochete *Borrelia*. *Borrelia garinii* and *Borrelia afzelii* are the predominant causes of the disease in Europe. *Borrelia burgdorferi* is the predominant cause in America. The disease usually begins with an expanding skin lesion, erythema migrans, at the site of the tick bite (early localized disease). Within days to weeks, the spirochete disseminates to the nervous system, heart, joints, and other organs. At this time, patients may develop acute neurologic abnormalities, atrioventricular block, myocarditis, and disseminated skin lesions of erythema migrans (early disseminated disease). Months later, untreated patients may develop arthritis, an encephalopathy, a neuropathy, and in Europe, acrodermatitis, chronica atrophicans (late disease). Less than 3.6% of patients with tick bites from *Ixodes scapularis*, the vector *of B. burgdorferi* in America, develop Lyme disease.

The Centers for Disease Control and Prevention case definition for Lyme disease for National Surveillance is as follows:

- Physician-observed erythema migrans. For surveillance, a solitary lesion must reach 5 cm in greatest diameter.

Or, at least one subsequent manifestation and laboratory evidence of infection:

- Nervous system: lymphocytic meningitis, cranial neuritis, radiculoneuropathy, or encephalomyelitis.
- Cardiovascular system: acute onset, second or third degree atrioventricular conduction defects that resolve in days or weeks.
- Musculoskeletal system: recurrent attacks lasting weeks to months of physician-confirmed joint swelling in one or few joints, sometimes followed by chronic arthritis.

- Laboratory: isolation of *B. burgdorferi* from tissue or body fluid or detection of diagnostic levels of antibody by the two-test approach of enzyme-linked immunosorbent assay and Western blotting.

Look For

Early Localized

Seven to fourteen days after the tick detaches (range, 3 to 30 days), a small red macule or papule appears at the site of the tick bite (in 50% to 80% of children). Gradually, the redness expands over several days with a slightly raised, warm, red to bluish-red border that lacks scale (erythema migrans) (Figs. 4-23 and 4-24). Central clearing may be present, and the diameter may reach 68 cm. Patients often have accompanying influenzalike symptoms.

Early Disseminated

Multiple erythematous, gradually expanding, blanching macules and minimally elevated plaques present in a generalized distribution (disseminated erythema migrans). These are often smaller than the primary lesion of erythema migrans.

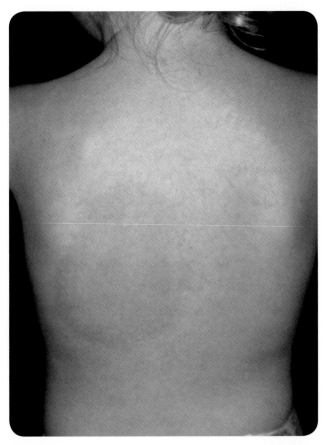

Figure 4-24 Lyme disease. Large lesion of erythema chronicum migrans with central hyperpigmentation and wide red annular border.

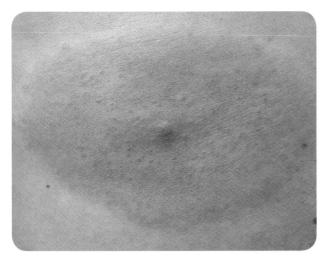

Figure 4-23 Early tick bite reaction consistent with early erythema migrans.

A *Borrelia* lymphocytoma can present as a bluish-red nodule or plaque on the ear lobe, nipples, or scrotum. Patients may have influenzalike symptoms, neurologic symptoms (15% of patients), oligoarticular arthritis (60% of patients), or signs of atrioventricular block (5% of patients).

Late

Acrodermatitis chronica atrophicans typically presents as erythematous, doughy, or indurated nodules or plaques that slowly expand over several months, leaving behind central atrophic changes. They are often associated with systemic signs of late Lyme disease, such as polyneuropathy, encephalomyelitis, cognitive abnormalities, dilated cardiomyopathy, or arthritis.

Diagnostic Pearls

- Mark the borders of skin lesions with ink and observe for 1 to 2 days without antibiotic therapy. Erythema migrans will expand beyond the markings, whereas tick bite reactions usually fade within 48 h.
- Transmission of Lyme borreliosis requires 24 to 48 h of attachment by an *Ixodes* sp. tick. Only black-legged adult *Ixodes* spp. are known to transmit Lyme disease. Entomologists can identify tick species, developmental stage, and the days of attachment by examining their level of engorgement.

?? Differential Diagnosis and Pitfalls

Early

Erythema annulare centrifugum—fine collarette of scale inside advancing border

Single Lesion

- Insect and tick bites—erythema migrans is typically not associated with significant pruritus and expands over days to weeks after a tick is removed, whereas insect and tick bite reactions are usually smaller than 5 cm in diameter, may appear urticarial, are often extremely pruritic, and typically resolve over 24 to 48 h of the bite. Erythema migrans also usually affects the axilla, popliteal fossae, and abdomen, whereas insect bites occur on exposed extremities.
- Fixed drug eruption—history of drug exposure, resolves with hyperpigmentation.
- Tinea corporis—associated scale, hyphal elements on skin scrapings.
- Contact dermatitis—well demarcated, pruritic, scaly, lichenified, or vesicular.
- Cellulitis—favors exposed sites, tender or painful.

Early Disseminated

Multiple Lesions

- Erythema multiforme—presents with target lesions and often coexisting herpes orolabialis
- Secondary syphilis—scale is typically more prominent in secondary syphilis
- Pityriasis rosea—presents with a trailing scale
- Urticaria—pruritic wheals that resolve within 24 h

Lymphocytoma

- A number of stimuli, including arthropod bites, can cause an inflammatory reaction pattern in the skin leading to the formation of nodular lesions clinically and histologically resembling cutaneous lymphoma, called pseudolymphoma. *Borrelia* lymphocytoma is a subset of pseudolymphomas.
- Scabies—nodular lesions in infants and young children with significant pruritus.
- Cutaneous metastases—less prevalent on the earlobe, nipple, and genitalia.
- Sarcoidosis—indurated papules and plaques favoring the face and scars.

Late

- Rheumatic diseases (juvenile idiopathic arthritis, systemic lupus erythematosus, or dermatomyositis)—negative *Borrelia* serologies, positive rheumatic serologies, no response to antibiotics
- Lichen sclerosus and morphea—negative *Borrelia* serologies, no response to antibiotics, not associated with systemic symptoms

✓ Best Tests

- It is important to remember that more than 4% of individuals in endemic areas have seropositivity but do not have Lyme disease. Seropositivity must be combined with characteristic clinical findings to be diagnostic. Also, erythema migrans is sufficiently distinctive to allow clinical diagnosis in the absence of further testing, and only 17% of the patients will have positive serologies for Lyme disease.
- Recommended CDC two-step testing regimen for suspected cases:
  (1) ELISA for either total or IgM or IgG antibodies. If there is a negative or equivocal result,
  (2) Perform Western blot (immunoblot) as a second line test.
- Tests can be negative if taken too early in infection and should be repeated between 2 and 4 weeks after the initial tick bite.
- Demonstrating the organism within lesions by histochemistry or polymerase chain reaction is currently a research procedure rather than a practical clinical diagnostic test.

▲▲ Management Pearls

- Parents of children with tick bites, but not erythema migrans, should be instructed to monitor for signs and symptoms of tick-borne illness (expanding skin lesions and viral-like illness) for up to 1 month after tick removal.
- In the United States, Lyme disease is reportable in the District of Columbia and all states **except** Hawaii.
- Per the CDC, Lyme disease is a nationally notifiable disease via the National Notifiable Diseases Surveillance System.

Therapy

Tick avoidance measures (avoiding tick-infested areas, using protective clothing, and using repellants such as DEET) and careful inspection following outdoor activities are the most effective preventative strategies. Ticks should be removed promptly with fine-tipped forceps.

Infectious Disease Society of America Guidelines

Prophylaxis*

Within 72 h of tick bite, doxycycline 4 mg/kg in children aged 8 years or older (maximum dose of 200 mg). Not recommended for children aged younger than 8 years.

*Prophylaxis is indicated only when *all* of the following conditions are met:

1. The attached tick is identified as an *I. scapularis* tick that has been attached for approximately 36 h (determined by the degree of engorgement of the tick with blood or certainty of the time of exposure).
2. Postexposure prophylaxis is started within 72 h of tick removal.
3. The local rate of tick infection with *B. burgdorferi* is 20%.
4. Doxycycline is not contraindicated.

Observation is recommended if these criteria are not met.

Treatment

Preferred Oral Regimens

- Amoxicillin 50 mg/kg/day in three divided doses (maximum, 500 mg per dose) for 14 to 21 days

or

- Doxycycline, for children aged 8 years or older, 4 mg/kg daily in two divided doses (maximum 100 mg per dose)

for 10 to 21 days (not recommended for children aged younger than 8 years)

or

- Cefuroxime axetil 30 mg/kg daily in two divided doses (maximum 500 mg per dose) for 14 to 21 days

Alternative Oral Regimens

- Azithromycin 10 mg/kg daily (maximum of 500 mg/day) for 7 to 10 days

or

- Clarithromycin 7.5 mg/kg twice daily (maximum of 500 mg per dose) for 14 to 21 days

or

- Erythromycin 12.5 mg/kg four times daily (maximum of 500 mg per dose) for 14 to 21 days

Preferred Parenteral Regimen

- Ceftriaxone 50 to 75 mg/kg IV daily in a single dose (maximum 2 g)

Alternative Parenteral Regimens

- Cefotaxime 150 to 200 mg/kg IV daily in three to four divided doses (maximum 6 g/day) (duration dependent upon severity of infection)
- Penicillin G 200,000 to 400,000 U/kg daily divided every 4 h (maximum 18 to 24 million U per day) (duration dependent upon severity of infection)

Suggested Readings

Bolognia JL, Jorizzo JL, Rapini RP, eds. *Dermatology*. Vol. 1. 2nd Ed. St Louis, MO: Mosby; 2008:282–284.

Bratton RL, Whiteside JW, Hovan MJ, et al. Diagnosis and treatment of Lyme disease. *Mayo Clin Proc*. 2008;83(5):566–571.

Centers for Disease Control and Prevention (CDC). Recommendations for test performance and interpretation from the Second National Conference on Serologic Diagnosis of Lyme Disease. *MMWR Morb Mortal Wkly Rep*. 1995;44:590–591.

James WD, Berger TG, Elston DM, eds. *Andrews' Diseases of the Skin*. 10th Ed. Philadelphia, PA: WB Saunders; 2006:291–293.

Steere AC. Lyme disease. *N Engl J Med*. 2001;345(2):115–125.

Steere AC, McHugh G, Damle N, et al. Prospective study of serologic tests for lyme disease. *Clin Infect Dis*. 2008;47(2):188–195.

Wharton M, Chorba TL, Vogt RL, et al. Case definitions for public health surveillance. *MMWR Morb Mortal Wkly Rep*. 1990;39(RR-13):1–43.

Wormser GP, Dattwyler RJ, Shapiro ED, et al. The clinical assessment, treatment, and prevention of lyme disease, human granulocytic anaplasmosis, and babesiosis: Clinical practice guidelines by the Infectious Diseases Society of America. *Clin Infect Dis*. 2006;43:1089–1134.

Urticaria

Diagnosis Synopsis

Urticaria is a group of conditions characterized by the wheal-and-flare reaction, which is a transient, local, intradermal edema (wheal) with surrounding erythema (flare). Urticaria is classified as acute for eruptions lasting <6 weeks or chronic for eruptions persisting longer than 6 weeks. A variety of factors, including systemic diseases, infections, drugs, food, insect bites, and physical agents, may cause urticaria. In children, viral infections are the most common cause of acute urticaria. Less common causes include food and drugs (especially the penicillins). Chronic urticaria is usually idiopathic.

Look For

Urticaria is characterized by well-circumscribed, blanching, erythematous, edematous, annular, or geographic papules and plaques (Figs. 4-25–4-28). Individual lesions resolve within 24h, leaving normal skin or a dusky appearance. Lesions vary in size from 2 to 5mm to over 30cm. Children are otherwise well and usually note significant pruritus. Lesions may occur anywhere on the body, but occur on the trunk with greater frequency.

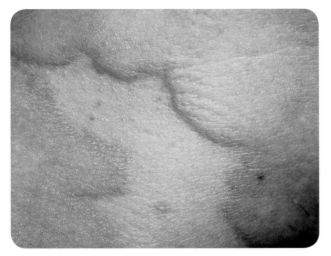

Figure 4-25 Urticaria with a large lesion with a polycyclic border.

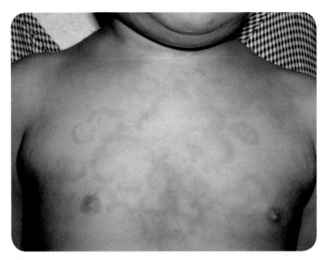

Figure 4-26 Urticaria. Multiple arcuate and annular lesions.

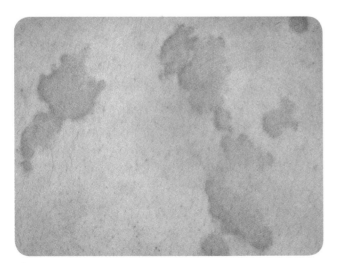

Figure 4-27 Urticaria. Multiple confluent wheals.

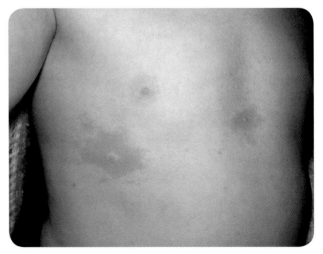

Figure 4-28 Urticaria pigmentosa is urticaria caused by a localized mast cell proliferation. Rubbing on a lesion causes a prominent urticarial wheal.

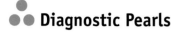

Diagnostic Pearls

- Although it may be extremely pruritic, unlike insect bites (papular urticaria), eczema, and most other pruritic dermatoses, the pruritus of urticaria rarely leads to excoriations.
- The duration of individual wheals can be helpful in eliciting a cause:
  - Ordinary urticaria (viral, food, or drug): 2 to 24 h
  - Contact urticaria (latex allergy): <2 h
  - Physical urticaria (heat, cold, water, and ultraviolet light): <1 h
  - Urticarial vasculitis: Several days
  - Angioedema: Several days
- If the duration is unclear by history, lesions can be circled with a pen and reassessed at a later time for clearing.

?? Differential Diagnosis and Pitfalls

Many serious illnesses present with urticarial lesions and should be considered with every case of urticaria. When in doubt, children should be observed for 2 to 4 h to monitor for disease progression.

Diseases with Urticarial Lesions Include

- Anaphylaxis—associated with angioedema and multiple systemic symptoms (especially respiratory and gastrointestinal) that usually begin within minutes of exposure
- Serum sickness/serum sicknesslike reaction—associated with fever, lymphadenopathy, arthralgias (refusal to use an extremity), dusky skin lesions, and recent drug (i.e., β-lactam) or sera exposure
- Kawasaki disease—the child appears ill and is febrile
- Urticarial vasculitis—individual lesions last longer than 24 h and are associated with purpura and arthralgias or arthritis (joint swelling or refusal to use extremities)
- Mastocytosis (urticaria pigmentosa)—has persistent yellow-brown macules and plaques that urticate with stroking
- Henoch–Schönlein purpura—associated with fever, edema, palpable purpura, renal, gastrointestinal, musculoskeletal, and central nervous system disease

Other Diseases with Urticarialike Lesions Include

- Angioedema—edema of the subcutaneous or submucosal tissues rather than edema of the dermis with urticaria, it is not pruritic, and it commonly affects the face (eyelids, earlobes, and lips); familial angioedema usually does not have individual small hives

- Erythema multiforme—fixed for several days; do not respond to antihistamines; and associated with dusky, necrotic centers (rather than the pale edematous center of urticaria)
- Papular urticaria/insect bites—often excoriated and lasts longer than 24 h
- Lupus erythematosus—often with epidermal changes (scaly, atrophic, or ulcerated)
- Herpes zoster—may also be urticarial but is painful and long lasting
- Erythema annulare centrifugum—often with epidermal changes (scale), and lesions persist for weeks
- Cellulitis
- Fixed drug eruption
- Morbilliform drug eruption
- Erythema migrans
- Erythema marginatum
- Juvenile idiopathic arthritis

✓ Best Tests

- Blood tests—an erythrocyte sedimentation rate and a C-reactive protein level may be helpful to rule out systemic disease in chronic urticaria.
- Urine tests—urinalysis for proteinuria is useful to rule out serum sickness and urinary tract infection as a source of the urticaria.
- Skin biopsy—useful to rule out urticarial vasculitis in lesions that are purpuric or persist for more than 24 h.
- Radioallergosorbent tests or fluoroimmunoassay may be considered in children to rule out potential food allergies.

▲▲ Management Pearls

- Within the first minutes of an initial episode, children with uncomplicated urticaria that responds to antihistamines should be observed by the caregiver for 30 min to 2 h for the development of signs of anaphylaxis. Children with coexisting facial angioedema or signs worrisome for anaphylaxis should be observed in an emergency room or outpatient clinic for several hours or overnight (in addition to appropriate therapy).
- If systemic signs of anaphylaxis have not developed within the first few hours of an urticarial episode, they are not likely to develop throughout the course of that episode.
- Oral and parenteral H1-antihistamines take at least 1 h to relieve skin symptoms. They are not effective against airway obstruction or shock from anaphylaxis.
- Allergist and pediatric dermatologic referral may be helpful in recurrent or chronic cases.

Therapy

All forms and etiologies of urticaria are treated by (i) eliminating the eliciting stimulus; (ii) inhibiting mast cell mediator release; and (iii) inhibiting the effect of mast cell mediators on target tissues.

Eliminating the eliciting stimulus will clear IgE-mediated urticaria within 48 h.

- Stop or substitute the offending drug.
- Treat the underlying infection.
- Elimination diets should be conducted under the guidance of a pediatric allergist.
- Avoid aspirin and other NSAIDs during an outbreak as they may exacerbate urticaria.

Inhibiting Mast Cell Mediator Release

For severe reactions (anaphylaxis, severe angioedema, serum sicknesslike reaction)—Solu-Medrol 1 to 2 mg/kg/day p.o. for 3 days.

Inhibiting the effect of mast cell mediators on target tissues is mainly achieved through H1-antihistamines.

- Diphenhydramine hydrochloride (Benadryl) 12.5 mg/5 mL (120 and 240 mL bottles; 25 and 50 mg capsules) 4 to 6 mg/kg/day divided four times daily
- Hydroxyzine (Atarax) 10 mg/5 mL, (240 mL bottle; 10 and 25 mg tablet) 2 mg/kg/day divided four times daily
- Cetirizine hydrochloride (Zyrtec) is given as a single daily dose, with or without food: 10 mg tabs, 5 mg/5 mL liquid
- Consider adding cimetidine (an H2-antihistamine) 10 to 20 mg/kg/day divided every 6 to 12 h in resistant urticaria

If Concern for Anaphylaxis

- Epinephrine 0.01 mg/kg intramuscularly
- Supplemental oxygen
- Establish intravenous access
- Institute continuous monitoring
- Intravenous methylprednisolone, repeat epinephrine, diphenhydramine, dopamine, Levophed, albuterol, and intubation as indicated by severity, degree of response, and the patient's course

Special Considerations in Infants

Unlike older children, infantile urticaria is often associated with two unique features:

(1) Infants often have hemorrhagic lesions or a cockade pattern, in which a bruised or dusky discoloration is left at sites of prior urtication. The purpuric discoloration may persist up to 2 days.
(2) Deep dermal or subcutaneous swellings of the eyelids, lips, and extremities (angioedema) are also common in infants.

Suggested Readings

Legrain V, Taïeb A, Sage T, et al. Urticaria in infants: A study of forty patients. *Pediatr Dermatol*. 1990;7(2):101–107.

Zuberbier T, Bindslev-Jensen C, Canonica W, et al. EAACI/GA2LEN/EDF guideline: Management of urticaria. *Allergy*. 2006;61(3):321–331.

Diagnosis Synopsis

Capillaritis, or pigmented purpura, refers to a group of benign conditions caused by inflammation of the superficial dermal capillaries. The disease is usually asymptomatic, but it may be pruritic. Names for the individual subtypes include Schamberg disease, Majocchi disease, lichen aureus, lichenoid pigmented purpura of Gougerot and Blum, and eczematoid purpura of Ducas and Kapetanakis. Proposed etiologies for capillaritis include capillary fragility, a hypersensitivity reaction, or a medication reaction. The course of the disease is unpredictable, with exacerbations and remissions lasting from several months to years.

Look For

Large numbers of uniform, nonpalpable, pinpoint petechiae in an otherwise well patient. The characteristic lesion is a red to yellow-brown macule with clusters of minute petechiae at its periphery ("cayenne pepper spots") (Figs. 4-29–4-32). Lesions do not blanch on diascopy.

Individual subtypes have characteristic features:

- Schamberg disease—asymptomatic, slowly developing, polymorphous macules of petechiae that typically affect the lower extremities symmetrically.
- Purpura annularis telangiectodes of Majocchi—annular with peripheral telangiectases.
- Lichen aureus—well-defined, static, rust-yellow papules and/or macules that coalesce into plaques of varying size. Lesions are often linear and favor the lower extremities.
- Eczematoid purpura of Ducas and Kapetanakis— generalized and pruritic with overlying eczematous change.

- Lichenoid pigmented purpura of Gougerot and Blum— polygonal, flat-topped papules and plaques; not reported in children.

Diagnostic Pearls

- Look closely at the lesions—there will be variation in color, reflecting different stages of hemosiderin resorption.
- The morphological variants may be hard to distinguish, hence the designation of capillaritis.
- Lichen aureus may closely resemble "hickeys," but lesions persist for months to years.

?? Differential Diagnosis and Pitfalls

- Minute leakage of red blood cells (RBCs) into an inflammatory rash such as dermatitis can sometimes cause similar skin lesions; however, the hemorrhage is an epiphenomena to the primary dermatitis
- Drug reaction
- Suction petechiae ("hickey")
- Fixed drug reaction

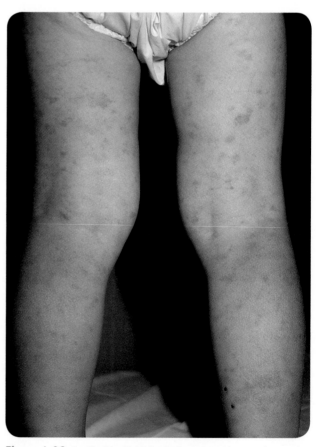

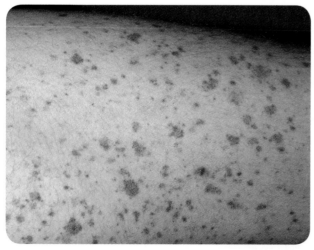

Figure 4-29 Capillaritis with small and large reddish-brown macules with peripheral petechiae.

Figure 4-30 Capillaritis. Multiple distinct nummular macules varying from bright red to brown.

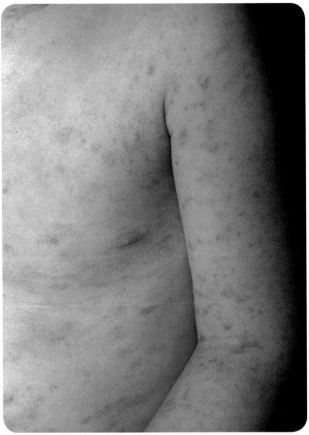

Figure 4-31 Capillaritis in a generalized distribution with discrete and confluent, yellow-to-orange, nonblanching macules.

- Kaposi sarcoma
- Lichen planus
- Mycosis fungoides
- Vasculitis
- Scurvy
- Thrombocytopenic purpura
- Trauma
- Venous stasis

✓ Best Tests

- Diascopy (viewing through a glass slide that is firmly pressed against the lesion) will reveal multiple, nonblanching pinpoint petechiae.
- Skin biopsy will reveal a superficial, perivascular lymphocytic infiltrate with RBC extravasation and melanophages.
- Platelet count and function, prothrombin time, bleeding time, and hemoglobin concentration will be normal.

▲▲ Management Pearls

- Midpotency topical steroids and antihistamines may provide some relief of itch if present.

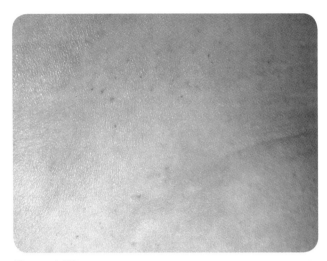

Figure 4-32 Capillaritis with pinhead-size reddish-brown macules resembling cayenne pepper grains.

- Consider a skin biopsy to rule out mycosis fungoides in unusually persistent or extensive disease.

Therapy

Some report success with a combination of vitamin C (500 mg p.o. twice daily) and rutoside (50 mg p.o. twice daily). If a medication is suspected (usually NSAIDs or acetaminophen), lesions may resolve within several months of discontinuing the offending agent.

Special Considerations in Infants

Capillaritis is extremely rare in infants, and one should rule out other causes of purpura with a thorough history and physical exam, evaluation for coagulopathy, and possible skin biopsy.

Suggested Readings

Paller AS, Mancini AJ. Vascular disorders of infancy and childhood. In: Paller AS, Mancini AJ, eds. *Hurwitz Clinical Pediatric Dermatology*. 3rd Ed. Philadelphia, PA: Elsevier Saunders; 2006:307–344.

Tristani-Firouzi P, Meadows KP, Vanderhooft S. Pigmented purpuric eruptions of childhood: A series of cases and review of literature. *Pediatr Dermatol*. 2001;18(4):299–304.

Weston WL, Orchard D. Vascular reactions. In: Schachner LA, Hansen RC, eds. *Pediatric Dermatology*. 3rd Ed. Edinburgh, Scotland: Mosby; 2003: 801–831.

Zvulunov A, Avinoach I, Hatsckelzon L, et al. Pigmented purpuric dermatosis (Schamberg's purpura) in an infant. *Dermatol Online J*. 1999;5(1):2. http://dermatology.cdlib.org/DOJvol5num1/case_reports/purpura.html. Accessed August 29, 2008.

Diagnosis Synopsis

Drug-induced pigmentation or dyspigmentation represents 10% to 20% of all cases of acquired hyperpigmentation. Mechanisms of drug-induced pigmentation include cutaneous deposition of the drug or its metabolites, accumulation of melanin, deposition of iron, or synthesis and deposition of special pigments such as lipofuscin. Increased melanin produces brown pigmentation. When medications are deposited in the dermis, they can cause blue-black or muddy-brown macules. Drugs commonly associated with hyperpigmentation include NSAIDs, antimalarials, psychotropic medications, amiodarone, bleomycin, tetracyclines (most commonly minocycline), and metals such as silver and gold.

Look For

Look for unusual colors of the pigmentation such as blue-gray, brown, yellow, or red-brown (Figs. 4-33–4-35). Color and distribution depend on the inciting medication.

Diagnostic Pearls

Diffuse hyperpigmentation may indicate systemic disease or a drug reaction to the following:

- Yellow—quinacrine
- Blue-black—antimalarials, chloroquine, hydroxychloroquine or hydroquinone, and minocycline
- Blue-gray—gold, minocycline
- Blue—amiodarone, mercury
- Purple—clofazimine
- Brown streaks (flagellate or linear)—bleomycin

?? Differential Diagnosis and Pitfalls

- Jaundice causes a yellow cast to the skin.
- Carotenemia causes an orange color.

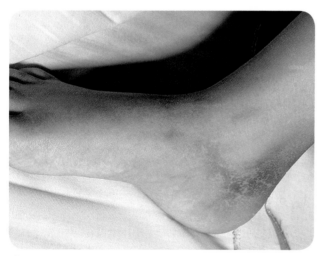

Figure 4-33 Drug-induced pigmentation.

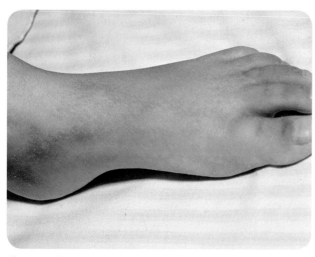

Figure 4-34 Drug-induced pigmention due to doxorubicin.

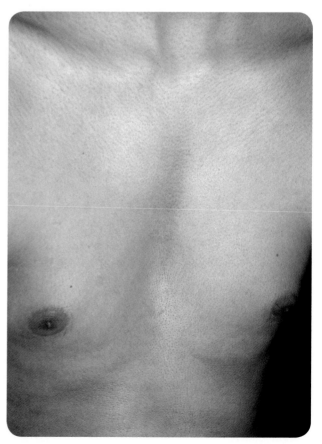

Figure 4-35 Drug-induced pigmentation due to sertraline.

- Generalized hyperpigmentation is also seen in Addison disease, Cushing syndrome, scleroderma, hemochromatosis, chronic renal failure, and porphyria cutanea tarda.
- Pellagra may also result in pigmentary change in a photodistribution.
- Postinflammatory hyperpigmentation has history of preceding inflammation.

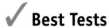

✓ Best Tests

Skin biopsy will often reveal the type of pigment in the skin, but is not generally helpful in pinpointing the causative agent.

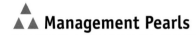

▲▲ Management Pearls

Identifying and discontinuing the responsible drug is the treatment of choice. It may take months to years for the pigment to resolve.

Therapy

Once the offending medication is discontinued, much of the pigmentation will improve with time.

As the hyperpigmentation can be worsened by sun exposure, sunscreens with UVB and UVA blockers may be helpful in preventing further darkening.

As the pigment is located in the dermis, bleaching agents are ineffective. Various lasers have been reported to be effective in the treatment of minocycline-induced hyperpigmentation.

Suggested Readings

Dereure O. Drug-induced skin pigmentation. Epidemiology, diagnosis and treatment. *Am J Clin Dermatol*. 2001;2(4):253–262.

Nikolaou V, Stratigos AJ, Katsambas AD. Established treatments of skin hypermelanosis. *J Cosmet Dermatol*. 2006;5(4):303–308.

◼◼ Diagnosis Synopsis

Fixed drug eruption (FDE) is an adverse drug reaction manifested by nonmigratory plaques. The plaques occur at the same body site each time the individual is re-exposed to a specific drug. Lesions are usually painful but infrequently cause burning or pruritus. Sometimes, these lesions will form blisters (bullous FDE) that eventually rupture.

Many different medications have been reported to cause FDE. Trimethoprim–sulfamethoxazole is the most frequently associated drug, but other drugs known to cause the condition are analgesics/antipyretics (aspirin and NSAIDs), other antibiotics (ampicillin, metronidazole, and tetracycline), as well as barbiturates, oral contraceptives, and quinine. Phenolphthalein (historically, a component of laxatives; replaced by senna) was found to be causative, but is no longer used.

◉ Look For

Solitary or multiple; sharply demarcated; round or oval; edematous; pink, red, or brown-red plaques begin anywhere from 30 min to 8 h after the drug is taken (Figs. 4-36–4-39).

Macules range in size from 2 to 10 cm and may intensify in inflammation with dusky or violaceous discoloration if exposure is continued. Once the offending agent is discontinued, the lesions usually resolve within 1 to 2 weeks but may leave hyperpigmented (gray-brown) patches that can last for months.

The most frequent locations are the trunk, limbs, lips, and genitals, but lesions can occur on any mucocutaneous surface, including the tongue.

●● Diagnostic Pearls

Suspect FDE in any patient who has recently started a new medication and presents with a single, well-defined, red plaque.

?? Differential Diagnosis and Pitfalls

- Insect bite reaction
- Urticaria
- Contact dermatitis
- Erythema multiforme
- Recurrent herpes simplex

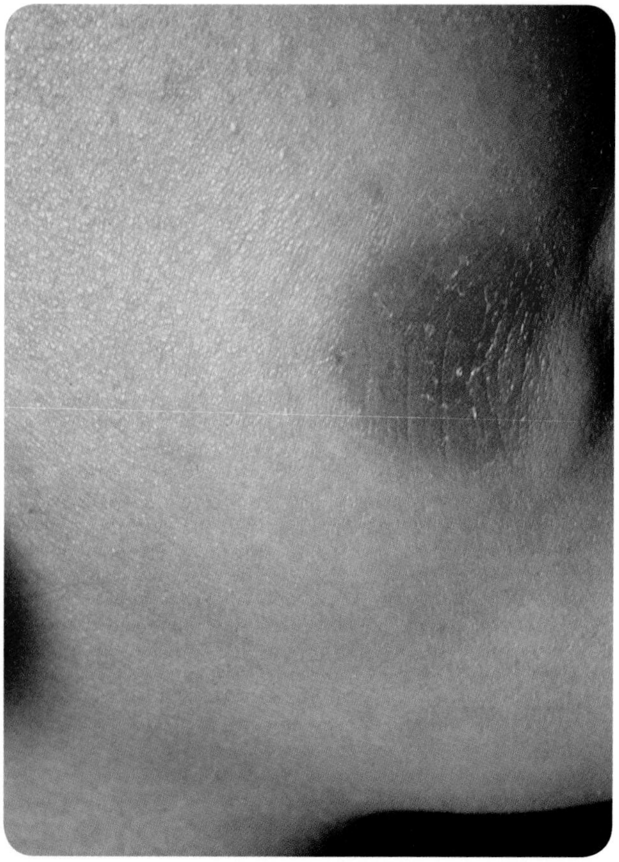

Figure 4-36 FDE. Round plaque with sharp borders and edema.

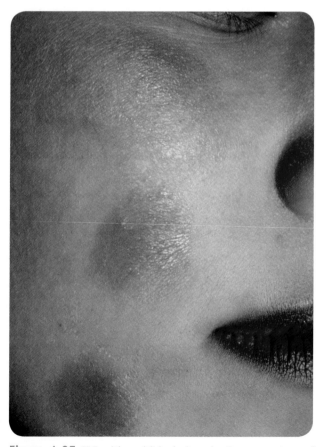

Figure 4-37 FDE with multiple lesions in the same stage of development.

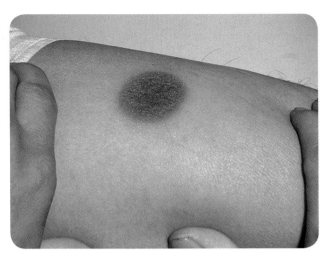

Figure 4-38 FDE due to amobarbital.

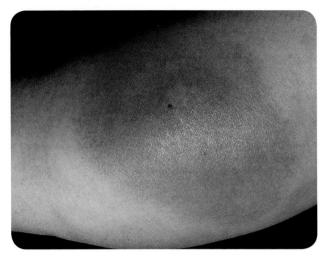

Figure 4-39 FDE due to cotrimoxazole.

✓ Best Tests

- A punch biopsy will reveal vacuolization along the dermoepidermal junction and melanophages, but it is not always necessary.
- If a vesicle is present, a Tzanck smear or viral PCR should be performed to rule out herpes simplex virus.

▲▲ Management Pearls

- The most important management issue is identifying the offending agent.
- A thorough medication history to include all over-the-counter medications as well as any herbal or vitamin supplements should be taken in all patients.

Therapy

Once the offending medication is discontinued, no other therapy is necessary. Topical corticosteroids may be helpful for treating pruritus if present.

Suggested Readings

Bolognia JL, Jorizzo JL, Rapini RP, eds. *Dermatology*. Vol. 1. 2nd Ed. St Louis, MO: Mosby; 2008:311–312.

Nussinovitch M, Prais D, Ben-Amitai D, et al. Fixed drug eruption in the genital area in 15 boys. *Pediatr Dermatol*. 2002;19(3):216–219.

Dermal Melanocytosis (Mongolian Spot)

■■ Diagnosis Synopsis

Mongolian spots, also known as blue-gray spots, are a congenital, benign, blue-to-gray hyperpigmentation caused by an excess quantity of dermal melanocytes. These spots are most commonly found on the sacrococcygeal area in infants of Asian or African decent but may be found on any cutaneous surface in infants of all races. The pigmentation becomes most intense at 1 year of age, reaches its peak diameter by 2 years of age, and usually fades completely by adulthood.

◉ Look For

Mongolian spots are evenly pigmented, blue to gray macules that range in size from 1 to >10 cm. They are typically round to oval but may be polymorphous. Infants may have one or multiple macules of varying shades of gray and blue. Borders are typically irregular to indistinct (Figs. 4-40–4-43).

●● Diagnostic Pearls

- The sacrococcygeal location of blue-gray patches at birth is highly suggestive of this diagnosis.
- Extensive Mongolian spots (covering the sacral to extrasacral area) have been described in GM1 gangliosidosis type 1, Hunter syndrome, and Hurler syndrome, but are typically an isolated finding.

?? Differential Diagnosis and Pitfalls

- Purpura and ecchymoses—changes color from blue to green to brown over days to weeks; uneven pigmentation; tender to palpation

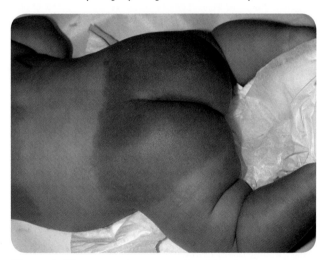

Figure 4-40 Dermal melanocytosis (Mongolian spot) in a typical location and larger than usual.

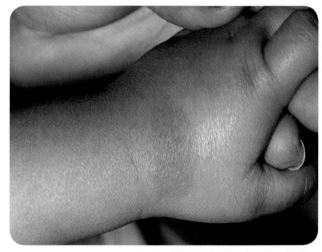

Figure 4-41 Dermal melanocytosis (Mongolian spot) may be anywhere on the skin.

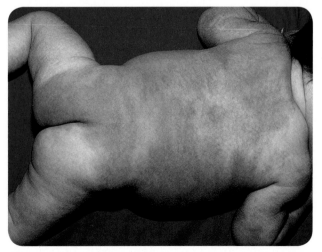

Figure 4-42 Dermal melanocytosis (Mongolian spot) can be confluent with variation in pigmentation.

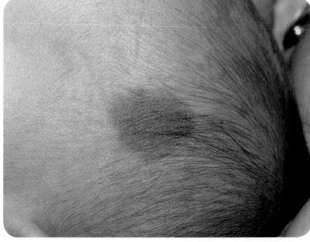

Figure 4-43 Dermal melanocytosis (Mongolian spot) can be limited to the scalp.

- Congenital melanocytic nevus—brown, well-defined, surface change (e.g., raised lesions)
- Blue nevus—usually smaller than 5 mm diameter, well-defined, surface change (e.g., raised lesions)
- Nevus of Ito—often speckled; progresses with age; located over the shoulder, clavicle, and scapular region
- Nevus of Ota—often speckled; progresses with age; located in the periorbital region
- Venous malformation—usually palpable; may swell or deepen in coloration when dependent or crying
- Infantile hemangioma—overlying telangiectases; may swell or deepen in coloration when dependent or crying; rapidly elevates over days to weeks

✓ Best Tests

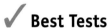

Skin biopsy will show increased numbers of melanocytes in the dermis; however, the diagnosis is usually made on clinical grounds.

▲▲▲ Management Pearls

- Document the presence of Mongolian spots to prevent false accusations of child abuse by unknowing persons.
- Mongolian spots have no increased risk for the development of melanoma or other skin cancers.

Therapy

Mongolian spots fade spontaneously during childhood, and therapy (lasers or excision) is not indicated prior to adulthood.

Suggested Readings

Kikuchi I. What is a Mongolian spot? *Int J Dermatol.* 1982;21(3):131–133.

Ochiai T, Ito K, Okada T, et al. Significance of extensive Mongolian spots in Hunter's syndrome. *Br J Dermatol.* 2003;148(6):1173–1178.

Vitiligo

Diagnosis Synopsis

Vitiligo is a relatively common idiopathic disorder affecting melanocytes, resulting in depigmented white patches of the skin. Vitiligo typically arises symmetrically in areas of frequent trauma, particularly on the face, upper chest, hands, elbows, knees, axillae, and perineum. Prevalence is estimated to be between 0.5% and 1%. Vitiligo often presents in childhood or young adulthood, with roughly half of cases beginning before the age of 20. While the exact etiology is not known, many consider vitiligo to be an autoimmune disease in which the melanocyte is targeted. Other autoimmune diseases are observed more frequently in patients with vitiligo, including diabetes mellitus type 1, pernicious anemia, Hashimoto thyroiditis, Graves disease, Addison disease, and alopecia areata.

The segmental form of the disease, which presents as an asymmetric, frequently dermatomal, depigmented band, disproportionally affects children. This form of the disease is less likely to be associated with coexisting autoimmune phenomena.

Look For

Sharply demarcated macules of depigmentation, typically beginning on the hands, face, or neck with no associated change in skin texture (Figs. 4-44–4-46). If the affected area bears hair, the hair can also turn white (poliosis) (Fig. 4-47). Lesions are often periorificial and at sites of trauma. Occasionally, tan zones of pigmentation may be observed between normal skin and depigmented lesions. This presentation is referred to as trichrome vitiligo.

The segmental variant of vitiligo presents as asymmetric macules arising within a dermatome.

Diagnostic Pearls

Use a Wood lamp (UVA light) to demonstrate depigmentation (very white) as opposed to hypopigmentation, which is less pronounced.

?? Differential Diagnosis and Pitfalls

- Note that albinism, piebaldism, and other genetic disorders begin in infancy.
- Pityriasis alba, typically affecting the cheeks of atopic individuals, presents with hypopigmented—not depigmented—macules with ill-defined borders.
- A history of prior trauma or skin inflammation can usually be elicited in cases of postinflammatory hypopigmentation. These lesions are not depigmented.
- Hypopigmented macules, also known as ash leaf spots, are typically the first cutaneous finding observed in patients with tuberous sclerosis. Wood lamp examination reveals hypopigmentation, not depigmentation. Lesions do not favor the face or areas of trauma, as may occur in vitiligo.
- Nevus depigmentosus are hypopigmented, usually present at birth, and usually do not extend or regress over time.
- Idiopathic guttate hypomelanosis presents as small 1 to 2 mm, hypopigmented macules arising in chronically sun-damaged skin.
- Pigmentary mosaicism, previously called hypomelanosis of Ito, presents as whorled areas of hypopigmentation following Blaschko lines.
- Chemical leukoderma arises following exposure to any of several depigmenting agents.

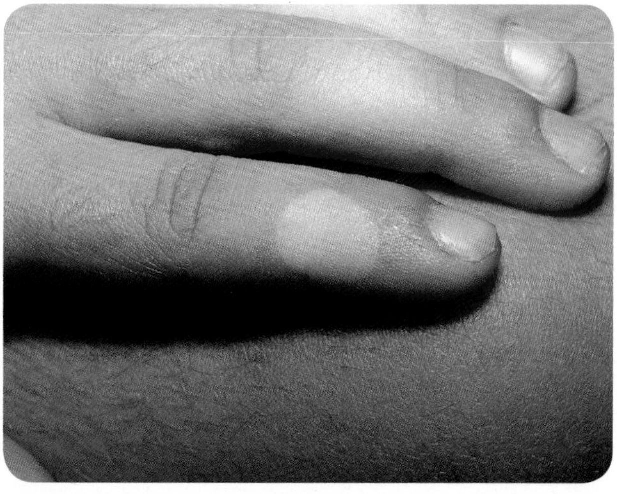

Figure 4-44

Figure 4-44 Vitiligo with depigmented macules in a common location.

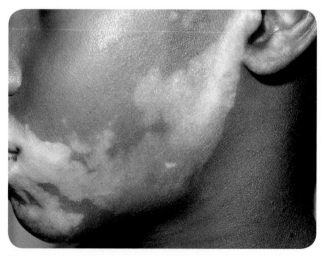

Figure 4-45 Vitiligo is common on the face.

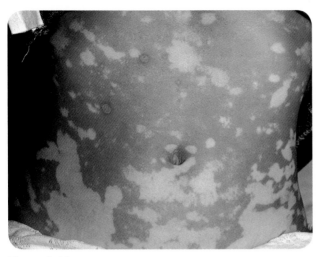

Figure 4-46 Vitiligo with multiple truncal depigmented macules.

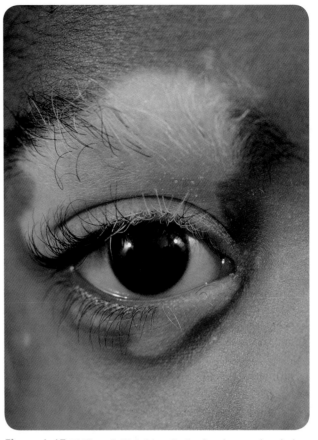

Figure 4-47 Vitiligo of skin with poliosis of eyebrow and eyelashes.

- Patients with Waardenburg syndrome may also present with heterochromia irides, deafness, limb defects, or Hirschsprung disease in addition to congenital pigmentary abnormalities.
- Lichen sclerosus can be depigmented but also has epidermal changes (atrophy, fissures, and petechiae).
- Lesions of tinea versicolor are located over the central upper chest and back and are hypopigmented and scaly. KOH examination can confirm the diagnosis.

✓ Best Tests

Diagnosis can usually be made clinically. Skin biopsy will reveal absence of melanocytes.

▲▲ Management Pearls

- Take a detailed personal and family history of autoimmune disease. Screening for coexisting autoimmune diseases should be guided by signs and symptoms. Vitiligo can be difficult to treat. Response to treatment can be subtle and slow. Tracking clinical response to treatment with serial photographs can be helpful to the patient, family, and treating clinician.
- Counsel patients and families about the importance of sun protection, as lesions of vitiligo are hypersensitive to UV light and burn easily.
- Facial and proximal extremities repigment more readily than acral locations.
- Total repigmentation is rare. With therapy, many patients will attain approximately 75% repigmentation.

Therapy

The appearance of vitiligo lesions can be extremely distressing. Patients frequently become anxious or depressed. Spontaneous repigmentation is rare, and response to treatment is slow. Several credible online resources are available to patients and families, including the National Vitiligo Foundation (http://www.nvfi.org/).

For patients with minimally pigmented, normal skin, lesions may be subtle and treatment with sun protection may be all that is necessary.

Several treatments have proven to be effective in partial repigmentation. Judicious use of topical steroids, with strength dependent upon anatomic location, has been successful. Close monitoring for signs of cutaneous atrophy is imperative. The topical immunomodulators tacrolimus and pimecrolimus are effective and are especially useful for the treatment of lesions in sites prone to atrophy, such as the face and eyelids. Narrowband UVB is another effective treatment option for more widespread cutaneous involvement. Patients should be counseled, however, that treatment may initially worsen the appearance of the disease due to increased pigmentation of surrounding normal skin, thus accentuating depigmented areas.

Additionally, several brands of makeup are available to temporarily conceal exposed lesions. Many light-skinned patients find application of sunless tanners containing dihydroxyacetone acceptable. Finally, patients with extensive disease that have failed other therapies may consider depigmentation of normal skin.

Special Considerations in Infants

Check for other stigmata or a family history of genetic pigmentary disorders such as oculocutaneous albinism, Waardenburg syndrome, or piebaldism, as they are more common to present at birth or in early infancy.

The natural course of vitiligo is slowly progressive, and most treatment options should be reserved for after infancy.

Suggested Readings

Bolognia JL, Jorizzo JL, Rapini RP, eds. *Dermatology*. Vol. 1. 2nd Ed. St. Louis, MO: Mosby; 2008:913–920.

Cohen BA, ed. *Pediatric Dermatology*. 3rd Ed. St. Louis, MO: Mosby; 2005: 153–155.

James WD, Berger TG, Elston DM, eds. *Andrews' Diseases of the Skin*. 10th Ed. Philadelphia, PA: WB Saunders; 2006:860–862.

Acne Vulgaris

■■ Diagnosis Synopsis

Acne vulgaris is a common condition in adolescents, affecting approximately 85% of patients aged 12 to 24. It begins most commonly at the onset of puberty and can last throughout adolescence and into adulthood. Acne is a result of androgen stimulation of the pilosebaceous unit and changes in the keratinization at the follicular orifice.

◉ Look For

Open comedones (blackheads), closed comedones (whiteheads), and red papules and pustules (Figs. 4-48–4-50). Nodules and cysts may be present in severe cases and can result in pitted or hypertrophic scars (Fig. 4-51). Acne most frequently targets the face, neck, upper trunk, and upper arms.

●● Diagnostic Pearls

- Differentiating between mainly comedonal and more inflammatory acne is important, as this will dictate treatment. Multiple ulcerative lesions in males in association with fever and joint pain are diagnostic of acne fulminans. Acne conglobata presents with cysts, abscesses, sinus tracts, and severe scarring without systemic symptoms.
- The combination of severe inflammatory acne in association with tender papules on the scalp and draining sinus tracts of axillae and/or perineum is often called the follicular occlusion complex. (Double comedones are frequently seen in this entity.)

?? Differential Diagnosis and Pitfalls

- Milia
- Periorificial dermatitis
- Folliculitis
- Benign appendageal lesions—e.g., syringomas
- Angiofibromas in tuberous sclerosis

✓ Best Tests

This is usually a clinical diagnosis. A skin biopsy will define the process but should be unnecessary. If folliculitis is suspected, a culture is helpful.

▲▲ Management Pearls

- Compliance is important with all treatment regimens and should be stressed at each visit. It is important that both patients and parents understand that acne may need to be treated throughout adolescence and that there is no quick cure. Acne can cause a great deal of psychosocial stress, especially in adolescents.
- As patients progress through teen years, acne can transition from comedonal to inflammatory.

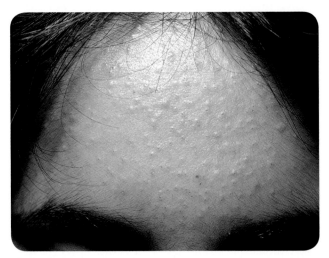

Figure 4-48 Acne vulgaris on forehead with multiple open comedones (*blackheads*).

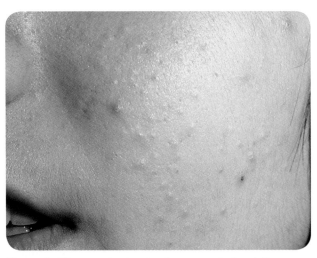

Figure 4-49 Acne vulgaris primarily composed of noninflammatory closed comedones (*whiteheads*).

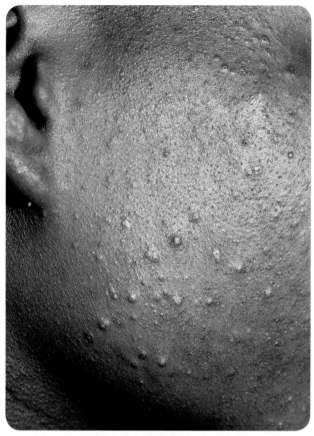

Figure 4-50 Acne vulgaris with inflammatory papules and postinflammatory hyperpigmentation often seen in those with darker skin pigmentation.

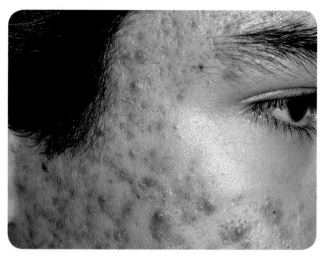

Figure 4-51 Acne vulgaris with multiple inflammatory papules and scarring. Several scars are from previous neonatal acne.

Therapy

Topical retinoids should be included in every acne regimen, as they normalize follicular keratinization and reduce inflammation. Side effects include irritation and dryness. Patients should be advised to use only a pea-size amount every night before bed and to treat their whole face, not just spot treat. It can take up to 3 months to see any benefit. Retinoids may be used as monotherapy or in conjunction with topical or oral antibiotics.

Topical antibiotics are useful in both comedonal and inflammatory acne. Examples include benzoyl peroxide, erythromycin, clindamycin, and sodium sulfacetamide. Monotherapy is not advised, with the exception of benzoyl peroxide, as this can lead to resistance. Many combination products are available. Benzoyl peroxide should not be applied at the same time as tretinoin.

Salicylic acid and azelaic acid may also be used topically. They are generally more effective when dosed in the morning in conjunction with a topical retinoid applied at night.

Oral antibiotics are used in inflammatory acne for their anti-inflammatory properties. The most commonly used antibiotics are minocycline and doxycycline. They should not be used in children aged younger than 8 years. Typical dosing regimens include twice daily use, though once daily dosing is also effective.

Oral isotretinoin is the only oral retinoid approved by the FDA for use in acne. This is tightly regulated, and both patients and providers must register with the iPLEDGE program (https://www.ipledgeprogram.com). Oral isotretinoin is associated with possible side effects including dryness, muscle and joint aches, gastrointestinal upset, pseudotumor cerebri (especially when used with oral tetracyclines), depression, and birth defects (if the pregnancy occurs while taking the medication or within 1 month of discontinuation).

Suggested Readings

Bolognia JL, Jorizzo JL, Rapini RP, eds. *Dermatology*. Vol. 1. 2nd Ed. St Louis, MO: Mosby; 2008:496–508.

Krakowski AC, Eichenfield LF. Pediatric acne: Clinical presentations, evaluation, and management. *J Drugs Dermatol.* 2007;6(6):589–593.

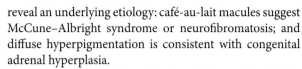

Acne, Neonatal (Benign Cephalic Pustulosis)

Diagnosis Synopsis

Neonatal acne, or neonatal cephalic pustulosis, is a very common acneiform eruption occurring on the face of neonates (aged 0 to 6 weeks). Many separate these two conditions as the following: neonatal cephalic pustulosis for a solely papulopustular eruption, often associated with *Malassezia* sp.; and neonatal acne for eruptions that include open comedones or nodulocystic lesions. This distinction is usually academic, as both tend to be very mild and spontaneously resolve by age 3 to 6 months without residual sequelae.

Look For

Neonatal cephalic pustulosis consists of erythematous papules and pustules, usually limited to the cheeks, chin, and forehead. Neonatal acne is diagnosed by the additional presence of open comedones (flat or elevated lesions with a central brown-to-black crater), closed comedones (tiny—<1 mm—flesh-colored papules), or nodulocystic lesions (erythematous nodules) (Figs. 4-52–4-55).

Diagnostic Pearls

- Neonatal cephalic pustulosis tends to be more erythematous and monomorphic than neonatal acne. Neonatal acne is also follicular based, whereas neonatal cephalic pustulosis is not.
- In cases of severe (nodulocystic or inflammatory and scarring) or recalcitrant neonatal acne, look for other signs of androgen excess such as axillary hair, pubic hair, testicular enlargement, clitoral enlargement, or ambiguous genitalia. Examination of skin pigmentation may

reveal an underlying etiology: café-au-lait macules suggest McCune–Albright syndrome or neurofibromatosis; and diffuse hyperpigmentation is consistent with congenital adrenal hyperplasia.

- A maternal prenatal medication history should be obtained to rule out acneiform drug reactions (i.e., phenytoin or lithium) when a neonate presents with an unusual acneiform eruption.

?? Differential Diagnosis and Pitfalls

- Miliaria rubra and pustulosa—identical to neonatal cephalic pustulosis but involves more of the skin folds (neck) and areas exposed to heat or occlusion
- Milia—more often on the nose and are white as opposed to erythematous
- Congenital candidiasis—more widespread and may be associated with infection of the mother, umbilical cord, or placenta
- Eosinophilic pustular folliculitis—more scalp involvement, rapidly crusts over, and is pruritic
- Staphylococcal folliculitis—more widespread and favors moist, occluded areas
- Scabies—pruritic and more widespread
- Keratosis pilaris—rough surfaced
- Nevus comedonicus—unilateral and linear
- Erythema toxicum neonatorum—more widespread and transient

✓ Best Tests

This is usually a clinical diagnosis; however, when the diagnosis is in doubt, direct microscopy with stains and culture of the pustular contents can be used to rule

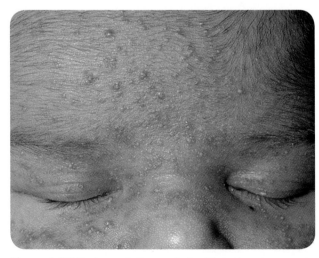

Figure 4-52 Benign cephalic pustulosis with erythematous papules and pustules in a typical location on the forehead.

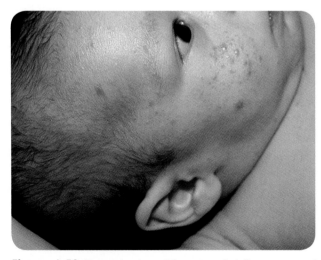

Figure 4-53 Neonatal acne with scattered inflammatory and noninflammatory papules.

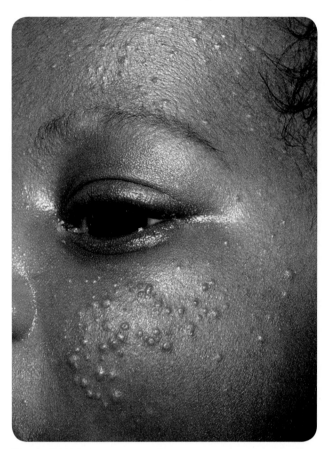

Figure 4-54 Neonatal acne with multiple papules with almost identical morphology.

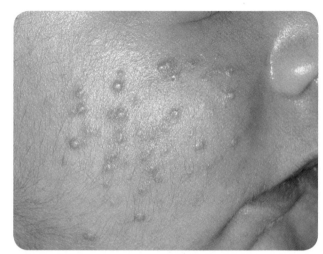

Figure 4-55 Neonatal acne with closely grouped, nearly identical papules.

out other diagnoses. Gram stain will rule out bacterial folliculitis, mineral oil to rule out scabies, or potassium hydroxide to rule out candidiasis. A Wright stain shows a preponderance of neutrophils as opposed to eosinophils in eosinophilic pustular folliculitis or erythema toxicum neonatorum. The results of direct microscopy would then be confirmed by cultures that either show no growth or are positive for *Malassezia* sp. (neonatal cephalic pustulosis, but these cultures are not commonly performed). Skin biopsies are rarely indicated.

▲▲ Management Pearls

- Parents should be reassured that the vast majority of neonatal acne and neonatal cephalic pustulosis are nonscarring and self-limited.
- An endocrinology referral should be considered for patients with severe or persistent neonatal acne. Additionally, a careful physical exam looking for signs of virilization and growth charts should be followed every 4 to 6 months to rule out evolving pathology in severely affected patients.

Therapy

Most cases of neonatal acne (and neonatal cephalic pustulosis) are mild and will resolve within 3 months without treatment. At most, parents should wash the child's face daily with soap (Dove or Cetaphil) and water. Occlusive baby oils and lotions should be avoided on the face, as they may exacerbate the disease.

For more moderate cases, one should attempt to distinguish between neonatal acne and neonatal cephalic pustulosis before beginning therapy:

- Neonatal acne can usually be managed with 2.5% to 5% benzoyl peroxide cream, topical clindamycin 1% cream, topical erythromycin 2% cream, or tretinoin 0.025% cream every other day to daily if there is no irritation. More severe cases require oral erythromycin or even isotretinoin to prevent scarring.
- Neonatal cephalic pustulosis is managed with either topical antifungal agents (ketoconazole cream) or hydrocortisone 1% to 2.5% cream twice daily as needed for flares.

Suggested Readings

Lucky AW. Transient benign cutaneous lesions in the newborn. In: Eichenfield LF, Frieden IJ, Esterly NB, eds. *Neonatal Dermatology*. 2nd Ed. Philadelphia, PA: WB Saunders; 2008:85–97.

Van Praag MC, Van Rooij RW, Folkers E, et al. Diagnosis and treatment of pustular disorders in the neonate. *Pediatr Dermatol*. 1997;14(2):131–143.

Wagner A. Distinguishing vesicular and pustular disorders in the neonate. *Curr Opin Pediatr*. 1997;9(4):396–405.

◼ Diagnosis Synopsis

Arthropods are invertebrate animals with a segmented body, jointed appendages, and hard exoskeleton. The most common biting arthropods of medical significance include organisms of the classes Insecta (lice, mosquitoes, flies, fleas, bedbugs, bees, wasps, and ants) and Arachnida (scabies, mites, ticks, and spiders). As there are multiple species of arthropods, bite reactions vary from mild local reactions to systemic illness depending on the characteristics of the host and species of the biting arthropod. Arthropod bite reactions are often seasonal depending on the organism's life cycle and habitat.

◉ Look For

Mosquito, fly, flea, chigger, and bedbug bites vary from pruritic erythematous papules and urticarial wheals to bullae that usually spontaneously subside over days (Figs. 4-56–4-59). Mosquito and fly bites have a predilection for exposed areas of the head, neck, and extremities. Flea and bedbug bites tend to be grouped in linear or irregular clusters ("breakfast, lunch, and dinner sign"). Chigger bites tend to cluster at areas where tight clothing meets the skin (below elastic diaper bands or above the sock line).

Wasp, bee, and fire ant stings are often painful and edematous. Fire ant stings may produce grouped painful papules that become vesicular within hours. In sensitized infants, anaphylactic reactions may develop (difficulty breathing, gastrointestinal disturbance, mental status change, generalized edema, and cardiovascular collapse).

Tick bites are often asymptomatic and only noticed when the attached tick is felt or seen during bathing. Occasionally, erythematous papules, nodules, edema, or ulcerations develop at the bite site.

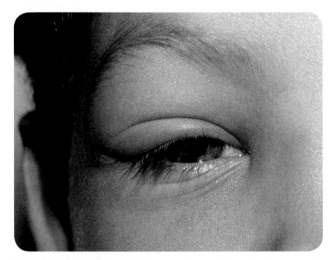

Figure 4-56 Arthropod bite around eye, where loose connective tissue is predisposed to extensive edema.

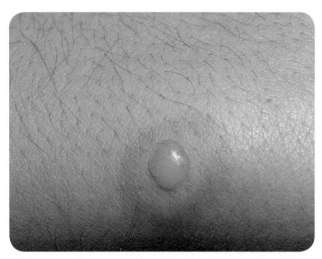

Figure 4-57 Arthropod bite with clear central vesicle and annular rim of erythema.

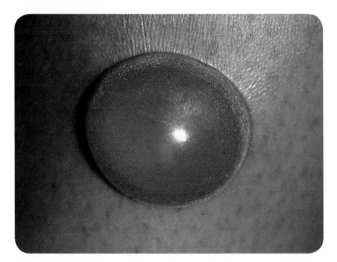

Figure 4-58 Arthropod bite with large bulla with clear fluid, as often seen in insect bites.

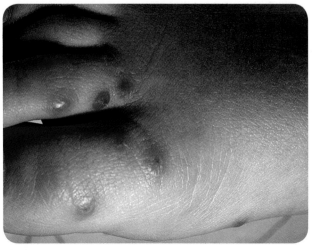

Figure 4-59 Arthropod bites on the feet from walking without socks in the grass are common in summer.

Diagnostic Pearls

- Do not discount an arthropod bite/sting because other family members do not have the same lesions, as not all individuals develop reactions to bug bites, and insects occasionally bite one family member preferentially.
- Arthropod bites should be considered in all individuals with otherwise unexplained pruritic papules.

?? Differential Diagnosis and Pitfalls

Bullous reactions to arthropod bites are often confused with bullous pemphigoid, linear IgA disease, cutaneous mastocytosis, and bullous impetigo. Tense bullae with a seasonal occurrence, a history of recent exposure to endemic areas, predilection for exposed sites, lack of significant surrounding inflammation, lack of systemic findings, and an absence of progression suggest arthropod bites over other diagnoses.

Urticarial/Papular Dermatoses

- Cutaneous mastocytosis (urticaria pigmentosa or mastocytoma)
- Urticaria
- Folliculitis
- Pityriasis lichenoides et varioliformis acuta
- Lymphomatoid papulosis
- Pseudolymphoma
- Papular acrodermatitis of childhood (Gianotti–Crosti syndrome)
- Cutaneous lymphoma/leukemia cutis
- Henoch–Schönlein purpura

Vesicular/Bullous Dermatoses

- Cutaneous mastocytosis (urticaria pigmentosa or mastocytoma)
- Bullous impetigo
- Linear IgA disease
- Varicella
- Bullous pemphigoid
- Acropustulosis of infancy
- Erythema multiforme

✓ Best Tests

Although usually unnecessary, skin biopsy of acute lesions will reveal a nonspecific superficial and deep, perivascular, and interstitial inflammatory infiltrate. Retained insect parts are occasionally seen.

▲▲ Management Pearls

- Avoid use of topical antihistamines, as sensitization may occur. Wear protective clothing (socks, shoes, hats, pants, and long-sleeve shirts), and avoid bright-colored clothing, perfumes, and scented hair and body lotions when visiting endemic areas.
- To prevent bites, parents should apply DEET (*N,N*-diethyl-3-methylbenzamide) at 20% to 30% concentration to all exposed skin (except the hands, eyes, mouth, or abraded skin). Alternatively, picaridin at 7% to 15% concentration may be used in children aged older than 2 years.
- Permethrin may provide protection from bites when applied to clothing, shoes, and camping gear, but it provides no protection from bites when applied directly to the skin.
- Parents should read all product labels and apply insect repellants only as directed by the manufacturer.

Therapy

All remaining arthropod parts (stingers and mouth parts) should be removed as soon as possible.

Cool compresses, topical antipruritic agents (calamine lotion and Sarna), midpotency topical steroids (Class II to V), and oral antihistamines (diphenhydramine and hydroxyzine) provide temporary relief from pruritus.

Thick ointments (Vaseline or bacitracin) should be applied multiple times daily to ulcerated lesions.

Secondary infections should be treated with appropriate antibiotics.

Tetanus prophylaxis should be considered for necrotic reactions.

Suggested Readings

American Academy of Pediatrics. Immunization in special clinical circumstances. In: Pickering LK, ed. *Red Book: 2003 Report of the Committee on Infectious Diseases.* 26th Ed. Elk Grove Village, IL: American Academy of Pediatrics; 2003:66–98.

Katz TM, Miller JH, Herbert AA. Insect repellents: Historical perspectives and new developments. *J Am Acad Dermatol.* 2008;58(5):865–871.

Paller AS, Mancini AJ. Bites and infestations. In: Paller AS, Mancini AJ, eds. *Hurwitz Clinical Pediatric Dermatology. A Textbook of Skin Disorders of Childhood and Adolescence.* 3rd Ed. Philadelphia, PA: Elsevier Saunders; 2006:479–502.

Steen CJ, Schwartz RA. Arthropod bites and stings. In: Wolff K, Goldsmith LA, Katz SI, Gilchrest BA, Paller AS, Leffell DJ, eds. *Fitzpatrick's Dermatology in General Medicine.* 7th Ed. New York, NY: McGraw-Hill; 2008: 2054–2063.

Diagnosis Synopsis

Erythema nodosum (EN) is the most common type of septal panniculitis (inflammation of the subcutaneous fat). EN has been associated with bacterial and viral infections (most commonly *Streptococcus* and Epstein–Barr, respectively), medications, malignancies, inflammatory bowel disease, and collagen vascular diseases. Various case reports have linked fungal and protozoal infections as well. However, in 33% to 50% of cases, no associations are found.

The eruption persists for 3 to 6 weeks (with a mean of 14 to 18 days in children) and spontaneously regresses without ulceration, scarring, or atrophy. In uncomplicated cases of EN, adenopathy, including hilar adenopathy, may occur.

EN occurs in boys and girls in equal proportions before puberty (it rarely occurs before age 2); however, after puberty, the female-to-male ratio is 5 to 10:1 as it is in the adult population, where most cases occur between the ages of 20 and 45. Recurrences with reappearance of the precipitating factors are reported.

Look For

Very tender, erythematous, warm, poorly defined nodules and plaques, usually 2 to 5 cm in diameter. The lesions are initially bright red nodules or plaques (Figs. 4-60 and 4-61). After a week or two, the lesions develop more of a yellow-green color, which resembles a bruise (*erythema contusiforme*) (Fig. 4-62). The lesions never ulcerate.

Lesions are most common on the shins and knees with a pretibial symmetric distribution being the most common distribution (Fig. 4-63). Small lesions may appear on the thighs, buttocks, or extensor arms and occasionally on

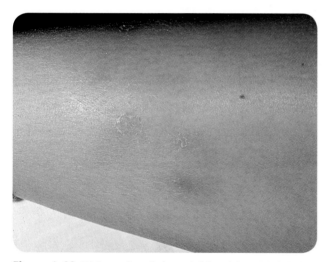

Figure 4-60 EN has red to dusky, painful nodules with indistinct borders.

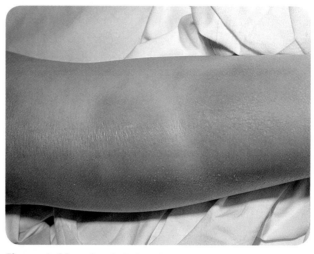

Figure 4-61 EN has indistinct borders, and lesions may become confluent.

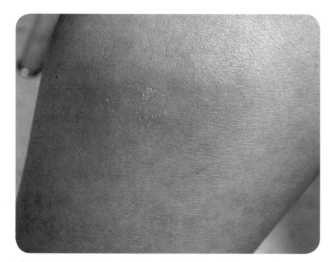

Figure 4-62 EN contusions often heal with a yellow-green hue.

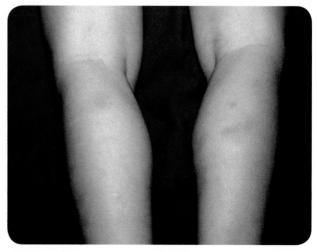

Figure 4-63 EN lesions are characteristically on the lower anterior leg but can be laterally as well.

the face and neck. Small conjunctival nodules may occur on the bulbar conjunctiva or other mucous membranes.

 ## Diagnostic Pearls

Tender lesions on the bilateral shins following an upper respiratory infection.

 ## Differential Diagnosis and Pitfalls

- Henoch–Schönlein purpura—generally not tender
- Child abuse
- Subcutaneous granuloma annulare
- Other panniculitides
- Nodular vasculitis

✓ ## Best Tests

Generally, this diagnosis is made clinically. When in doubt, a punch biopsy, which must include subcutaneous fat, should be diagnostic. Throat culture, ASO titer, or EBV (Epstein–Barr virus) titer may help identify the underlying etiology.

 ## Management Pearls

Management includes analgesics for pain relief. If any underlying etiology can be found, it should be treated appropriately. Referrals are generally not required for straightforward EN.

Therapy

As EN is a self-resolving condition, generally no treatment is required. NSAIDs may be used for symptom relief. Potassium iodine may be used for persistent cases. Intralesional or systemic corticosteroids are rarely required.

Suggested Readings

Labbé L, Perel Y, Maleville J, et al. Erythema nodosum in children: A study of 27 patients. *Pediatr Dermatol*. 1996;13(6):447–550.

Requena L, Requena C. Erythema nodosum. *Dermatol Online J*. 2002;8:4.

Folliculitis

■■ Diagnosis Synopsis

Folliculitis (staphylococcal folliculitis) is a localized infection of the hair follicle, most often caused by *Staphylococcus aureus*. It typically occurs on areas of occlusion, friction, and irritation such as sites rubbed by clothing or sporting equipment, or on occluded skin areas of a hospitalized patient. The lesions of folliculitis are often pruritic. Obese, diabetic, and immunocompromised patients are at increased risk for episodes of bacterial folliculitis.

(◉) Look For

Follicular-centered pustules of varying size (Figs. 4-64–4-67). A halo of perifollicular erythema is typical, and pustules may erupt to form crusts on the surface of the skin. The eruption is often regionalized.

The most common presentation of community-acquired MRSA is as an abscess. Surrounding cellulitis may be present.

●● Diagnostic Pearls

Folliculitis occurs more frequently among diabetics and teenagers who exercise daily.

?? Differential Diagnosis and Pitfalls

- Molluscum contagiosum
- Keratosis pilaris

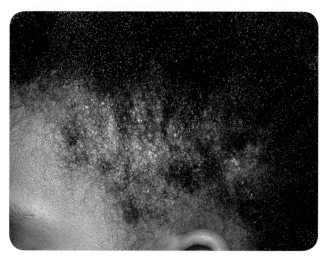

Figure 4-64 Folliculitis grouped on the scalp.

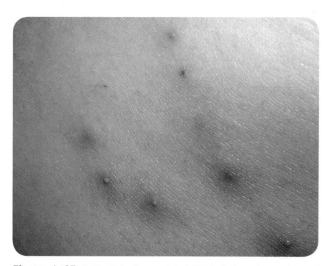

Figure 4-65 Folliculitis. Some with follicularly based pustules and rim of erythema.

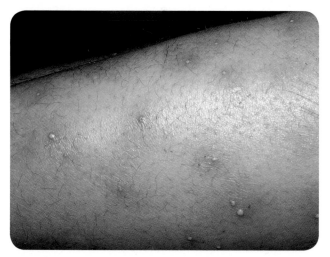

Figure 4-66 Folliculitis with pustules and wide rim of erythema.

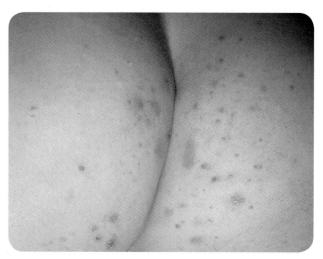

Figure 4-67 Folliculitis in common location, possibly related to occlusion.

- *Pseudomonas* folliculitis (hot tub folliculitis)
- *Pityrosporum* folliculitis
- Candidiasis
- Scabies
- Acne
- Miliaria rubra
- *Tinea* corporis

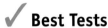 Best Tests

Given the prevalence of MRSA, a culture and sensitivity should be considered in all patients. If scale is present and tinea is suspected, a KOH should be performed. A punch biopsy will show neutrophils within the hair follicle.

 Management Pearls

- Changing the skin care routine of the patient might suffice. In teenagers, identify habits, such as shaving, as playing a role. Antibacterial soaps can be helpful.
- Given the prevalence of MRSA, maintain a high index of suspicion for this diagnosis and make the initial choice of empiric antibiotic therapy based on patterns of antimicrobial resistance within your community.
- Eradication of MRSA nasal carriage may be accomplished with application of 2% mupirocin ointment twice daily for 5 days to the nares.
- **Precautions:** Standard and contact (Isolate patient, wear gloves and a gown, limit patient transport, and avoid sharing patient care equipment).
- Per the CDC, infections due to vancomycin-intermediate *S. aureus* and VRSA (Vancomycin resistant *S. aureus*) are Nationally Notifiable via the National Notifiable Diseases Surveillance System.

Therapy

Abscesses should be incised and drained. The choice of antibiotic should be based on sensitivity results when available.

For uncomplicated infections not caused by MRSA, topical mupirocin may be used twice daily. If the involvement is more widespread, oral antibiotics should be used. First-generation cephalosporins, penicillin, and amoxicillin/clavulanic acid are good options.

Infections caused by MRSA can be more difficult to treat. While first-generation cephalosporins, penicillin, and β-lactamase stable penicillins such as amoxicillin/clavulanic acid may be used, other antibiotics should also be considered. Trimethoprim/sulfamethoxazole and clindamycin are often effective. Tetracyclines are effective in adults but should be avoided in children aged younger than 9 years. For more serious infections, patients may require hospitalization. Vancomycin and linezolid are effective in most cases.

Special Considerations in Infants

Consider bacterial folliculitis when pustules in the diaper area fail to respond to anticandidal/yeast therapies.

Suggested Readings

Cohen PR. Community-acquired methicillin-resistant *Staphylococcus aureus* skin infections: Implications for patients and practitioners. *Am J Clin Dermatol.* 2007;8(5):259–270.

Ladhani S, Garbash M. Staphylococcal skin infections in children: Rational drug therapy recommendations. *Paediatr Drugs.* 2005;7(2):77–102.

Granuloma Annulare

■ Diagnosis Synopsis

Granuloma annulare is a common inflammatory skin disorder of unknown etiology targeting the dermis or subcutaneous tissues. The disease is seen in children and adults, most frequently in children from age 2 to puberty, and more frequently in girls than boys.

The disorder is usually localized when it occurs in children, but a generalized variant can occur.

Typically, the disease has a prolonged course, but lesions usually resolve spontaneously over time without scarring.

◉ Look For

Ring-shaped (annular) or arcuate (arclike), reddish-brown, indurated plaques (Fig. 4-68). The overlying skin appears normal and lacks scale (Fig. 4-69). The center of the annular plaques can have normal or hyperpigmented skin (Fig. 4-70). They are commonly localized on the dorsum of the fingers and hands, elbows, feet, or ankles (Fig. 4-71).

Subcutaneous lesions may be up to 4 to 5 cm in diameter and are most frequently found on the shins, palms, buttocks, and scalp, and they may be mistaken for rheumatoid nodules, bone, or malignancy. Patients with this form often have coexisting papular or annular lesions elsewhere. In the disseminated or generalized form, hundreds of smaller papular lesions can be widely distributed.

Occasionally, granuloma annulare presents as small papules with central umbilications, crusts, or focal ulcerations. This form, called perforating granuloma annulare, exhibits extrusion of degenerated collagen through the epidermis when examined histologically.

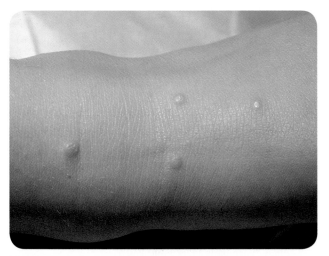

Figure 4-68 Granuloma annulare. Discrete, smooth papules.

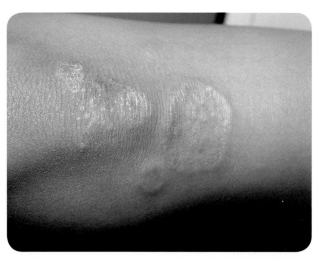

Figure 4-69 Granuloma annulare. Raised erythematous border consisting of ringed papules that lack scale.

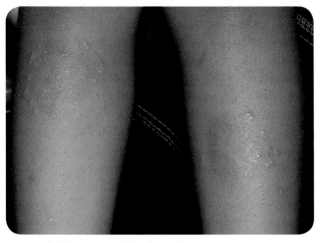

Figure 4-70 Granuloma annulare with central hyperpigmentation, composed of annularly arranged discrete papules.

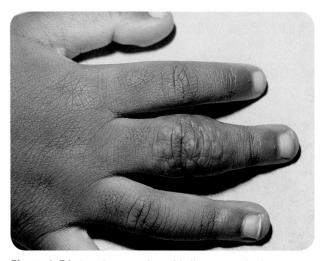

Figure 4-71 Granuloma annulare with discrete papules in a common location, on the hand.

Diagnostic Pearls

The ring-shaped or arclike lesions lack overlying scale. When stretched, larger annular lesions show individual papules in a ring. The association with small papules will establish the diagnosis. Subcutaneous granuloma annulare presents as firm, bonelike lesions on the dorsal feet and anterior lower legs.

?? Differential Diagnosis and Pitfalls

- Granuloma annulare is most often mistaken for dermatophyte infection (ringworm and tinea corporis). The presence of scaling in the annular plaques of a dermatophyte infection should allow the distinction. Additionally, dermatophyte infection can be established by KOH examination of associated scale.
- Sarcoidosis can be annular and similar in appearance.
- Subcutaneous lesions are often mistaken for rheumatoid nodules, malignancy, or lymphadenopathy.
- Erythema annulare centrifugum may be distinguished from granuloma annulare by characteristic trailing scale at the inner border of the annular erythema.
- Lichen planus may occasionally present with annular lesions. However, these lesions tend to be flat topped and violaceous with an overlying network of fine white lines (Wickham striae).
- Necrobiosis lipoidica diabeticorum presents as violaceous to red-brown plaques with atrophic yellow-brown centers on the shins.
- Perforating granuloma annulare may occasionally be mistaken for other perforating dermatoses or molluscum contagiosum.
- Subcutaneous granuloma annulare is frequently mistaken for rheumatoid nodules. Coexisting papular or annular lesions are frequently seen in patients with this form of granuloma annulare.

 Best Tests

A KOH preparation of scrapings, if negative, will support the diagnosis of granuloma annulare. Skin biopsy will confirm the diagnosis, but a clinical diagnosis is often made in the localized form by lesional morphology and distribution.

▲▲ Management Pearls

There are no clear-cut successful therapies. Lesions are usually asymptomatic and in children, almost always resolve spontaneously. Patients often report that a biopsy of a lesion results in its resolution. Intralesional triamcinolone suspension is effective for individual lesions, but cases frequently relapse after several months. Superpotent topical steroids are effective in some patients. Parental reassurance and education about the benign nature of this disease is key.

Therapy

Topical corticosteroids with or without occlusion have limited benefits. Intralesional corticosteroids infiltrated into the elevated thickened plaque can flatten the lesions (triamcinolone 3 mg/mL) but should be used for symptomatic plaques only. Note: Skin atrophy is a potential side effect.

If the patient has pruritus, or for those parents who are anxious, a short course of topical corticosteroids may have limited benefit. Monitor for epidermal atrophy.

High-potency topical corticosteroids (Class 2) should not be used for more than 1 to 2 weeks:

- Fluocinonide cream, ointment (Lidex) apply twice daily
- Desoximetasone cream, ointment (Topicort) apply twice daily

Midpotency topical corticosteroids (Classes 3 and 4):

- Triamcinolone cream, ointment (Kenalog, Aristocort) apply twice daily in 120 and 240 g
- Mometasone cream, ointment (Elocon) apply twice daily
- Fluocinolone ointment, cream (Synalar) apply twice daily

Suggested Readings

Bolognia JL, Jorizzo JL, Rapini RP, eds. *Dermatology*. Vol. 2. 2nd Ed. St Louis, MO: Mosby; 2008:1460–1463.

Cohen BA, ed. *Pediatric Dermatology*. 3rd Ed. St Louis, MO: Mosby; 2005:128.

James WD, Berger TG, Elston DM, eds. *Andrews' Diseases of the Skin*. 10th Ed. Philadelphia, PA: WB Saunders; 2006:703–706.

Histiocytosis, Langerhans Cell

■ Diagnosis Synopsis

Langerhans cell histiocytosis (LCH) is a group of rare idiopathic disorders in which dendritic histiocytes accumulate in one or many organs. Patients have previously been classified as having histiocytosis X, Hand–Schüller–Christian syndrome, Letterer–Siwe disease, Hashimoto–Pritzker disease, self-healing reticulohistiocytosis, or eosinophilic granuloma; however, patients are now classified based on the number of organ systems involved (i.e., single-system or multisystem LCH). Organs may include the skin, oral mucosa, bone, bone marrow, lungs, liver, spleen, gastrointestinal tract, lymph nodes, or central nervous system. LCH most commonly affects children aged 1 to 4 years, but may present from birth to adulthood. The 3-year survival rate is approximately 80% with age under 2 years, multiorgan involvement, and organ dysfunction portraying a worse prognosis.

◉ Look For

LHC typically affects the scalp and skin folds with subtle erythematous to brown papules and plaques that become scaly, crusted, and/or petechial (Figs. 4-72–4-74). With further progression, they may appear verrucous and waxy, become ulcerative and weeping, and/or develop hemorrhagic crusts (scabs). However, any cutaneous surface may be involved with almost any primary lesion including papules, vesicles, nodules, ulcers, crusted plaques, purple nodules, and purpura. Lesions are typically painful rather than pruritic.

Systemic involvement may be asymptomatic or manifest by constitutional symptoms (i.e., fever, weight loss, and failure to thrive) and signs of organ dysfunction. Typical extracutaneous organs include the bones (painful swelling), lymph nodes (lymphadenopathy), liver and spleen (hepatosplenomegaly, jaundice, prolonged prothrombin time) (Fig. 4-75),

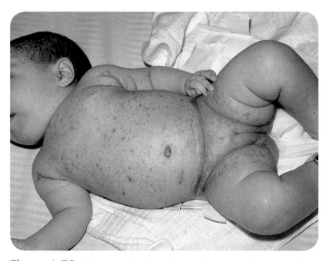

Figure 4-72 LCH generalized with involvement of common locations: scalp and skin folds.

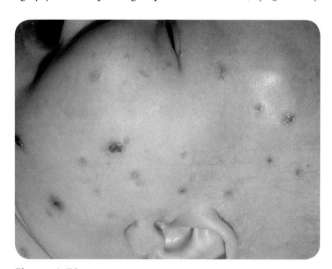

Figure 4-73 LCH with characteristic papulonodules with necrotic centers and rolled borders.

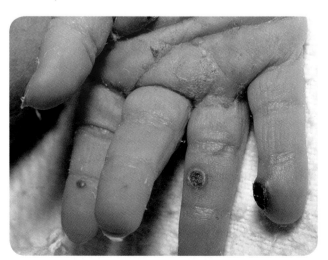

Figure 4-74 LCH with necrotic papules and scale.

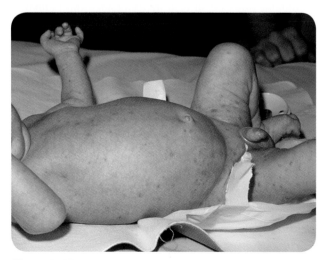

Figure 4-75 LCH with disseminated papules and enlarged abdomen consistent with hepatosplenomegaly.

lungs (tachypnea, retractions), gastrointestinal tract (malabsorption, vomiting, and diarrhea), and central nervous system (diabetes insipidus, progressive encephalopathy, and cranial nerve deficits).

Diagnostic Pearls

Seborrheic or diaper dermatitis with atypical features, such as resistance to therapy, presence of underlying petechiae, or progressive development of oozing and crusting should prompt consideration for LCH.

?? Differential Diagnosis and Pitfalls

- Benign cephalic histiocytosis is a non-LCH presenting as a self-healing papular eruption in children aged younger than 3 years. Histology with immunohistochemistry will differentiate it from LCH.
- Seborrheic dermatitis usually lacks distinct papules. The presence of eroded, ulcerated, or purpuric lesions in an infant thought to have seborrheic dermatitis should prompt a biopsy to rule out LCH.
- Scabies may resemble LCH clinically and histologically. Inquire about potentially affected family members.
- Atopic dermatitis is much more pruritic and rapidly responds to topical steroids.
- Diaper dermatitis is localized to the diaper area and responds to gentle skin care and topical steroids.

✓ Best Tests

- Skin biopsy for histology and immunohistochemistry, which will reveal an infiltrate of CD1a and S100 positive histiocytic cells.
- Multiple other organ biopsies, laboratory and radiologic tests as directed by a pediatric oncologist, are required to determine the extent of the disease.

▲▲ Management Pearls

As LCH commonly recurs after resolution and has an unpredictable course, all patients require regular long-term follow-up by a pediatric oncologist even if the disease was localized and spontaneously resolving.

Therapy

Therapy depends upon the degree of systemic involvement. If histiocytosis has extensive organ involvement, chemotherapy is indicated and the need for multispecialist management is needed. Isolated cutaneous disease may be treated with topical steroids, topical nitrogen mustard, or systemic therapy. Responsive cutaneous lesions generally resolve within 3 weeks of therapy.

Suggested Readings

Bolognia JL, Jorizzo JL, Rapini RP, eds. *Dermatology*. Vol. 2. 2nd Ed. St Louis, MO: Mosby; 2008:1395–1400.

Cohen BA, ed. *Pediatric Dermatology*. 3rd Ed. St Louis, MO: Mosby; 2005:33.

Gadner H, Grois N, Arico M, et al. A randomized trial of treatment for multisystem Langerhans' cell histiocytosis. *J Pediatr*. 2001;138(5):728–734.

James WD, Berger TG, Elston DM, eds. *Andrews' Diseases of the Skin*. 10th Ed. Philadelphia, PA: WB Saunders; 2006:721–724.

Longaker MA, Frieden IJ, LeBoit PE, et al. Congenital "self-healing" Langerhans cell histiocytosis: The need for long-term follow-up. *J Am Acad Dermatol*. 1994;31(5 Pt 2):910–916.

Minkov M, Steiner M, Pötschger U. Reactivations in multisystem Langerhans cell histiocytosis: data of the International LCH Registry. *J Pediatr*. 2008 Nov; 153(5):700–705, 705.e1–2.

Satter EK, High WA. Langerhans cell histiocytosis: A review of the current recommendations of the Histiocyte Society. *Pediatr Dermatol*. 2008;25(3):291–295.

Juvenile Xanthogranuloma

▪▪ Diagnosis Synopsis

Juvenile xanthogranulomas (JXG) are benign, spontaneously regressing histiocytic tumors. Lesions most often appear at birth or within the first year of life. Their number and size may increase over the first 18 months of life. Lesions usually regress over 3 to 6 years, leaving behind persistent pigmentary change or atrophy. Systemic involvement is rare, with the most common site of extracutaneous involvement being the eye (0.3% to 0.5%). Multiple cutaneous lesions in infants is a risk factor for ocular involvement.

◉ Look For

JXGs present as well-demarcated, dome-shaped, red-orange to tan papules or nodules that gradually become more yellow over time (Figs. 4-76–4-79). Lesions are typically 0.5 to 2 cm in diameter and favor the head and neck. Larger JXGs often ulcerate or crust centrally. Most children have a solitary lesion, but some are affected by hundreds of JXGs.

Ocular involvement may present as an asymptomatic mass in the iris, glaucoma, spontaneous hyphema, or a change in iris color. Significant involvement of other extracutaneous organs will present with clinical findings consistent with mass effects from the nodular lesion.

●● Diagnostic Pearls

There should be no pigment in a JXG. If any pigmented globules or a pigmented network is found on magnification (i.e., dermoscopy), a Spitz nevus is favored over JXG.

?? Differential Diagnosis and Pitfalls

- The primary differential of red-to-yellow papules on an infant are JXG, Spitz nevus, and mastocytoma. Mastocytomas have a similar color to JXGs, but they urticate when rubbed. Spitz nevi are pigmented and do not regress over time.
- Mastocytoma
- Spitz nevus
- Xanthomas
- Langerhans cell histiocytosis
- Dermatofibroma

✓ Best Tests

Skin biopsy shows a dense infiltrate of foamy macrophages and Touton giant cells. Immunohistochemistry is negative for S100 and CD1a, and is positive for factor XIIIa and CD68.

▲▲ Management Pearls

- Referral for ophthalmologic examination should be obtained in patients presenting with multiple JXGs.
- Specific tests for internal lesions are not necessary unless clinically significant signs and symptoms develop.
- There is a reported association between the coexistence of JXGs and neurofibromatosis predisposing patients for childhood leukemia. This association has been debated in larger population studies. At this time, patients with multiple JXGs, a family history of neurofibromatosis, or multiple café-au-lait macules should have regular

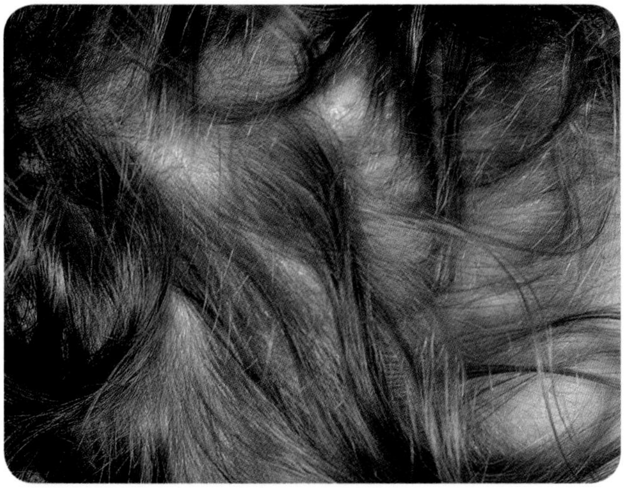

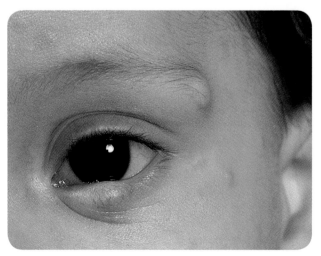

Figure 4-76 Juvenile xanthogranuloma with multiple yellow scalp nodules.

Figure 4-77 Juvenile xanthogranuloma. Yellow nodules with overlying telangiectases.

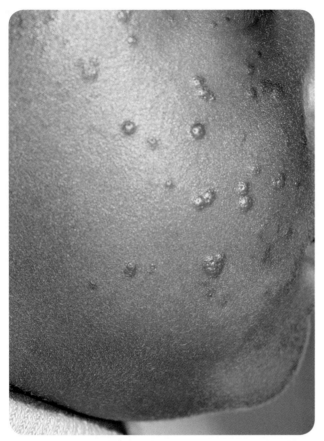

Figure 4-78 Juvenile xanthogranuloma with multiple yellow and red-brown papules.

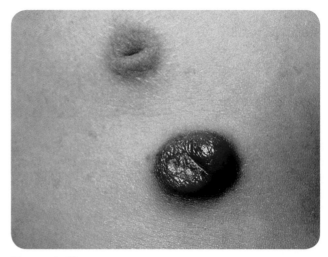

Figure 4-79 Juvenile xanthogranuloma. Red and yellow dome-shaped nodule.

Special Considerations in Infants

Although JXGs resolve spontaneously, they often leave texture and pigmentary changes behind. Hence, facial lesions on infants should be followed for growth and considered for excision during infancy if significant cosmetic deformity is deemed likely.

physical examinations with special attention to signs and symptoms of childhood leukemia. CBC (complete blood count), however, is unnecessary in the absence of signs and symptoms.

Suggested Readings

Hernandez-Martin A, Baselga E, Drolet BA, et al. Juvenile xanthogranuloma. *J Am Acad Dermatol.* 1997;36(3 Pt 1):355–367.

Karcioglu ZA, Mullaney PB. Diagnosis and management of iris juvenile xanthogranuloma. *J Pediatr Ophthalmol Strabismus.* 1997;34:44–51.

Strover DG, Alapati S, Regueira O, et al. Treatment of juvenile xanthogranuloma. *Pediatr Blood Cancer.* 2008;51:130–133.

Therapy

Unless symptomatic, no treatment is necessary. Parents should be reassured that lesions resolve spontaneously. Symptomatic cutaneous lesions may be excised. Symptomatic ocular lesions may be treated with corticosteroids, radiation therapy, or excision. Symptomatic internal organ lesions may be treated with a combination of systemic corticosteroids and vinca alkaloids.

Keratosis Pilaris

◾◾ Diagnosis Synopsis

Keratosis pilaris is an exceedingly common skin condition with retention of keratin at follicular openings. The condition most commonly presents within the first 2 years of life. Dry wintertime temperature and humidity often worsen the condition. Keratosis pilaris is more common in atopic individuals and, frequently, there is a family history of the condition.

◉ Look For

Keratosis pilaris has rough, about 1 mm diameter, firm, follicular papules, especially on the cheeks, extensor arms, and anterior thighs (Figs. 4-80–4-83). Surrounding erythema, especially on the cheeks, is often the presenting complaint. Associated xerosis, atopic dermatitis, or ichthyosis vulgaris is common.

●● Diagnostic Pearls

- As keratosis pilaris is often familial, parents and siblings are often affected.

- The symmetry of follicular papules on the cheeks, arms, and/or legs is another clue to the diagnosis.

?? Differential Diagnosis and Pitfalls

- Lichen spinulosus—grouped keratotic, spiny, follicular papules coalescing to form nummular or circular plaques on the trunk and extremities.
- Phrynoderma—tiny–to-large individual keratotic horny papules on the buttocks, shoulders, and around the elbows and knees; there is usually an obvious underlying nutritional deficiency.
- Lichen nitidus—small, tiny, dome-shaped, smooth-surfaced, nonfollicular papules on the extremities, abdomen, and penis; koebnerization is present.
- Lichen scrofulosorum (tuberculids)—asymptomatic, yellow-brown lichenoid, firm follicular papules (flat-topped or spiny) on the trunk.
- Folliculitis—inflammatory, tender follicular papules/pustules (with perilesional erythema).
- Miliaria—inflammatory follicular papules, vesicles, or pustules on the trunk or proximal extremities; keratosis pilaris is noninflammatory.

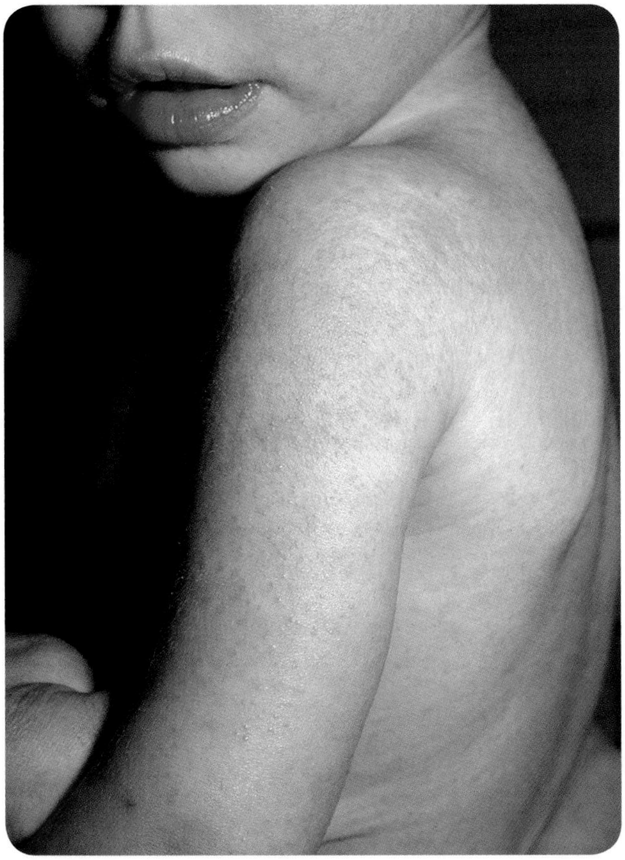

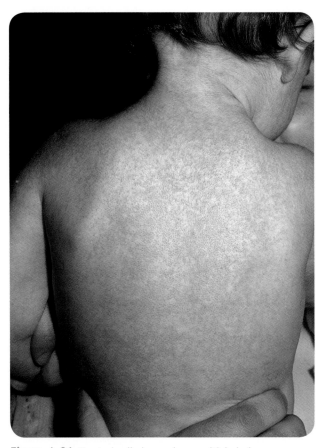

Figure 4-80 Keratosis pilaris with rough red papules in a common location on extensor extremities and cheeks.

Figure 4-81 Keratosis pilaris may have multiple lesions, even on a less common location like the trunk.

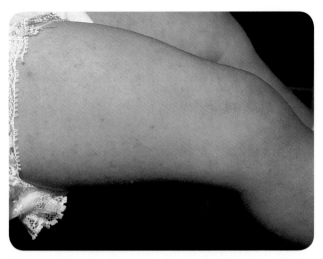

Figure 4-82 Keratosis pilaris is common on the anterior thighs.

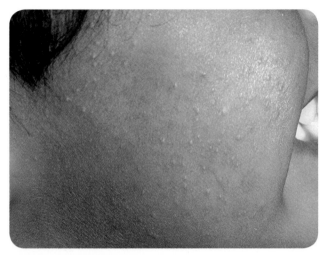

Figure 4-83 Keratosis pilaris on the face may be confused with acne or appendageal tumors.

- Facial lesions may be confused with milia or acne: Milia are yellow-white, tiny, nonfollicular, hemispherical, smooth-surfaced papules, and acne is characterized by comedones, inflammatory papules, and pustules.

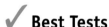 **Best Tests**

This is a clinical diagnosis.

▲▲ **Management Pearls**

Parents should be reassured that keratosis pilaris is not scarring and usually completely clears from the face around puberty without any treatment. It should also be emphasized that keratosis pilaris is familial and that it can be improved, but it cannot be cured by intensive medical or surgical (laser) therapy without scarring.

Therapy

Therapy is directed at reducing the rough texture or erythema of individual lesions rather than "curing" the patient. Roughness may be reduced by moisturizing the skin by using soft soaps (e.g., Dove, Olay, or Basis) or soapless cleansers (e.g., Cetaphil or Aquanil); limiting bathing to 5 to 10 min daily in warm water; and applying thick ointments or creams (Vaseline, Aquaphor, Cetaphil, and CeraVe) immediately after bathing. Keratolytics such as urea 10%, lactic acid, or salicylic acid 4% to 12% lotions or creams may also diminish the thickness of the papules.

Special Considerations in Infants

The cheeks are more often involved in infants than older children and adolescents.

Keratosis pilaris atrophicans (atrophoderma vermiculata, keratosis follicularis spinulosa decalvans, ulerythema ophryogenes) should be considered when keratosis pilaris is present at birth; located in the scalp, eyebrows, or other unusual locations; or is associated with alopecia or scarring.

Suggested Readings

Baden HP, Byers HR. Clinical findings, cutaneous pathology, and response to therapy in 21 patients with keratosis pilaris atrophicans. *Arch Dermatol.* 1994;130(4):469–475.

Marqueling AL, Gilliam AE, Prendiville J, et al. Keratosis pilaris rubra: A common but underrecognized condition. *Arch Dermatol.* 2006;142(12):1611–1616.

Oranje A, Van Gysel D. Keratosis pilaris. In: Harper J, Oranje A, Prose N, eds. *Textbook of Pediatric Dermatology.* 2nd Ed. Malden, MA: Wiley-Blackwell; 2006:1390–1394.

Poskitt L, Wilkinson JD. Natural history of keratosis pilaris. *Br J Dermatol.* 1994;130(6):711–713.

Milia

■■ Diagnosis Synopsis

Milia (singular, milium) are minute epidermal cysts. Primary milia are extremely common on the face of newborns in whom they usually spontaneously resolve by the end of the first month of life. Secondary milia occur after injury to the skin, such as from burns or subepidermal blistering disorders (epidermolysis bullosa).

(◉) Look For

Milia are firm, 1 to 2 mm, white, pearly papules (Figs. 4-84–4-87). Primary milia appear predominantly on the face of newborns but may affect the trunk, genitalia, and extremities as well. Secondary milia occur within areas of chronic skin injury.

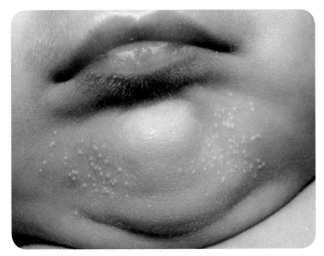

Figure 4-84 Milia with grouped small papules.

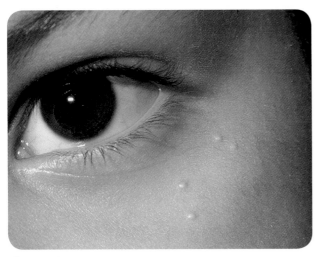

Figure 4-85 Milia with a few small white papules.

●● Diagnostic Pearls

Milia that are widespread, in unusual locations, or persist over several months should alert one to the possibility of an associated syndrome (Marie-Unna hypotrichosis, Bazex–Dupré–Christol disease, or orofaciodigital syndrome type 1).

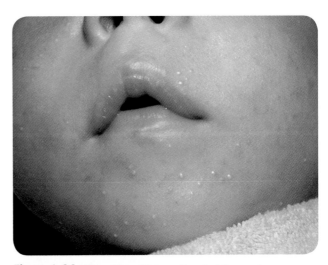

Figure 4-86 Milia with multiple scattered white papules.

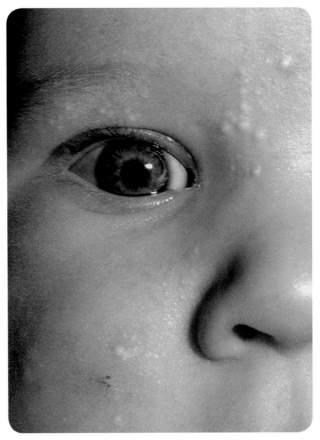

Figure 4-87 Milia with papules that are slightly larger than typical milia in addition to small milia.

73

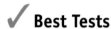 Differential Diagnosis and Pitfalls

- Closed comedones (neonatal acne)
- Molluscum contagiosum
- Sebaceous hyperplasia
- Keratosis pilaris
- Milialike calcinosis cutis
- Eruptive vellus hair cysts
- Syringomas
- Nevus comedonicus

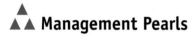 Best Tests

This is a clinical diagnosis. However, the diagnosis can be confirmed by incising the stratum corneum above the cyst using a no. 11 blade or large bore needle and expressing the cyst, which will appear as a hard, white sphere.

▲▲ Management Pearls

Parents should be reassured that milia are nonscarring and almost always spontaneously resolve within a month.

Therapy

Treatment in newborns is not necessary, as lesions resolve spontaneously. Tretinoin (0.025% cream every other night) may be considered to hasten the resolution of persistent milia.

Suggested Readings

Mallory SB. Neonatal skin disorders. *Pediatr Clin North Am.* 1991;38(4): 745–761.

O'Connor NR, McLaughlin MR, Ham P. Newborn skin: Part I. Common rashes. *Am Fam Physician.* 2008;77(1):47–52.

Paller AS, Mancini AJ. Cutaneous disorders of the newborn. In: Paller AS, Mancini AJ, eds. *Hurwitz Clinical Pediatric Dermatology. A Textbook of Skin Disorders of Childhood and Adolescence.* 3rd Ed. Philadelphia, PA: Elsevier Saunders; 2006:17–47.

▪▪ Diagnosis Synopsis

Miliaria rubra, also known as prickly heat or heat rash, is the most common form of miliaria. Miliaria rubra is due to the obstruction of the intraepidermal eccrine sweat ducts. The resultant sweat retention and the escape of sweat into the dermis evokes an inflammatory response that manifests as papules.

The predisposing factors are hot and humid conditions, febrile illnesses, and occlusive clothing, dressing, or ointments (e.g., Aquaphor).

◉ Look For

Small, 1 to 3 mm, erythematous, nonfollicular papules on the upper trunk, back, and flexor aspect of the arms and body folds (Figs. 4-88–4-91).

Miliaria rubra is usually most prominent in occluded areas, such as the back of a hospitalized patient or nonambulatory child.

Miliaria pustulosa is a variant of miliaria rubra that consists of superficial (nonfollicular) pustules.

●● Diagnostic Pearls

There is acral sparing, and the palms and soles are never involved.

?? Differential Diagnosis and Pitfalls

- Candidiasis—usually affects the warm, moist areas, such as groin, axillae, and neck. The lesion consists of beefy red, moist erythema with satellite pustules. A KOH scraping from the pustules demonstrates pseudohyphae and spores.
- Herpes simplex infection—characteristic grouped vesicles on an erythematous base.
- Scabies—pruritic papules, papulovesicles, nodules, and linear burrows on the palms, soles, wrists, ankles, axillae, groin, and genitals. Family history is often present.
- Varicella—initial prodromal symptoms followed by the polymorphic lesions (lesions in different stages) consisting of erythematous macules, vesicles, pustules, and crusts. Tzanck smear from a vesicle shows multinucleated giant cells.
- Acne—open and closed comedones along with inflammatory papules and pustules on the face and chest.
- Folliculitis—follicular-based pustules with perilesional erythema on the gluteal region and extremities.

✓ Best Tests

This is a clinical diagnosis that rarely needs to be confirmed by skin biopsy.

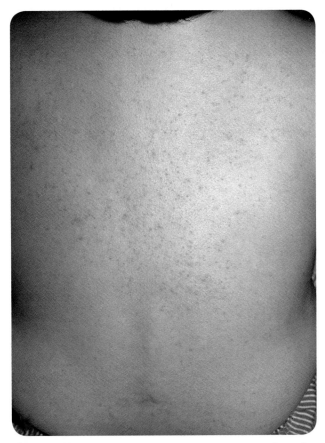

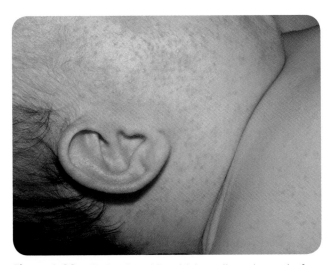

Figure 4-88 Miliaria rubra with multiple small papules on the face.

Figure 4-89 Miliaria rubra with multiple nonfollicular, small papules.

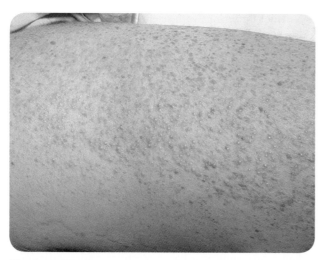

Figure 4-90 Miliaria rubra with red and brown papules and some pustules.

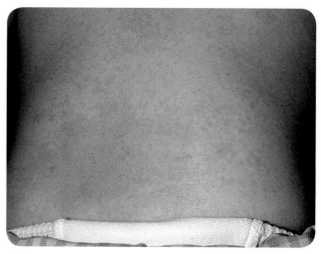

Figure 4-91 Miliaria rubra with varying sizes of papules and no vesicles.

▲▲ Management Pearls

Reassure parents that it is a benign condition that will resolve in several days.

Therapy

Avoidance of heat, humidity, occlusive clothing, and ointments.

Suggested Readings

Van Praag MC, Van Rooij RW, Folkers E, et al. Diagnosis and treatment of pustular disorders in the neonate. *Pediatr Dermatol.* 1997;14:131–143.

Wagner A. Distinguishing vesicular and pustular disorders in the neonate. *Curr Opin Pediatr.* 1997;9:396–405.

Molluscum Contagiosum

■ Diagnosis Synopsis

Molluscum contagiosum is caused by poxviruses and is spread by direct skin-to-skin contact. Infection is worldwide. School-aged children, sexually active adults, and the immunosuppressed are the three groups that are primarily affected. In children, underlying atopic dermatitis, swimming in public pools, and sharing of fomites appear to be associated with higher rates of infection. The exact incubation period is unknown but is estimated to be between 2 and 6 weeks. Though self-limited, the infection is often chronic and can range from a few months to 4 years before disappearing. In a recent survey, 82% of parents of affected children reported that molluscum contagiosum infection concerned them moderately or greatly.

◉ Look For

Smooth, skin-colored, 2 to 6 mm, domed papules with central umbilication (depression). Lesions may occur on any cutaneous or mucosal surface but are typically found on the face, trunk, and extremities, clustered near each other (Figs. 4-92–4-95). A predilection for skin folds (axillae and groin) is frequently present. Central umbilication is seen in a minority of lesions and is not a required morphologic feature. Lesions frequently become inflamed with a surrounding pruritic, eczematous eruption (molluscum dermatitis) or pustulation (simulating secondary bacterial infection). While this host inflammatory response heralds impending resolution of individual lesions, the appearance and associated pruritus can be distressing and alarming to both the patient and parents.

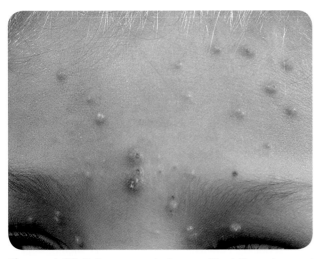

Figure 4-92 Molluscum contagiosum with inflammatory and noninflammatory papules.

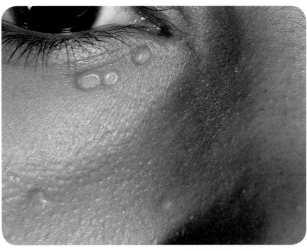

Figure 4-93 Molluscum contagiosum with prominent keratotic papules.

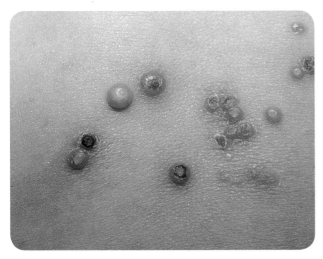

Figure 4-94 Molluscum contagiosum with grouped and scattered papules.

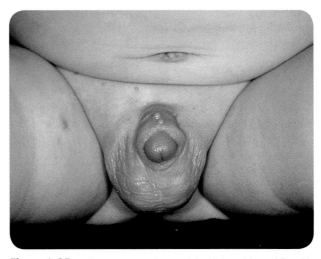

Figure 4-95 Molluscum contagiosum with thigh, pubic, and foreskin lesions with secondary edema.

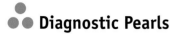

Diagnostic Pearls

- The central umbilication within a firm domed papule is highly suggestive of molluscum. The umbilicated portion may be difficult to see but becomes more obvious when the lesion is frozen with liquid nitrogen. Larger lesions will frequently have more than one umbilication.
- Lesions may have a linear distribution due to local inoculation and spread.
- Lesions can become inflamed (and resemble secondary infection) as the host immune system recognizes the infection.

?? Differential Diagnosis and Pitfalls

- Herpes virus infection—systemic symptoms, pain, and fluid-filled grouped vesicles and erosions rather than firm papules
- Warts—verrucous or flat-topped rather than smooth and dome-shaped with a central umbilication
- Milia—small keratinous cysts typically seen on the face
- Folliculitis—follicularly centered pustules

✓ Best Tests

Skin biopsies have a very characteristic histopathologic appearance with large eosinophilic cytoplasmic inclusions. Molluscum bodies can be seen under light microscopy following extraction of the central core of a lesion. However, the diagnosis is ordinarily a clinical one.

▲▲ Management Pearls

- Because lesions arising in immunocompetent children eventually heal spontaneously without scarring, aggressive treatment that may be emotionally traumatic and potentially lead to scarring should be avoided. However, as noted above, the presence of visible contagious skin lesions can be distressing to both child and parent, and multiple effective treatments are available. Additionally, early treatment can prevent autoinoculation and further spread.

- While genital lesions occurring as part of a more widespread eruption are common, the possibility of sexual abuse should be considered in children with lesions restricted to the genitals.

Therapy

Cantharidin (an extract from the blister beetle) is an effective, yet off-label, well-tolerated method of treating molluscum lesions. At the patient's first visit, a thin film is applied to the surface of five to seven noninflamed extrafacial lesions. Parents are instructed to remove the extract with soap and warm water 3 to 4 h after application or earlier with blister appearance. Response is measured at 1 month. If deemed effective and well tolerated, the remaining nonfacial lesions are treated in the same manner.

Molluscum lesions also respond to cryotherapy with liquid nitrogen as well as extraction with a sharp curette. These methods are painful, however, and not well tolerated by children. Cryotherapy may result in temporary hypopigmentation.

For lesions on the face, topical tretinoin cream 0.025% and imiquimod 5% cream have been used off-label with variable efficacy.

Special Considerations for Neonates/Infants

Infection is infrequent in newborns and infants. The rarity of the condition in those aged younger than one year is thought to reflect transmitted immunity through maternal antibodies.

Suggested Readings

Bolognia JL, Jorizzo JL, Rapini RP, eds. *Dermatology.* Vol. 1. 2nd Ed. St Louis, MO: Mosby; 2008:1229–1233.

Braue A, Ross G, Varigos G, et al. Epidemiology and impact of childhood molluscum contagiosum: A case series and critical review of the literature. *Pediatr Dermatol.* 2005;22(4):287–294.

James WD, Berger TG, Elston DM, eds. *Andrews' Diseases of the Skin.* 10th Ed. Philadelphia, PA: WB Saunders; 2006:394–397.

Diagnosis Synopsis

Morphea is a localized form of scleroderma without systemic involvement. The etiology is unknown; an association with *Borrelia burgdorferi* has been suggested but not conclusively proven. Trauma, sunburn, and lichen striatus were reported as possible triggers in 1 review of 136 patients. Morphea can be divided into subcategories: plaque (which includes guttate, bullous, and keloidal), generalized, morphea profunda, and linear (which includes en coup de sabre and progressive hemifacial atrophy).

The linear subtype represents the most common subtype in children, followed by plaque type. Morphea associated with systemic symptoms is uncommon in children. There is a 2:1 female-to-male ratio.

Look For

The most common presenting lesions are firm ivory plaques with a purple-to-brown halo **(Figs. 4-96 and 4-97)**.

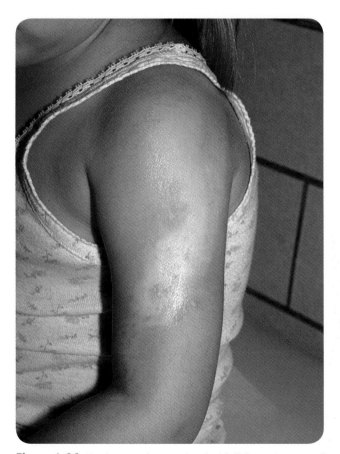

Figure 4-96 Morphea may be associated with lichen sclerosus and has a more ivorylike color than usual.

The linear variant is most common on the extremities **(Fig. 4-98)** and face. When the extremities are involved, the presentation is usually unilateral. Facial involvement of the linear variant (en coup de sabre) may involve the forehead and frontal scalp **(Fig. 4-99)**. The Parry–Romberg variant involves hemifacial atrophy that may include the entire distribution of the trigeminal nerve including the tongue and eye.

Diagnostic Pearls

- Contractures may occur if morphea occurs over a joint. Patients with the generalized variant may have systemic symptoms to include headaches and arthralgias.
- "Burned out" areas will be soft and hyperpigmented.

Differential Diagnosis and Pitfalls

- Morphea and lichen sclerosus may present together. This presentation is known as LS/morphea overlap
- Lipoatrophy
- Panniculitis

Best Tests

- This diagnosis is usually made clinically.
- A punch biopsy may be helpful if the diagnosis is in doubt.
- Eosinophilia is commonly seen on CBC.
- Antibodies include ANA, rheumatoid factor, scl-70, anticentromere, anti-dsDNA, and anti-U1RNP have all been reported to be positive in various cases.

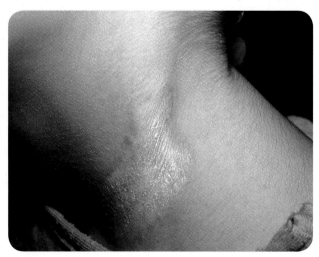

Figure 4-97 Morphea is firm and has an ivorylike color, with obliteration of normal skin markings.

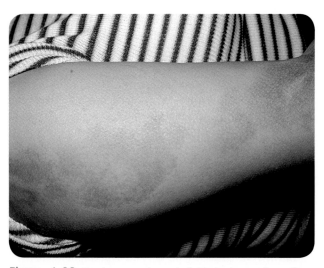

Figure 4-98 Morphea may have individual plaques in a linear configuration.

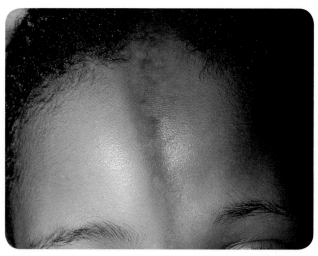

Figure 4-99 Morphea in an *en coup de sabre* configuration with deep atrophy.

▲▲ Management Pearls

· ·

- Early diagnosis and treatment are important to prevent joint involvement when the extremities are affected.
- Traditionally, inflammation/induration lasts 3 to 5 years, leaving postinflammatory hyperpigmented.

Therapy

Most cases can be treated with topical corticosteroids and calcipotriene. If this is unsuccessful or if there is extensive involvement, oral corticosteroids and methotrexate may be considered. A recent review initiated methotrexate at a dose of 0.3 to 0.5 mg/kg/week. Oral corticosteroids, in this same review, were initiated at a dose of 1 mg/kg/day in conjunction with the methotrexate and tapered to a dose of 0.5 mg/kg/day before discontinuation. Folic acid at 1 mg/day was used with the methotrexate. Calcitriol was also used orally at a dose of 0.025 μg/day in a few cases, with a maximum dose of 1.5 μg/day. If calcitriol is used, calcium intake should be restricted, and 24-h calcium/creatinine ratios should be performed for monitoring.

Suggested Readings

Christen-Zaech S, Hakim MD, Afsar FS, Paller AS. Pediatric morphea (localized scleroderma): Review of 136 patients. *J Am Acad Dermatol.* 2008 Sep; 59(3):385–396.

Liou JS, Morrell DS. Firm and dyspigmented linear plaques: Childhood linear morphea. *Pediatr Ann.* 2007;36(12):792–794.

Diagnosis Synopsis

The neurofibromatoses comprise several syndromes in which nerves become surrounded by tumors. The most common type is neurofibromatosis type 1 (NF1 or von Recklinghausen disease), an autosomal dominant condition with variable clinical expression. When evaluating a child, it is important to remember that several of the cardinal features of NF1 have age-related penetrance, and, therefore, many young children will need to be followed over time to make a clinical diagnosis. By age 11, 95% of children can be diagnosed by clinical criteria alone.

Look For

A clinical diagnosis requires any two or more of the NIH diagnostic criteria for NF1. All children with a high suspicion for NF1 should be evaluated by a dermatologist, ophthalmologist, orthopedic surgeon, neurologist, and pediatrician.

NIH Diagnostic Criteria for Neurofibromatosis Type 1

- More than five café-au-lait macules (CALMs) larger than 5 mm in greatest diameter before puberty or 15 mm after puberty
- More than one neurofibroma of any type or one plexiform neurofibroma
- Axillary or inguinal freckling
- Optic glioma
- More than one Lisch nodule (iris hamartoma) (Fig. 4-100)
- Distinctive osseous lesions (sphenoid dysplasia or pseudo-arthrosis)
- First-degree relative with NF1

Intertriginous freckling consists of 1 to 4 mm tan to red-brown, well-defined macules (Fig. 4-101).

The CALMs of NF1 are tan to brown, smooth-bordered, ovoid macules (Figs. 4-102 and 4-103).

Dermal neurofibromas are soft papules with an overlying pink to violaceous hue that can characteristically be pushed into the lower dermis and subcutaneous tissue (buttonhole sign).

Plexiform neurofibromas tend to present under the skin surface, and initial diagnosis requires a combination of palpation, evaluation of asymmetry, and recognition of alterations in pigmentation and hair patterns. Lesions may feel like the classic "bag of worms," present as a hard mass, or be barely palpable. Asymmetry may manifest as bony overgrowth, soft tissue hyperplasia, scoliosis, exophthalmos, or vertical dystopia. The overlying skin often appears like a CALM but with unusual features, such as large size, irregular boarders, hypertrichosis, or location on the face (an unusual location for CALMs).

Diagnostic Pearls

When applying diagnostic criteria or evaluating a child, it is important to remember the age-related penetrance of manifestations of NF1:
- Sphenoid wing dysplasia—birth
- Long-bone bowing—birth to early childhood
- Optic pathway tumors—birth to early childhood
- CALMs—birth to childhood
- Plexiform neurofibromas—birth to adulthood

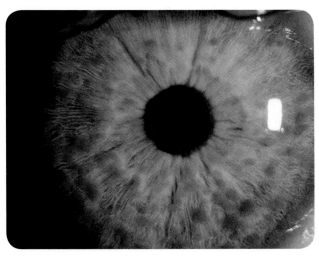

Figure 4-100 Neurofibromatosis with multiple Lisch nodules in iris.

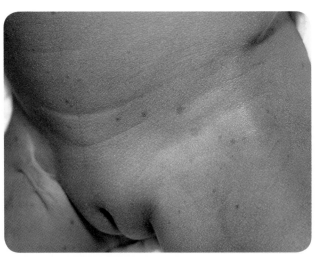

Figure 4-101 Neurofibromatosis with multiple small, hyperpigmented macules.

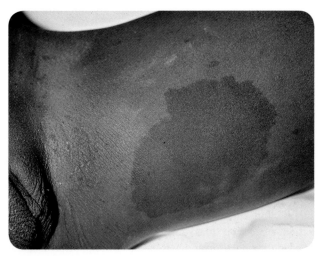

Figure 4-102 Neurofibromatosis with multiple small and some larger CALMs.

- Hypertension—lifelong
- Intertriginous freckling—childhood
- Scoliosis—childhood
- Neurofibromas—late childhood to adolescence
- Nerve sheath tumors—adolescence to adulthood

?? Differential Diagnosis and Pitfalls

Syndromes with Café-au-lait Macules

- Watson syndrome—associated with pulmonic stenosis
- Autosomal dominant CALMs—no other findings of NF1
- Neurofibromatosis type 2—associated with central nervous syndrome tumors
- McCune–Albright syndrome—often unilateral, irregularly shaped CALMs

Syndromes with other Pigmentary Abnormalities

- LEOPARD syndrome—hundreds of lentigines rather than few CALMs
- Peutz–Jeghers syndrome—dark macules on lips, oral mucosa, fingers, and soles
- Pigmentary mosaicism—pigmentation follows lines of Blaschko

Syndromes with Tumors Similar to Neurofibromas

- Lipomatosis—rubbery, homogenous, and cannot be pushed into the lower dermis and subcutaneous tissue (negative buttonhole sign)
- Bannayan–Riley–Ruvalcaba syndrome—macules on penis with lipomas (negative buttonhole sign)

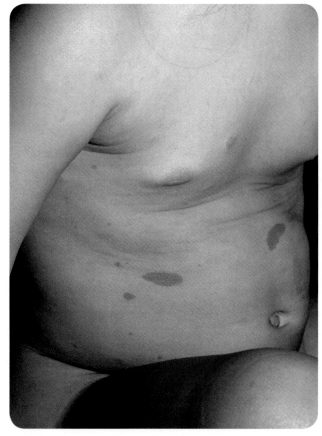

Figure 4-103 Neurofibromatosis with café-au-lait spots on the trunk.

- Gardner syndrome—well-defined, firm cysts and other tumors with negative buttonhole sign

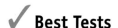 Best Tests

NF1 is a clinical diagnosis. Testing should be individualized and only considered based on symptoms:
- Increased growth velocity or precocious puberty—cranial imaging for optic pathway gliomas
- Painful or rapidly growing mass—magnetic resonance imaging (MRI) and possible biopsy for malignant peripheral nerve sheath tumor or other tumors
- Tibial bowing—X-ray for pseudoarthrosis
- Increased curvature of the spine—spine radiographs for scoliosis
- Dystopia—MRI for plexiform neurofibroma
- Hypertension—abdominal MRI or angiography for renovascular disease or pheochromocytoma; and 24-h urine catecholamines, homovanillic acid, and vanillylmandelic acid for pheochromocytoma
- Significant weight loss and constitutional symptoms—blood smear and bone marrow evaluation for juvenile chronic myelogenous leukemia

▲▲ Management Pearls

Children with NF1 should have the following evaluated annually:

- Height and weight—precocious puberty (optic pathway glioma)
- Blood pressure—hypertension
- Skin examination—dermal and plexiform neurofibromas
- Bone examination—scoliosis
- Neurologic examination—developmental delays and learning disabilities
- Vision screen—optic pathway gliomas
- Sexual maturation—delayed/precocious puberty (optic pathway glioma)
- Psychological/social adjustment—self-esteem problems

Therapy

All children should be referred to a neurofibromatosis clinic or a specialist with significant experience with NF1.

Most plexiform neurofibromas are asymptomatic and require no further treatment other than regular evaluation of growth. Painful or functionally impairing plexiform neurofibromas, however, should be imaged by MRI and considered for excision by a soft-tissue tumor oncology team. All orbitotemporal plexiform neurofibromas should be evaluated by a plastic surgeon and/or soft-tissue tumor oncology team for possible early excision to prevent future disfiguring and vision-threatening growth.

Symptomatic dermal neurofibromas can be excised.

Laser therapy of CALMs has produced mixed results with up to a 67% recurrence rate.

Special Considerations in Infants

Infants and neonates with NF1 most commonly present with multiple CALMs and intertriginous (axillary and inguinal) freckling. However, only 70% of these infants will be able to be diagnosed clinically. When an infant does not meet diagnostic criteria but clinical suspicion is high, annual re-evaluation of the diagnostic criteria by a physician familiar with NF1 and ophthalmology evaluations should suffice. Genetic testing is rarely necessary.

Although the NIH diagnostic criteria require CALMs to be larger than 5 mm in greatest diameter in prepubescent children, skin lesions present at birth are estimated to grow eight times their size by adulthood. Hence, macules smaller than 5 mm in infants may meet the criteria for size.

Suggested Readings

Alper JC, Holmes LB. The incidence and significance of birthmarks in a cohort of 4,641 newborns. *Pediatr Dermatol.* 1983;1(1):58–68.

American Academy of Pediatrics Committee on Genetics. Health supervision for children with neurofibromatosis. *Pediatrics.* 1995;96(2):368–372.

DeBella K, Szudek J, Friedman JM. Use of the National Institutes of Health criteria for diagnosis of neurofibromatosis 1 in children. *Pediatrics.* 2000;105:608–614.

Ferner RE, Huson SM, Thomas N, et al. Guidelines for the diagnosis and management of individuals with neurofibromatosis 1. *J Med Genet.* 2007;44:81–88.

Korf BR. Plexiform neurofibromas. *Am J Med Genet.* 1999;89(1):31–37.

Listernick R, Charrow J. The neurofibromatoses. In: Wolff K, Goldsmith LA, Katz SI, et al. *Fitzpatrick's Dermatology in General Medicine.* Vol 1. 7th Ed. New York: McGraw-Hill; 2008:1331–1338.

Viskochil D. Neurofibromatosis type 1. In: Cassidy SB, Allanson JE, eds. *Management of Genetic Syndromes.* 2nd Ed. Hoboken, NJ: John Wiley & Sons; 2005:229–252.

Trichoepithelioma

■■ Diagnosis Synopsis

Trichoepithelioma is a benign cutaneous tumor of hair follicle origin. The lesion typically occurs as an isolated papule on the face of a young adult but may occur as multiple lesions in children and adolescents as part of one of several autosomal dominant disorders (i.e., Brooke disease, Brooke–Spiegler syndrome, Rombo syndrome, or Bazex–Dupré–Christol syndrome). Malignant degeneration does not occur, but early onset of associated basal cell carcinomas may occur in patients with multiple trichoepitheliomas (i.e., Rombo syndrome or Bazex–Dupré–Christol syndrome).

● Look For

Multiple firm, skin-colored or slightly pink papules (1 to 5 mm in diameter) with a shiny to translucent surface, usually involving the upper lip and cheeks, favoring the paranasal region, are seen in the familial form (Figs. 4-104–4-107). Isolated lesions appear identical to the hereditary form but are usually larger (5 mm or more in diameter).

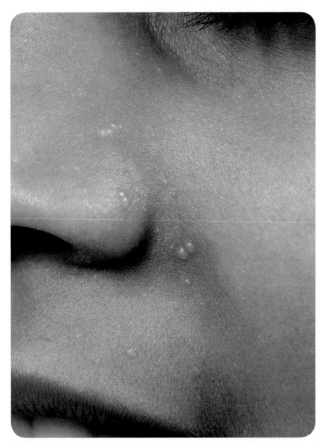

Figure 4-104 Trichoepitheliomas presenting as flesh-colored papules.

●● Diagnostic Pearls

Trichoepithelioma commonly involves the upper lip, which is a site frequently spared in the angiofibromas of tuberous sclerosis.

?? Differential Diagnosis and Pitfalls

- Clinically, trichoepithelioma may appear similar to a number of other adnexal neoplasms, including trichoblastoma, tricholemmomas, and syringomas. Occasionally, lesions may mimic molluscum contagiosum, milia, sebaceous hyperplasia, or basal cell carcinoma. The clustering of multiple papules within the nasolabial folds of multiple family members is highly suggestive of trichoepitheliomas over other diagnoses.
- Histologically, trichoepithelioma may be difficult to distinguish between basal cell carcinoma and microcystic adnexal carcinoma.

✓ Best Tests

Biopsy is necessary to confirm the diagnosis in nonfamilial, isolated lesions.

▲▲ Management Pearls

Patients with multiple trichoepitheliomas should be followed periodically for the development of other adnexal tumors and basal cell carcinomas.

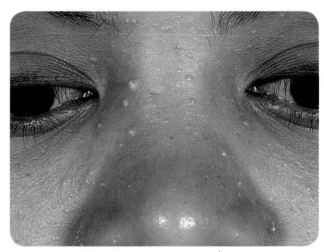

Figure 4-105 Trichoepithelioma with distribution of multiple lesions.

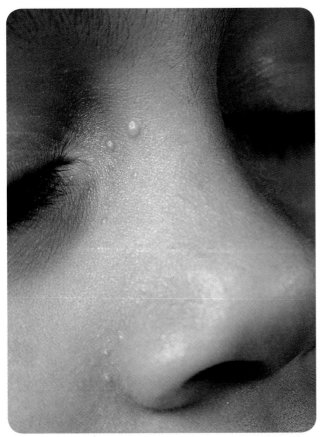

Figure 4-106 Trichoepithelioma presenting as flesh-colored papules.

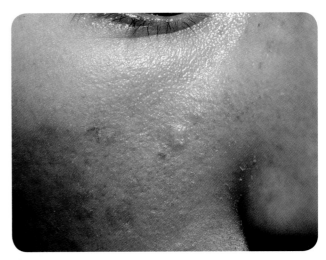

Figure 4-107 Trichoepithelioma in a 6-year-old with an affected mother.

Suggested Readings

Bolognia JL, Jorizzo JL, Rapini RP, eds. *Dermatology*. Vol. 1. 2nd Ed. St Louis, MO: Mosby; 2008:1697–1698.

Cohen BA, ed. *Pediatric Dermatology*. 3rd Ed. St Louis, MO: Mosby; 2005:131.

James WD, Berger TG, Elston DM, eds. *Andrews' Diseases of the Skin*. 10th Ed. Philadelphia, PA: WB Saunders; 2006:672.

Therapy

Biopsy is usually curative, but lesions may recur requiring re-excision, electrosurgery, or laser surgery (CO_2 laser). The immediate benefits from these destructive therapies should be weighed with the long-term risks of scarring and dyspigmentation. Patients with multiple familial trichoepitheliomas should be informed that multiple treatments may be necessary as they develop more lesions over time.

Tuberous Sclerosis

◼◼ Diagnosis Synopsis

Tuberous sclerosis (tuberous sclerosis complex, TSC) is a multisystem autosomal dominant disorder caused by mutations in the genes for the proteins hamartin and tuberin. Approximately, 60% of patients have no family history of TSC. It is characterized by tumorlike growths, or hamartomas, in almost every organ. It is often associated with epilepsy, mental retardation, and autism. Diagnosis is challenging due to the wide variation in severity and age-related penetrance of individual manifestations.

Clinical Diagnostic Criteria for Tuberous Sclerosis: Definite TSC requires two major features or one major and two minor features; may not be diagnosed until adulthood.

Major Features

- Facial angiofibromas or forehead plaque
- Ungual fibroma
- Three or more hypomelanotic macules
- Shagreen patch
- Multiple retinal nodular hamartomas
- Cortical tuber
- Subependymal nodule
- Subependymal giant cell astrocytoma
- Cardiac rhabdomyoma (usually asymptomatic)
- Renal angiomyolipoma or pulmonary lymphangiomyomatosis

Minor Features

- Multiple pits in dental enamel
- Hamartomatous rectal polyps
- Bone cysts
- Cerebral white-matter radial migration lines
- Gingival fibromas
- Nonrenal hamartoma
- Multiple renal cysts
- Retinal achromic patch
- "Confetti" skin lesions

◉ Look For

Hypomelanotic macules ("ash-leaf spots") are round, oval, linear, or lance-ovate-shaped, well-defined macules of decreased pigmentation. Although usually obvious under natural light, occasional fair-skinned infants require Wood lamp examination in a completely darkened room to accentuate the macules.

Angiofibromas are 1 to 4 mm, flesh-colored, pink, or red papules with a smooth surface located over the nasolabial folds, medial cheeks, and chin (**Figs. 4-108–4-110**). The upper lip and sides of the face are usually spared.

Forehead plaques are flesh-colored, pink, or red plaques with irregular outlines and an uneven surface usually located on the forehead or scalp. They may be soft, doughy, or hard.

Shagreen patches are flesh-colored, pink, or brown plaques that range in size from 1 to several centimeters. They

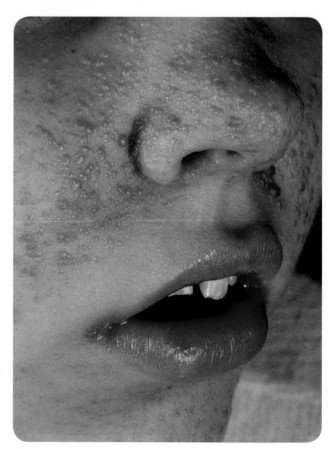

Figure 4-109 Tuberous sclerosis with multiple angiofibromas that are often reddish.

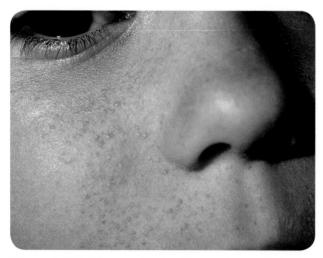

Figure 4-108 Tuberous sclerosis with multiple angiofibromas in typical distribution.

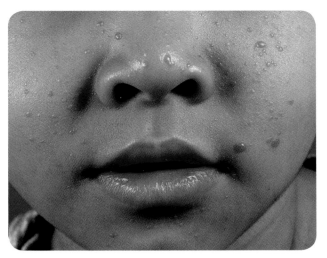

Figure 4-110 Tuberous sclerosis with multiple angiofibromas in a slightly asymmetric distribution.

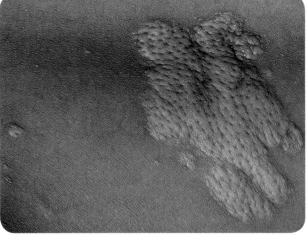

Figure 4-111 Tuberous sclerosis with *peau d'orange*-appearing plaque (shagreen patch).

may have depressions at follicular orifices, giving them the appearance of an orange peel (peau d'orange) or an irregular and cobbled surface (Fig. 4-111). Usually, palpation reveals a firm to rubbery texture. In addition to the large solitary plaque, shagreen patches may present as a localized collection of smaller plaques.

Ungual or periungual fibromas are skin-colored to reddish nodules that appear on top of nails and are often associated with deep grooves.

Confettilike lesions are grouped, 1 to 3 mm hypopigmented macules that are usually found on the extremities.

Diagnostic Pearls

Age of Onset of Cutaneous Signs of Tuberous Sclerosis Complex

- Hypomelanotic macule—infancy to childhood
- Fibrous forehead plaque—infancy to childhood
- Facial angiofibroma—infancy to adulthood
- Shagreen patch—childhood
- Ungual fibroma—adolescence to adulthood
- Confettilike lesions—adolescence to adulthood

?? Differential Diagnosis and Pitfalls

Angiofibromas

- Acne vulgaris—deep nodules, pustules, and open and closed comedones instead of smooth papules.
- Periorificial dermatitis—concentrated periorificially rather than over the central face, often affects the upper lip, and waxes and wanes over time.

- Keratosis pilaris—pinpoint and rough rather than dome-shaped and smooth.
- Trichoepitheliomas—often familial (Brooke tumor), smooth, and translucent, may require biopsy to distinguish.

Hypomelanotic Macule

- Pigmentary mosaicism (nevus depigmentosus)—follows lines of Blaschko, often with irregular borders rather than randomly distributed and smooth.
- Nevus anemicus—disappears on diascopy, does not fluoresce under Wood lamp.
- Vitiligo—progressive, depigmented, and symmetric.

Ungual Fibroma

Traumatic ungual fibroma—often solitary with a history of nail trauma

Connective Tissue Nevi (Shagreen Patch and Fibrous Forehead Plaque)

- Smooth muscle hamartoma—hypertrichosis, piloerection on rubbing
- Leiomyoma—intermittently painful, brown-to-blue, with translucent appearance
- Elastoma—increased elastic tissue on histochemistry
- Plexiform neurofibroma—hyperpigmentation, hypertrichosis, "bag of worms" consistency, underlying soft tissue or bony hypertrophy
- Lipoma—rubbery and well-defined
- Hemangioma—history of rapid growth in first year of life followed by gradual resolution

✓ Best Tests

Consider skin biopsy to confirm angiofibromas and connective tissue nevi.

Tuberous Sclerosis Consensus Conference Guidelines for the Evaluation of Newly Diagnosed Children

- Funduscopy by an ophthalmologist—retinal hamartomas
- Cranial imaging (CT or MRI)—cortical tubers, subependymal nodules, and subependymal giant cell astrocytomas
- Electroencephalography (EEG)—if seizures occur
- Cardiac EKG—arrhythmias (Wolff–Parkinson–White syndrome)
- Echocardiography—if evidence of cardiac dysfunction
- Renal ultrasound—renal angiomyolipomas
- Neurodevelopmental testing—need for early intervention

▲▲▲ Management Pearls

Tuberous Sclerosis Consensus Conference Guidelines for the Ongoing Evaluation of Established Patients

- Cranial imaging (CT or MRI)—every 1 to 3 years
- Neurodevelopmental testing—at the time child enters school and periodically if educational or behavioral concerns
- EEG—as indicated for seizure management
- Renal ultrasonography—every 1 to 3 years
- Chest CT—only women upon reaching adulthood
- Dermatologic exam—yearly in patients who may benefit from laser surgery

Therapy

Disfiguring facial angiofibromas may be treated with cryosurgery, curettage, dermabrasion, chemical peels, excision, and laser surgery. Laser surgery is currently the most popular treatment option. Multiple treatments are often needed, as lesions are variably recurrent.

Special Considerations in Infants

In infants, it is usually seizures (infantile spasms) or discovery of cardiac rhabdomyomas (benign cardiac tumors) on routine antenatal scanning that suggests the diagnosis; after that, characteristic skin lesions are noted. Potential skin lesions in infants with TSC are hypomelanotic macules, facial angiofibromas, forehead plaque, or shagreen patch. Periungual fibromas and "confetti" skin lesions (small hypopigmented lesions) do not appear until childhood or later. Questionable patients should be re-evaluated periodically for the development of new cutaneous and systemic signs of TSC.

Suggested Readings

Crino PB, Nathanson KL, Henske EP. The tuberous sclerosis complex. *N Engl J Med.* 2006;355(13):1345–1356.

Józwiak S, Schwartz RA, Janniger CK, et al. Usefulness of diagnostic criteria of tuberous sclerosis complex in pediatric patients. *J Child Neurol.* 2000;15(10):652–659.

Roach ES, DiMario FJ, Kandt RS, et al. Tuberous Sclerosis Consensus Conference: Recommendations for diagnostic evaluation. National Tuberous Sclerosis Association. *J Child Neurol.* 1999;14(6):401–407.

Schwartz RA, Fernández G, Kotulska K, et al. Tuberous sclerosis complex: Advances in diagnosis, genetics, and management. *J Am Acad Dermatol.* 2007;57(2):189–202.

Tuberous Sclerosis Alliance. http://www.tsalliance.org. Accessed May 22, 2009.

Wart, Flat

■ Diagnosis Synopsis

Flat warts, also known as verrucae planae or plane warts, like all other warts, are caused by human papillomavirus, usually types 3 and 10. They are mostly seen in older children and young adults.

◉ Look For

Minimally elevated, flat-topped, usually skin-colored or reddish papules that have a tendency to occur in groups or in a linear distribution due to autoinoculation (Figs. 4-112–4-115). The warts are most commonly seen on the face, neck, wrists, or legs of girls who shave.

●● Diagnostic Pearls

- Flat warts can be subtle. The surface may have a faint velvety feel.
- If flat warts are found, also examine the forehead, chin, and dorsal hands.

?? Differential Diagnosis and Pitfalls

- Lichen planus also presents with pruritic, flat-topped papules on the hands and wrists. A violaceous hue and the presence of overlying whitish, lacy, reticulated markings (Wickham striae) are helpful clues to this diagnosis.

- Lichen nitidus presents as tiny, uniform, pinhead-sized papules.
- The lesions of molluscum contagiosum are usually more significantly raised (dome-shaped) and may have a central dell.
- Lichen striatus presents unilaterally with pink to skin-colored, flat-topped papules in a linear distribution along the lines of Blaschko. If digital involvement is present, an associated nail dystrophy is a helpful clue to the diagnosis.

✓ Best Tests

This is usually a clinical diagnosis, though biopsy will confirm the diagnosis.

▲▲ Management Pearls

- This type of wart, like many other warts, typically enters remission spontaneously. Therefore, observation is a valid treatment option.
- The infection of flat warts may be more superficial than common warts. Therefore, liquid nitrogen application can be administered for a shorter duration.

Therapy

Destructive Therapies
- Liquid nitrogen
- Pulsed dye laser

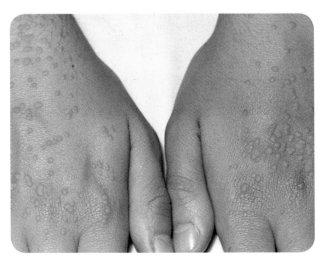

Figure 4-112 Flat warts are usually multiple and symmetrical on the extremities.

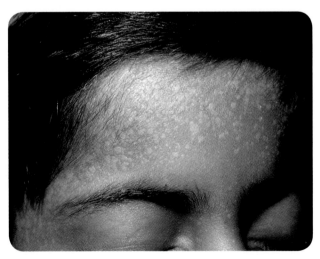

Figure 4-113 Flat warts on the forehead are often multiple and do not scale. They appear hypopigmented in those with dark skin.

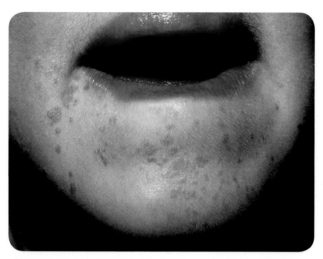

Figure 4-114 Flat warts can be hyperpigmented in lighter skin.

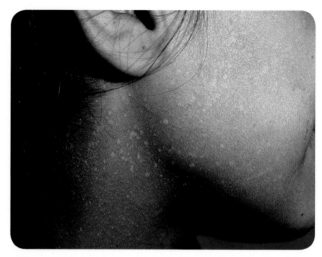

Figure 4-115 Flat warts that are hypopigmented on the face and neck.

Medical Therapies

- 5-Fluorouracil (Efudex 5% cream or Fluoroplex 1% cream) applied once to twice daily
- Retin-A 0.1% cream applied once to twice daily as tolerated
- Retin-A 0.1% plus imiquimod cream (Aldara) at bedtime until clear

Suggested Readings

Bolognia JL, Jorizzo JL, Rapini RP, eds. *Dermatology.* Vol. 1. 2nd Ed. St Louis, MO: Mosby; 2008:1183–1198.

James WD, Berger TG, Elston DM, eds. *Andrews' Diseases of the Skin.* 10th Ed. Philadelphia, PA: WB Saunders; 2006:404–406.

▪▪ Diagnosis Synopsis

Acanthosis nigricans (AN) is a localized skin disorder most commonly associated with obesity and insulin resistance. One recent study found that up to 90% of youth with AN also carried a diagnosis of type 2 diabetes mellitus. AN may be associated with various syndromes, malignancy, medications, or it may be congenital.

◉ Look For

Hyperpigmented and velvety thickening, usually on the back of the neck, axillae, and inguinal and inframammary folds (Figs. 4-116–4-119). In darker-skinned individuals, the plaques can be densely pigmented, appearing dark brown to black. The plaques are almost always symmetrical. Severe forms may show velvety plaques on the knuckles and extensor surfaces as well as the palms, soles, and mucosal surfaces. Acrochordons (small, dark, warty growths) are frequently present within neck and intertriginous locations. Very mild forms of this condition present as darkened areas of skin. AN is almost always asymptomatic.

●● Diagnostic Pearls

The plaques of AN are almost always symmetrical. AN does not rub off with an alcohol wipe as in retention hyperkeratosis.

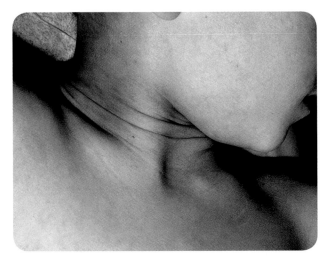

Figure 4-116 AN in a typical locus on neck; often confused with infrequent washing.

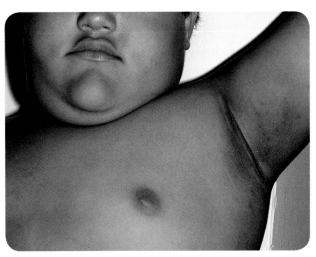

Figure 4-117 AN in a typical locus in axilla; borders are often indistinct.

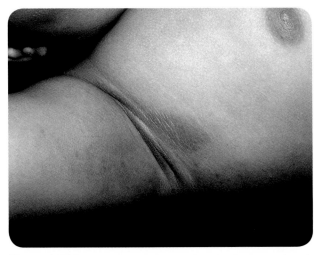

Figure 4-118 AN with hyperpigmented and velvety rugations in axilla.

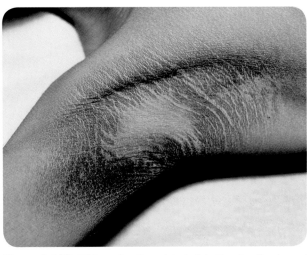

Figure 4-119 AN in an insulin-resistant diabetic extending beyond axilla.

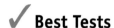 **Differential Diagnosis and Pitfalls**

- Tinea infection
- Candidiasis
- Atopic dermatitis
- Confluent and reticulated papillomatosis

 Best Tests

This is usually a clinical diagnosis. Biopsy would be helpful if an alternative diagnosis was being considered. Fasting glucose and hemoglobin A_1C may be helpful if insulin resistance is suspected.

▲▲ **Management Pearls**

As AN is most commonly associated with obesity, patients should be counseled on weight loss and the role their weight plays in their conditions.

Therapy

In patients with AN associated with obesity, weight reduction is the most important treatment. The association with diabetes and the corresponding health risks should be stressed to both patients and their parents. As patients dislike the appearance of AN, explaining that the condition may improve with weight loss can be a motivating factor.

Medications most commonly associated include nicotinic acid, oral contraceptives, and corticosteroids. Identifying and discontinuing the offending medication will result in clearance.

Malignancy is rarely associated with pediatric AN; this is more common in adults. Nevertheless, gastric adenocarcinoma, Wilms tumor, and osteogenic sarcoma have been associated with AN in the pediatric population. If a malignancy is suspected, proper workup should be initiated. In most cases, treatment of the underlying malignancy is curative.

Topical tretinoin in combination with 12% ammonium lactate may be helpful in obesity associated AN. Topical and oral retinoids may also be used as monotherapy. Other potential treatments include podophyllin, urea, and salicylic acid. Various lasers have also been reported to be effective.

Suggested Readings

Brickman WJ, Binns HJ, Jovanovic BD, et al. Acanthosis nigricans: A common finding in overweight youth. *Pediatr Dermatol.* 2007;24(6):601–606.

Sinha S, Schwartz RA. Juvenile acanthosis nigricans. *J Am Acad Dermatol.* 2007;57(3):502–508.

Acne Excoriée

Diagnosis Synopsis

Acne excoriée is an inflammatory disease that occurs when the affected individual compulsively squeezes and picks at minor superficial acne lesions. As a result of the mechanical trauma caused by the picking, scarring can occur. It is considered a form of factitial dermatitis and may be a sign of an underlying psychological disorder (obsessive-compulsive disorder).

Look For

You can see excoriated red papules, small pitted scars, and papules with small hemorrhagic and dark crusts (Figs. 4-120–4-123). In severe cases, small ulcers, hypertrophied scars, and keloids can be present.

Diagnostic Pearls

This is typically seen in adolescent females. Patients may have very few acne lesions.

?? Differential Diagnosis and Pitfalls

Herpes simplex if there are multiple erosions or crusted lesions.

✓ Best Tests

This is primarily a clinical diagnosis.

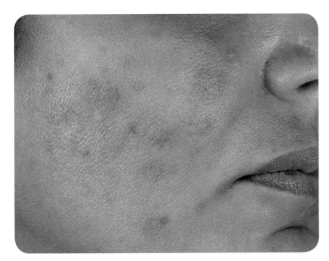

Figure 4-120 Acne excoriée with marked erythema and irregular erosions.

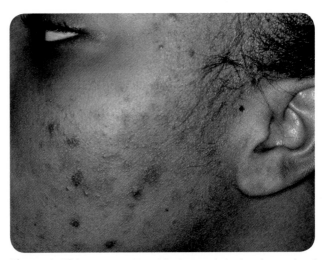

Figure 4-121 Acne excoriée with characteristic sharply angulated erosions and postinflammatory pigmentation.

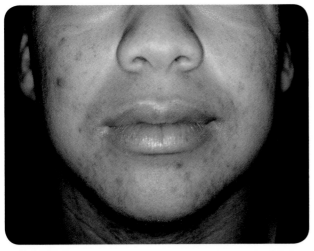

Figure 4-122 Acne excoriée with irregular scar from picking and squeezing.

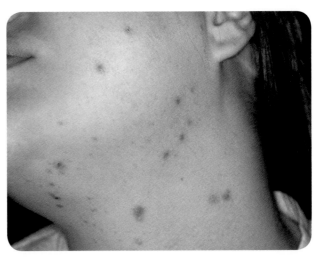

Figure 4-123 Acne excoriée with erosions on neck, a less typical area for early acne vulgaris.

▲▲ Management Pearls

These adolescents should be seen frequently, as a trusting physician–patient–parent relationship is important.

Therapy

The acne should be treated appropriately to diminish the patient's available lesions to pick. If acne is clear and excoriated lesions persist, referral to a psychiatrist may be helpful if the condition is severe enough or if it is felt there is an underlying psychological disorder. Various reports have noted different techniques such as behavioral and cognitive therapy to be effective. Antidepressants and hypnosis have also been used with success in some cases.

Suggested Readings

Shah KN, Fried RG. Factitial dermatoses in children. *Curr Opin Pediatr.* 2006;18(4):403–409.

Shenefelt PD. Hypnosis in dermatology. *Arch Dermatol.* 2000;136(3): 393–399.

Diagnosis Synopsis

Candidal diaper dermatitis develops when sufficient moisture in the diaper area allows *Candida albicans* to proliferate and invade the stratum corneum. The dermatitis usually begins around 6 weeks of age and is often associated with recent antibiotic use or diarrhea. *Candida* may also secondarily infect and exacerbate irritant diaper dermatitis.

Look For

Classically, candidal diaper dermatitis presents as a sharply demarcated, beefy-red diaper area; satellite pustules are uncommon (Figs. 4-124–4-126). Most commonly, there is diffuse erythema with peripheral scale or pink scaly papules that coalesce into plaques. The skin folds and the entire scrotum or labia may be confluently involved. In severe cases, there may be large erosions within the diaper area or there may be psoriasiform skin lesions on the trunk and extremities, which is known as candidal diaper dermatitis with psoriasiform id reaction.

Diagnostic Pearls

- Candidiasis should be strongly considered in any irritant diaper dermatitis that does not respond to standard therapies.
- Peripheral papulopustules and involvement of the deep skin fold is highly suggestive of candidal diaper dermatitis.
- A recent history of antibiotic use is highly suggestive of candidal diaper dermatitis.

- When candidiasis involves the genitalia, lesions are confluent, as opposed to psoriasis, in which lesions are more localized and sharply demarcated.

Differential Diagnosis and Pitfalls

The diaper area and distant skin should be examined for signs of other dermatoses. *Candida* may superinfect any diaper dermatitis that persists longer than 72 h (especially, irritant diaper dermatitis). Therefore, isolated candidal diaper dermatitis should be considered only when other possibly coexistent dermatoses have been ruled out.

Other diaper area dermatoses include the following:

Diaper-induced or Exacerbated Dermatoses

- Seborrheic dermatitis
- Psoriasis
- Irritant diaper dermatitis
- Allergic contact dermatitis

Dermatoses Unrelated to the Presence of a Diaper

- Acrodermatitis enteropathica
- Cystic fibrosis
- Langerhans cell histiocytosis
- Lichen sclerosus
- Kawasaki disease
- Perianal streptococcal dermatitis
- Congenital syphilis

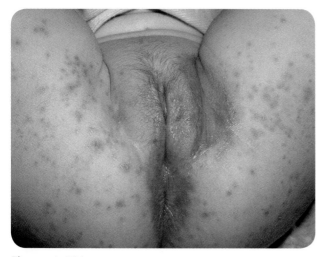

Figure 4-124 Candidal diaper dermatitis often has associated inflammatory vesiculopustules beyond the diaper area.

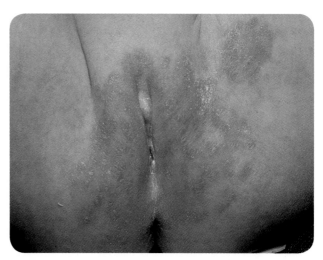

Figure 4-125 Candidal diaper dermatitis with pustules and erythema.

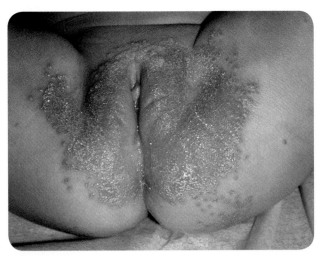

Figure 4-126 Candidal diaper dermatitis with multiple pustules and satellite lesions.

✓ Best Tests

Potassium hydroxide preparations will reveal budding yeasts, hyphae, and pseudohyphae. Cultures on Sabouraud medium will grow yeast within 72 h.

▲▲ Management Pearls

- Candidal diaper dermatitis will quickly recur if other concurrent diaper dermatoses are not treated simultaneously.
- Every infant should be examined for coexisting oral thrush.

Therapy

Candidal diaper dermatitis is treated topically with either nystatin; an azole antifungal (i.e., clotrimazole, miconazole, econazole, etc.); or ciclopirox twice daily for 2 to 3 weeks, or until 1 week after the rash has cleared.

If thrush is also present, oral nystatin suspension should be applied to the mucosa dosed at 1 mL four times daily until 2 to 3 days after resolution.

Suggested Readings

Honig PJ, Gribetz B, Leyden JJ, et al. Amoxicillin in diaper dermatitis. *J Am Acad Dermatol.* 1988;19(2 Pt 2): 275–279.

Dermatitis, Atopic (Eczema)

Diagnosis Synopsis

Atopic dermatitis (eczema) is a chronic relapsing, itchy dermatitis often associated with allergic rhinitis and/or asthma. Infants and children are most frequently affected, but the condition may persist into adulthood in some individuals.

In childhood, the disease involves the flexural aspects of extremities. The exact cause of the condition is unknown, with likely multiple genetic and environmental predisposing factors. A family history of atopic dermatitis is frequent. Most patients have marked xerosis and an inability to retain moisture in the skin. Environmental triggers such as heat, humidity, detergents/soaps, abrasive clothing, chemicals, and smoke, along with stress, tend to aggravate this disorder.

The hallmark of atopic dermatitis is intense itching. Scratching induces lichenification, and along with an impaired barrier function of the skin, increases the incidence of cutaneous infections. Cutaneous lesions in atopic dermatitis are prone to impetiginization with *Staphylococcus aureus*. Additionally, patients are at risk for generalized cutaneous infection with herpes simplex virus (eczema herpeticum) as well as widespread vaccinia infection (eczema vaccinatum).

Look For

Atopics sleep poorly due to itching. In childhood, plaques tend to involve the extensor legs and arms (Fig. 4-127). There is generally sparing of the diaper area and nasal tip. Less-involved skin is frequently dry, slightly erythematous, and may be scaly (Figs. 4-128–4-130).

Children can develop slightly scaly hypopigmented patches (pityriasis alba) on the cheeks, upper arms, and trunk. This condition is more apparent in highly pigmented skin, in which case there may also be extensive follicular accentuation without obvious lichenified plaques.

In older children and teenagers, there are thickened, scaly, erythematous papules and plaques involving the flexural surfaces. Lesions are less likely to be exudative and are most prominent on the posterior neck, antecubital fossae, popliteal fossa, and extremities in general. Look for hyperlinear palms and accentuation of the follicles. Impetiginized plaques can develop yellow or hemorrhagic (red) crusts. Keratotic follicular lesions of the outer aspects of the upper arms, legs, cheeks, and buttocks (keratosis pilaris) are frequently observed. Impetiginized plaques can develop thick crusts.

Diagnostic Pearls

- Additional cutaneous stigmata of atopic dermatitis include linear transverse folds just below the edge of the lower eyelids (Dennie–Morgan folds), paranasal and periorbital pallor ("headlight sign"), thinning of the lateral eyebrows (Hertoghe sign), and hyperkeratosis and hyperpigmentation producing a "dirty neck" appearance.
- Multiple lichenified papules on the elbows, knees, and dorsal hands should elicit a search for nickel allergy (periumbilical or earlobe dermatitis) as an exacerbating factor to the patient's atopic dermatitis.

Differential Diagnosis and Pitfalls

- An atopiclike eczematous dermatitis may be observed in patients with Wiskott–Aldrich syndrome, hyperimmunoglobulinemia E syndrome (Job syndrome), and Netherton syndrome.

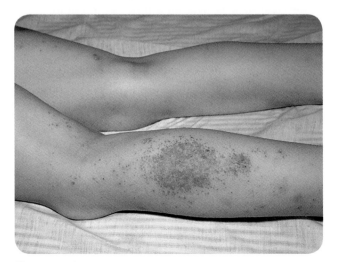

Figure 4-127 Atopic dermatitis. Both scattered lesions and confluent lesions with crusting on the posterior leg.

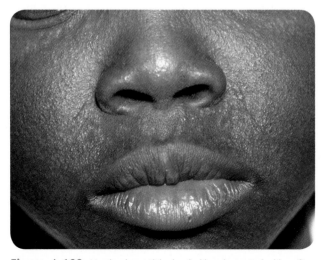

Figure 4-128 Atopic dermatitis in darkly pigmented skin often appears as closely aggregated skin-colored papules.

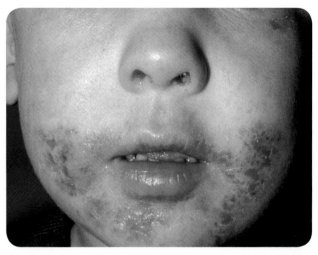

Figure 4-129 Atopic dermatitis in a common periorbital location with prominent erosions.

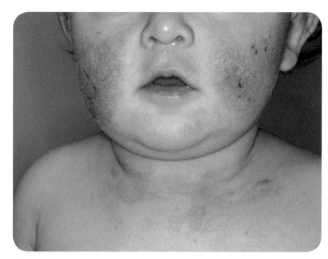

Figure 4-130 Atopic dermatitis in a symmetric involvement of cheeks with scaling and redness.

- Disorders of keratinization (i.e., nonbullous congenital ichthyosiform erythroderma, Netherton syndrome) may appear similar but present at birth rather than 3 to 6 months of age.
- Nutritional deficiencies (i.e., phenylketonuria, multiple carboxylase deficiency, zinc deficiency, and essential fatty acid deficiency) may appear identical to atopic dermatitis, but are usually associated with failure to thrive and systemic symptoms.
- Seborrheic dermatitis tends to involve the scalp and groin in infants and has greasy scale as opposed to dry scale seen in atopic dermatitis.
- The impaired cutaneous barrier in patients with atopic dermatitis makes them more prone to irritant contact dermatitis. Allergic contact dermatitis is also frequently encountered in atopic patients.
- Lichen simplex chronicus is composed of isolated, hyperpigmented, leathery plaques, frequently seen on the posterior neck, genitals, and extensor forearms and lower legs. Xerosis and atopy may be exacerbating factors in this condition.
- Scabies is also intensely pruritic, classically accentuated at night. Typical sites of involvement include the interdigital web spaces, axillae, wrists, belt area, buttocks, and feet. The pathognomic sign is the burrow.
- Lesions in tinea corporis are typically annular or arcuate. Fungal elements can be demonstrated using a KOH preparation.
- Classic lesions in psoriasis vulgaris are well-defined erythematous plaques involving the scalp and extensor elbows and knees with overlying silvery scale.

✓ Best Tests

- Take a careful history; this is primarily a clinical diagnosis. Serum IgE level is elevated in 80% of patients.

- Bacterial culture should be sent if lesions appear impetiginized. A Tzanck smear, viral culture, and/or viral PCR should be performed if eczema herpeticum is considered.
- Skin scrapings for scabies should be performed on any lesion that resembles a burrow.

▲▲ Management Pearls

- Emphasizing good sensitive skin care is very important. Emollients and moisturizing skin care routines are essential. Recommend nonsoap cleansers, such as Cetaphil, or moisturizing soaps, such as Dove. Have the patient apply fragrance-free and dye-free emollients, such as petroleum jelly, Aquaphor ointment, Eucerin cream, and Cetaphil cream to the skin after bathing. A fragrance-free/dye-free laundry detergent is also recommended.
- The child should follow up if there is concern for infection or if previously controlled dermatitis cannot be controlled. Multiple hemorrhagic crusts (scabs) associated with dermatitis often signify staphylococcal colonization or superinfection. In younger children, adequate control of cutaneous inflammation will eliminate pruritus and make oral antihistamines unnecessary.

Therapy

Intermittent use of topical corticosteroids to treat active, inflamed, palpable plaques. Once the areas are smooth, discontinue the use of topical steroids. In general, use low- to mid-potency topical steroids on the face and mid- to high-potency steroids on the trunk and extremities. The goal of treatment is to quickly achieve clearance of dermatitis with the lowest-strength effective topical steroid and maintain clearance without steroids for 1 week before dermatitis recurs and needs retreatment. Be careful of atrophy from steroids in skin folds and occluded areas. Try to use ointments, which usually require fewer preservatives and stabilizers. Topical nonsteroidal agents, including tacrolimus (Protopic) and pimecrolimus (Elidel), are typically less effective than topical corticosteroids and frequently elicit a burning sensation with application and are not indicated in children aged younger than 2 years.

Localized Body

Midpotency topical corticosteroids (Classes 3 and 4) need supervision with scheduled follow-up to monitor use, control, and response to therapy.

- Triamcinolone ointment (Kenalog and Aristocort)—apply twice daily (15, 30, 60, 120, and 240 g)
- Mometasone ointment (Elocon)—apply twice daily (15 and 45 g)
- Fluocinolone ointment (Synalar)—apply twice daily (15, 30, and 60 g)

Intertriginous and Facial

Use low-potency topical steroids on thinner skin areas of the face and intertriginous areas.

Desonide (DesOwen) or Aclovate ointment 30 g twice daily.

Extensive

Cyclosporin, azathioprine, tacrolimus, and mycophenolate mofetil have all been used to treat extensive, resistant disease with varying degrees of success. Phototherapy—including UVB, PUVA, and, most recently, narrow band UVB—has also been used successfully in many patients. These treatments are best administered by a dermatologist familiar with their use.

Pruritus

Antihistamine therapy can be a helpful component of treatment if pruritus continues after dermatitis is well controlled, the patient displays significant dermatographism, or the patient has a seasonal component to atopy. Consider one of the following antihistamines:

- Diphenhydramine hydrochloride (Benadryl): 5 mg/kg/ day every 6 h, as needed, for itching

- Hydroxyzine (Atarax):
  - Children aged 6 and older: 12.5 to 25 mg every 6 h as needed
  - Children up to age 6: 2 mg/kg/day three times daily
- Cetirizine hydrochloride (Zyrtec) is given as a single daily dose, with or without food:
  - Children aged 6 and older (and adults): 5 or 10 mg per day
  - Children aged 2 to 5: 2.5 mg once daily
- Loratadine (Claritin):
  - Children aged 6 and older (and adults): 10 mg once daily
  - Children aged 2 to 5: syrup, 5 mg once daily

Antibiotic therapy is beneficial when there is evidence of impetiginization (honey-colored crust, denuded skin, or oozing). Treat with a 10-day course of oral antibiotics to cover *S. aureus* infection. As MRSA becomes more prevalent in the community, therapy should be appropriately tailored. Bleach baths (1/4 to 1/2 cup Clorox bleach diluted in a full bath tub of water before the child enters the tub) one to three times weekly may be useful in a patient with multiple open areas (excoriations) or a history of multiple superinfections. Secondary infection due to herpes simplex should be treated with oral acyclovir.

Special Considerations in Infants

In infancy, the disease tends to primarily involve the face, scalp, and torso. Infantile atopic dermatitis is often exudative, consisting of erythematous, weeping plaques with variable degrees of crusting on the face and scalp. Alopecia and facial rash can result from the infant rubbing the scalp against the crib sheet to alleviate itch. In infants, there is usually sparing of the diaper area, in contrast to seborrheic dermatitis.

Suggested Readings

Bolognia JL, Jorizzo JL, Rapini RP, eds. *Dermatology*. Vol. 1. 2nd Ed. St Louis, MO: Mosby; 2008:181–195.

Cohen BA, ed. *Pediatric Dermatology*. 3rd Ed. St Louis, MO: Mosby; 2005:77–85.

James WD, Berger TG, Elston DM, eds. *Andrews' Diseases of the Skin*. 10th Ed. Philadelphia, PA: WB Saunders; 2006:69–77.

Diagnosis Synopsis

Allergic contact dermatitis is a cutaneous inflammatory process (type IV cell-mediated or delayed hypersensitivity reaction) localized to areas where allergens contact the skin. Initial sensitization and development of cutaneous inflammation takes 1 to 4 weeks; however, repeat exposure produces reactions within 48 h. As in adults, the most common contact allergens in children are urushiol (poison ivy, oak, or sumac), nickel, fragrance, cobalt (a metal), chromates (leather products), neomycin, thimerosal (ophthalmic preparations and vaccines), and adhesives. The distribution and geometry of lesions are important clues to diagnosis.

Look For

The clinical findings in acute cases range from scaling erythematous papules and plaques to vesicles and bullae in areas where the skin has contacted the allergen (Figs. 4-131–4-134). Lesions often have well-demarcated borders and geometric shapes coinciding with areas in contact with the allergen. As the dermatitis becomes chronic, plaques develop hyperpigmentation and lichenification. Allergic contact dermatitis is highly pruritic.

Diagnostic Pearls

The shape and distribution of the rash are highly suggestive of an etiology:

- Earlobes—nickel in earrings
- Lower abdomen—nickel in clothing snaps or belt buckles
- Diffuse lichenified papules on the torso and extremities—nickel

- Dorsal feet (toe webs spared)—rubber components or chromates in leather shoes
- Eyelids—thimerosal or nail products
- Well-demarcated eruption under a bandage—adhesive or rubber compounds
- Well-demarcated eruption around a cut—neomycin
- Linear streaks on exposed areas—plants (poison ivy)
- Linear on the central chest and abdomen—nickel in clothing snaps
- Margins of diaper—diaper dyes
- Entire diaper region—topically applied allergen (neomycin)
- Outer buttocks and hips—rubber components in elastic bands ("Lucky Luke Dermatitis")

Differential Diagnosis and Pitfalls

- Tinea pedis—affects toe webs, asymmetric.
- Seborrheic dermatitis—less pruritic, localized to seborrheic areas.
- Irritant contact dermatitis—history of irritant exposure, resolves with low- to mid-potency steroids and gentle skin care (use of barrier ointments and avoiding detergents, wet work, and saliva).
- Atopic dermatitis—history of atopy, characteristic location of lesions (flexures, face, and acral extremities).
- Impetigo—flaccid bullae, honey-colored crust, with ill-defined nongeometric borders.
- Facial cellulitis is accompanied by pain, fever, and systemic symptoms.
- Mycosis fungoides is very rare in children, but consider when lesions are unresponsive to therapy, often with atrophy, hypopigmentation and hyperpigmentation, and telangiectases. Biopsy is required to establish this diagnosis.

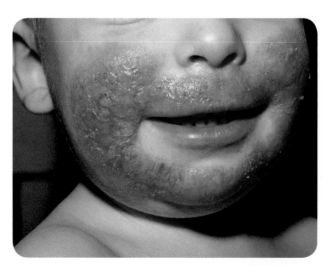

Figure 4-131 Contact dermatitis to a topical medication, as suggested by sharp borders.

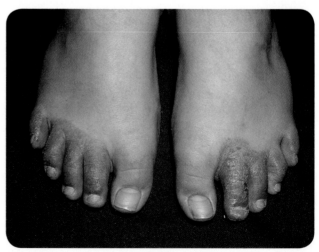

Figure 4-132 Contact dermatitis from shoes. Many chemicals in rubber, cement, and leather can cause contact dermatitis.

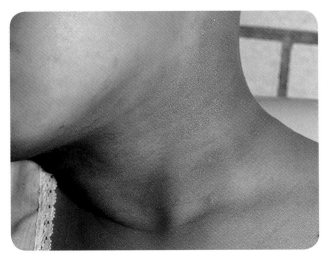

Figure 4-133 Contact dermatitis from a plant.

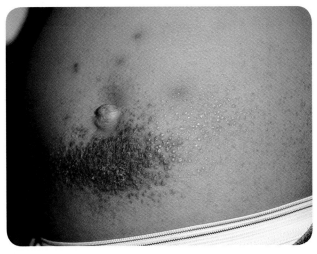

Figure 4-134 Contact dermatitis from nickel in a blue jeans button or belt buckle.

✓ Best Tests

Skin patch tests (i.e., T.R.U.E. TEST) will confirm allergy to individual chemicals. Skin biopsies are generally nonspecific but may be helpful to rule out other diagnoses.

▲▲ Management Pearls

- Ointment-based steroid preparations are preferred over creams, lotions, and solutions, as they enhance delivery of the active steroid and do not sting on application.
- The delayed hypersensitivity reaction is at least a 2-week process, and shorter courses of oral steroids will result in rebound of the dermatitis.
- Short-acting oral antihistamines (hydroxyzine and diphenhydramine) do not speed resolution of allergic contact dermatitis but may be used to induce drowsiness when pruritus interferes with sleep. Topical antihistamines should not be used because they are known contact sensitizers.

Therapy

The first goal of therapy is to remove the allergen. Then, inflammation is treated with topical or systemic steroids. Systemic steroids should be considered when the eruption is extensive or bullous. When the dermatitis is more localized, the choice of topical steroids is decided by the location and severity of the dermatitis. In general, low-potency steroids (alclometasone dipropionate 0.05%, desonide 0.05%, or hydrocortisone 2.5%) are appropriate for the face, groin, and axilla; midpotency steroids (fluocinolone acetonide 0.025% or hydrocortisone valerate 0.2%) are appropriate for the trunk and proximal extremities; and high-potency steroids (triamcinolone 0.1% or fluticasone propionate 0.0005%) are appropriate for the hands and feet. These steroid ointments can be safely used on localized areas twice daily for 2 weeks. More severe dermatitis may require more potent steroid ointments.

Special Considerations in Infants

The most common allergens in infants include nickel (earrings and snaps on clothing), dichromate (leather products, [e.g., straps, shoes]), and neomycin (topical antibiotic).

Suggested Readings

Mortz CG, Andersen KE. Allergic contact dermatitis in children and adolescents. *Contact Dermatitis*. 1999;41(3):121–130.

Weston WL. Contact dermatitis in children. *Curr Opin Pediatr*. 1997;9(4): 372–376.

Weston WL, Weston JA, Kinoshita J, et al. Prevalence of positive epicutaneous tests among infants, children, and adolescents. *Pediatrics*. 1986;78(6):1070–1074.

Wohrl S, Hemmer W, Focke M, et al. Patch testing in children, adults, and the elderly: Influence of age and sex on sensitization patterns. *Pediatr Dermatol*. 2003;20(2):119–123.

Dermatitis, Diaper Irritant

Diagnosis Synopsis

Irritant diaper dermatitis is a term for dermatitis caused by the occlusion, moisture, and friction produced by diapers. Once the skin barrier is compromised by this environment, secondary factors such as urinary ammonia, increased urine pH, fecal proteases and lipases, *Candida albicans*, bacterial overgrowth, and detergent soaps exacerbate the dermatitis.

Look For

Irritant diaper dermatitis presents as confluent erythema covering areas in greatest contact with the diaper (i.e., the convexities of the buttocks, lower abdomen, medial thighs, mons pubis, scrotum, and labia majora) (Figs. 4-135–4-138). Early or mild disease may only manifest as perianal erythema. More severe cases appear glazed with edema and erythematous papules in the involved skin. A wrinkled surface and postinflammatory hyperpigmentation may develop as the inflammation resolves.

Alternative presentations of irritant diaper dermatitis may include bandlike erythema and maceration along the diaper margins (tidewater mark dermatitis) or severe dermatitis with punched out ulcerations (Jacquet dermatitis and erosive perianal eruption).

Diagnostic Pearls

- Sparing of the skin folds is often seen.
- Irritant diaper dermatitis is rare in infants under 3 weeks of age, and other etiologies should be strongly considered when dermatitis occurs in the diaper area in this age group.

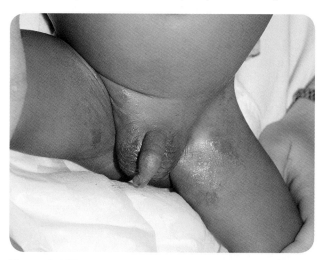

Figure 4-135 Diaper irritant dermatitis with prominent erosions.

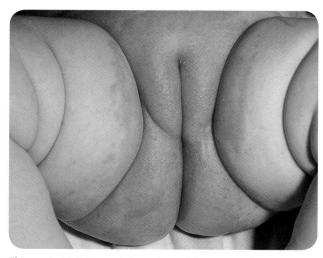

Figure 4-136 Diaper irritant dermatitis with confluent erythema and no discrete vesicular or pustular lesions.

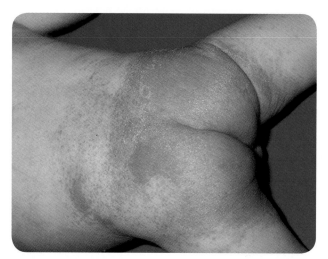

Figure 4-137 Diaper irritant dermatitis with extensive erythema and very tiny papular lesions.

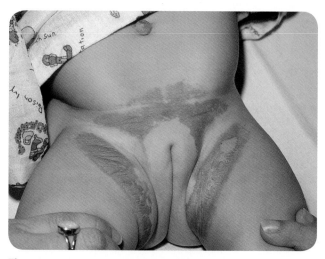

Figure 4-138 Diaper irritant dermatitis with prominent areas of sparing.

?? Differential Diagnosis and Pitfalls

Irritant diaper dermatitis often coexists with and exacerbates other dermatoses, and the presence of another dermatosis does not exclude concurrent irritant diaper dermatitis.

Diaper-Induced or Exacerbated Dermatoses

- Seborrheic dermatitis
- Psoriasis
- Candidiasis
- Allergic contact dermatitis

Dermatoses Unrelated to the Presence of a Diaper

- Acrodermatitis enteropathica
- Cystic fibrosis
- Langerhans cell histiocytosis
- Lichen sclerosus
- Kawasaki disease
- Perianal streptococcal dermatitis
- Congenital syphilis

✓ Best Tests

This is a clinical diagnosis. Potassium hydroxide preparations and fungal cultures (Sabouraud medium is usually positive by 3 days) may reveal secondary candidal infection.

▲▲ Management Pearls

- Irritant diaper dermatitis is frequently superinfected with *C. albicans,* and one should consider adding anticandidal agents when the rash is severe; when there is a history of coexistent pustules; or when response to therapy takes longer than 3 days. If the dermatitis is unresponsive to concurrent treatment of irritant dermatitis and candidiasis, other diagnoses should be considered.
- Parents should be reassured that irritant diaper dermatitis is not the result of improper or negligent care of the infant. Instead, they should be educated that irritant diaper dermatitis is an almost inevitable consequence of diapering, for which multiple treatment strategies exist.

Therapy

Diapers should be changed immediately after urinating or defecating (usually hourly for neonates and every 3 to 4 h for infants). Infants with diarrhea or who are otherwise ill will require more frequent diaper changes. Superabsorbent disposable diapers with multilayered acrylate gelling material are preferable to cloth diapers. Diapers 1 to 2 sizes larger than the infant's normal size are preferable to tight-fitting diapers.

Improving the Skin Barrier

Thick ointments and pastes, such as petrolatum and zinc oxide preparations, should be applied with every diaper change.

- Avoid harsh soaps and alcohol and instead use plain water or unscented diaper wipes.
- Avoid scrubbing and instead use mineral oil or Vaseline on a cotton ball to remove thick pastes and dried feces.
- Pat the diaper area dry instead of rubbing.
- Avoid using hair dryers in the diaper area.

Reducing Inflammation

Apply low-potency topical steroids ointments, such as 1% hydrocortisone, 0.05% alclometasone dipropionate, or 0.05% desonide ointment twice daily for inflamed areas. Alternatively, one may consider tacrolimus ointment twice daily for inflamed areas.

Treat Secondary Candidiasis

If there is any suspicion of candidiasis (pustules or rash longer than 3 days), apply nystatin, an azole antifungal (i.e., clotrimazole, miconazole, econazole, etc.), or ciclopirox twice daily for 2 to 3 weeks or until 1 week after the rash has cleared.

If the patient also has thrush, consider 1 mL of oral nystatin suspension four times daily for 1 week.

Suggested Readings

Harper J, Oranje A, Prose NS, eds. *Textbook of Pediatric Dermatology.* 2nd Ed. Malden, MA: Wiley-Blackwell; 2006:161–172.

Kazaks EL, Lane AT. Diaper dermatitis. *Pediatr Clin North Am.* 2000; 47(4):909–919.

Wolf R, Wolf D, Tüzün B, et al. Diaper dermatitis. *Clin Dermatol.* 2000; 18(6):657–660.

Dermatitis, Dyshidrotic

Diagnosis Synopsis

Dyshidrotic dermatitis, or pompholyx, is generally defined as an acute vesicular dermatitis limited to the hands (usually the palms and sides of the digits) and sometimes the feet. Its cause is unknown; no causal relationship with sweating has been shown.

Dyshidrotic dermatitis is rare in younger children. When arising in the pediatric population, it is generally seen after the age of 10.

The lesions of dyshidrotic dermatitis are extremely pruritic, and the condition often presents episodically, more commonly in warm weather.

Look For

Small, tense, clear, fluid-filled vesicles bilaterally on palmar/plantar surfaces and the lateral aspects of the digits. These vesicles can appear "deep-seated" (tapioca-like) due to the thickness of the palmar skin (Figs. 4-139–4-142). In severe cases, lesions can become confluent and present as large bullae. Erythema is mild to absent.

Diagnostic Pearls

To rule out inflammatory tinea infection with KOH examination, scrape the undersurface of the roof of the bullae for the greatest yield.

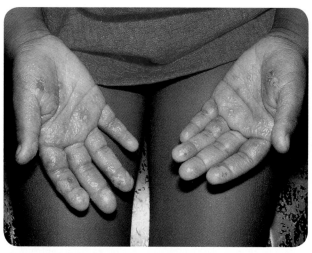

Figure 4-139 Dyshidrotic dermatitis with symmetric, discrete, and multilocular palmar vesicles; pustules may form when blisters become superinfected.

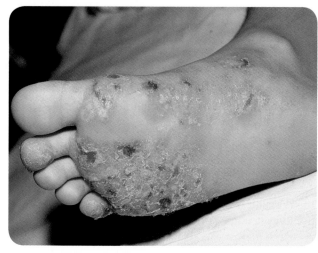

Figure 4-140 Dyshidrotic dermatitis may become eroded, crusted, and secondarily infected, requiring antibiotics.

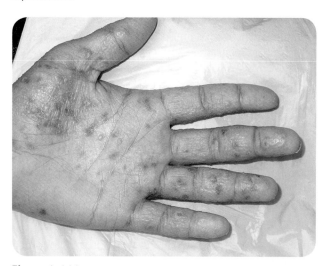

Figure 4-141 Dyshidrotic dermatitis with vesicles and hypopigmentation from previous lesions.

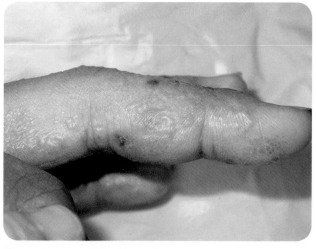

Figure 4-142 Dyshidrotic dermatitis with clear and deep tapioca-like vesicles on the lateral fingers being characteristic of this condition.

?? Differential Diagnosis and Pitfalls

- When limited to the feet, all efforts to exclude a bullous dermatophyte infection should be made.
- Distinguishing idiopathic dyshidrotic dermatitis from allergic contact dermatitis can be difficult, although contact dermatitis often involves the dorsum of the hand. An extensive history of environmental exposure should be gathered and patch testing considered when a vesicular hand rash is present.
- Hand-foot-and-mouth disease causes cutaneous oval-shaped vesicles as well as concomitant oral mucosal vesicles or erosions.
- Palmoplantar psoriasis starts with pustules, not vesicles. Pruritus is not a characteristic feature of this condition.
- Scabies is associated with superficial vesicles, pustules, and burrows; often has coexistent lesions on the wrists, waist, and axillae; and is diffusely pruritic.
- Id reaction is associated with additional lesions on the trunk and extremities and is associated with exacerbation of a pre-existing dermatitis or in response to a bacterial or dermatophyte infection.

✓ Best Tests

Biopsy will confirm the eruption as an acute spongiotic dermatitis but will not help establish the etiology.

▲▲ Management Pearls

- Warm saline compresses may be soothing and induce drainage of vesicles.
- Parents should be educated that dyshidrotic dermatitis is a chronic relapsing disease and that current therapies ameliorate but do not cure the dermatitis.
- Avoiding wet-work; using soft soaps (Dove, Cetaphil, and Oil of Olay); and application of moisturizers (Cetaphil cream, Aquaphor, and Eucerin) immediately after washing are all helpful.
- Although not caused by sweating, topical aluminum chloride (Certain Dri or Drysol) is helpful in some instances.
- Oral steroids should be considered only in recalcitrant, severe cases. Patch testing for the presence of a contact allergy should be considered.

Therapy

Initially, use a high-potency topical steroid (Classes 2 and 3).

High-potency (Class 2)
- Fluocinonide ointment (Lidex)—apply twice daily (15, 30, 60, and 120 g)
- Desoximetasone ointment (Topicort)—apply twice daily (15, 60, and 120 g)
- Halcinonide ointment (Halog)—apply twice daily (15, 60, and 240 g)
- Amcinonide ointment (Cyclocort)—apply twice daily (15, 30, and 60 g)

Midpotency (Classes 3 and 4)
- Triamcinolone ointment (Kenalog and Aristocort)—apply twice daily (15, 30, 60, 120, and 240 g)
- Mometasone ointment (Elocon)—apply twice daily (15 and 45 g)
- Fluocinolone ointment (Synalar)—apply twice daily (15, 30, and 60 g)

If severe, use a superpotent topical steroid for a short 2-week course and schedule close follow-up.

Superpotent (Class 1)
- Clobetasol 0.05% ointment—apply twice daily (15, 30, and 45 g)
- Betamethasone (Diprolene) 0.05% ointment—apply twice daily (15, 30, and 45 g).
- Diflorasone (Psorcon) 0.05% ointment—apply twice daily (15, 30, and 60 g)
- Halobetasol (Ultravate) ointment—apply twice daily (15 and 50 g)

Caution: Beware of skin atrophy over dorsal hands/feet with potent and superpotent steroids.

Suggested Readings

Bolognia JL, Jorizzo JL, Rapini RP, eds. *Dermatology.* Vol. 1. 2nd Ed. St Louis, MO: Mosby; 2008:543.

James WD, Berger TG, Elston DM, eds. *Andrews' Diseases of the Skin.* 10th Ed. Philadelphia, PA: WB Saunders; 2006:79–80.

Diagnosis Synopsis

Nummular dermatitis is a form of dermatitis characterized by coin-shaped scaly plaques. It is of uncertain etiology, but it is associated with triggers such as frequent bathing with irritating and drying soap and exposure to irritating fabrics such as wool. Patients often have some of the signs and symptoms typically associated with atopic dermatitis. Pruritus can be severe, and affected children can be irritable.

Winter is usually the time of onset and exacerbation. Nummular dermatitis can be chronic with a waxing and waning course.

Some experts consider childhood nummular dermatitis as a subtype of atopic dermatitis.

Look For

Several to multiple, round or coin-shaped, well-defined, erythematous scaly plaques, often with overlying fissures, erosions, and crusts (Figs. 4-143–4-146). Lesions tend to be 2 to 5 cm in size. Plaques are scattered over the trunk and/or extremities.

Diagnostic Pearls

The discrete coin-shaped morphology helps to distinguish nummular dermatitis from atopic dermatitis. After treatment, postinflammatory pigmentary changes are common.

Differential Diagnosis and Pitfalls

- Tinea corporis
- Impetigo
- Psoriasis
- Contact dermatitis
- Small plaque parapsoriasis
- Pityriasis rosea
- Seborrheic dermatitis
- Atopic dermatitis

Best Tests

Swab crusted plaques for bacterial culture. Rule out dermatophytosis with a KOH smear of scale. A skin biopsy can support the clinical diagnosis of an eczematous eruption.

Management Pearls

Look for signs of secondary bacterial infection, and treat with antistaphylococcal antibiotics if indicated. Moisturizing creams and ointments are key. If pruritus is severe, use systemic antihistamines. Potent topical steroids are necessary to address cutaneous inflammation.

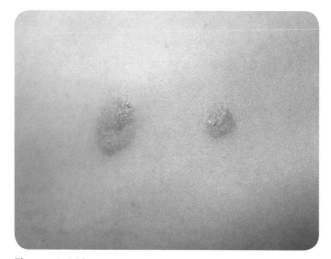

Figure 4-143 Nummular dermatitis with a characteristic coin-shaped lesion with some erosions and scale.

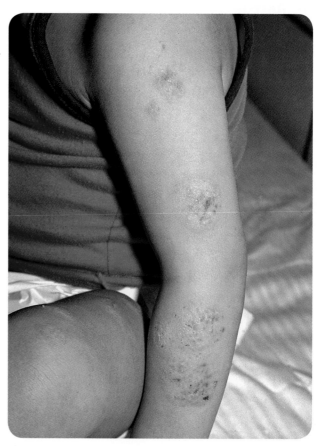

Figure 4-144 Nummular dermatitis with lesions in several locations favoring the extensor extremities.

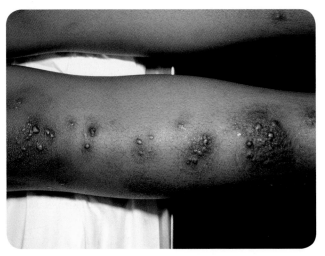

Figure 4-145 Nummular dermatitis with multiple relatively discrete lesions.

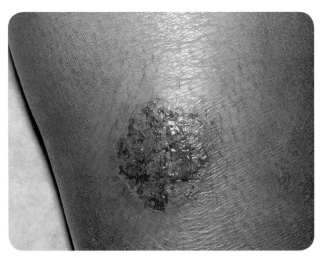

Figure 4-146 Nummular dermatitis. A discrete coin-shaped, oozing plaque.

Therapy

Use systemic antibiotics when indicated.

Appropriate skin care includes daily lukewarm baths or showers; use of mild soaps (Dove, Cetaphil, and Purpose); and use of copious amounts of thick emollients (Eucerin or Cetaphil cream, white petrolatum) applied while the skin is wet. Use a mid- to high-potency (Classes 2 to 5) topical corticosteroid twice daily on lesions, with close follow-up (2 to 4 weeks).

Class 2

Fluocinonide ointment (Lidex)—apply twice daily

Desoximetasone ointment (Topicort)—apply twice daily

Halcinonide ointment (Halog)—apply twice daily

Amcinonide ointment (Cyclocort)—apply twice daily

Classes 3 to 4

Triamcinolone ointment (Kenalog and Aristocort)—apply twice daily

Mometasone ointment (Elocon)—apply twice daily

Fluocinolone ointment (Synalar)—apply twice daily

Suggested Readings

Gutman AB, Kligman AM, Sciacca J, et al. Soak and smear: A standard technique revisited. *Arch Dermatol.* 2005;141(12):1556–1559.

Krol A, Krafchik B. The differential diagnosis of atopic dermatitis in childhood. *Dermatol Ther.* 2006;19(2):73–82.

Shaw M, Morrell DS, Goldsmith LA. The study of targeted enhanced patient care for pediatric atopic dermatitis (STEP PAD). *Pediatr Dermatol.* 2008;25:19–24.

Diagnosis Synopsis

Seborrheic dermatitis is an idiopathic inflammatory disease of the scalp, nasolabial folds, eyebrows, ears, and presternal and intertriginous areas (the "seborrheic areas"). It is believed to be caused by some combination of abnormalities in sebum production or composition, altered immune response, and the presence of *Malassezia furfur*. As such, the disease typically appears at the time of puberty (presence of sebum), is highly prevalent in individuals with HIV infection (altered immunity), and is often associated with Tinea versicolor and *Pityrosporum folliculitis* (presence of *M. furfur*). Neurologic disease also predisposes to seborrheic dermatitis.

Look For

Loose, often greasy scale within well-defined erythematous macules or plaques symmetrically involving the scalp (dandruff), eyebrows, nasolabial folds, pinna, postauricular skin, aural canal, and central chest (**Figs. 4-147–4-149**). In children with darker skin, facial lesions may be arcuate or annular, have discrete papules, and have moderate hypopigmentation.

Diagnostic Pearls

- Severe, resistant, or rapidly progressive seborrheic dermatitis is suspicious for immunodeficiency (especially HIV infection).
- Purpura in seborrheic lesions on the scalp or in the groin should raise the suspicion of Langerhans cell histiocytosis.
- Scaling of the eyebrows, nasolabial, or postauricular folds is highly characteristic.

Differential Diagnosis and Pitfalls

- In the absence of risk factors, seborrheic dermatitis should be questioned in the prepubescent patient
- Psoriasis—adherent dry scales, knee and elbow involvement, and nail changes
- Tinea capitis—favors preadolescent children, significantly pruritic, associated with lymphadenopathy and alopecia
- Tinea corporis—dry scale and asymmetric distribution
- Contact dermatitis—pruritic and burning, less well-demarcated, not confined to seborrheic areas
- Darier disease—composed of papules that coalesce into plaques, associated with acral skin and nail changes
- Discoid lupus erythematosus—atrophic and hyper-pigmented
- Pemphigus foliaceous—moist, oozing crust
- Perioral dermatitis—erythematous scaling papules in the nasolabial creases without associated scalp, eyebrow, or periauricular involvement

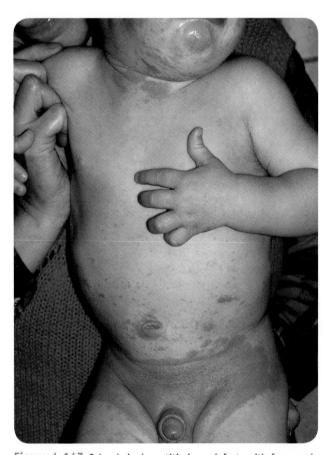

Figure 4-147 Seborrheic dermatitis in an infant, with face, neck, and diaper area involvement.

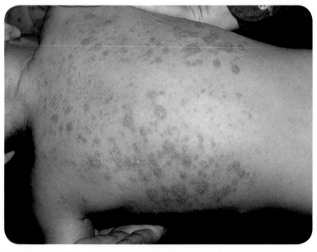

Figure 4-148 Seborrheic dermatitis in an infant, with extensive truncal involvement.

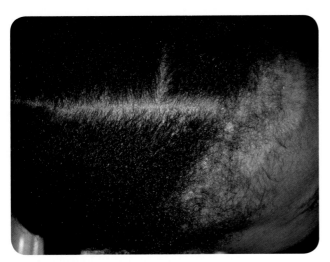

Figure 4-149 Seborrheic dermatitis with mild scaling. Culture for fungus was negative.

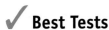 Best Tests

This is a clinical diagnosis. A skin biopsy is not diagnostic but can be used to rule out other diagnoses.

Management Pearls

It should be emphasized to parents and adolescents that there is no cure for seborrheic dermatitis. The condition intermittently waxes and wanes, and patients should be educated to restart therapy at the first sign of recurrent disease. Rotational use of shampoo preparations is often helpful to prevent development of tolerance.

Therapy

Scalp

- Ketoconazole 2% shampoo should be applied to the wet scalp and rinsed off in shower twice weekly as needed. The lather should also be used to cleanse the face and any other involved areas.

- 2% pyrithione zinc shampoos (Head & Shoulders, DHS Zinc, Sebulon, etc.) twice weekly to daily as needed.
- Tar- and salicylic-acid-based preparations (e.g., Neutrogena T/Gel, Neutrogena T/Sal) twice weekly to daily as needed.
- Selenium sulfide 2.5% shampoo daily as needed.
- Mid- to high-potency topical steroid solution, shampoo or foam such as betamethasone valerate 0.12% foam (Luxiq) or fluocinonide 0.05% solution (Lidex), fluocinolone shampoo (Capex) daily as needed.
- For dense scalp scale or in African–American patients, consider oil-based products: fluocinolone acetonide 0.01% in peanut oil (Derma-Smoothe F/S oil) or nonsteroid mineral oil preparations (P&S liquid) applied nighty.

Face and Body

- Ketoconazole 2% cream (Nizoral) twice daily until clear.
- Mild topical steroids (Classes 6 and 7) such as desonide (DesOwen or Desonate gel) or hydrocortisone 2.5% cream (Hytone) twice daily as needed for flares.
- Topical immunomodulators, such as tacrolimus 0.1% (Protopic) or pimecrolimus (Elidel) may be used twice daily as needed in place of topical steroids.

Suggested Readings

Gupta AK, Batra R, Bluhm R, et al. Skin diseases associated with Malassezia species. *J Am Acad Dermatol.* 2004;51(5):785–798.

Gupta AK, Bluhm R, Cooper EA, et al. Seborrheic dermatitis. *Dermatol Clin.* 2003;21(3):401–412.

Henderson CA, Taylor J, Cunliffe WJ. Sebum excretion rates in mothers and neonates. *Br J Dermatol.* 2000;142(1):110–111.

Plewig G, Jansen T. Seborrheic dermatitis. In: Wolff K, Goldsmith LA, Katz SI, Gilchrest BA, Paller AS, Leffell DJ, eds. *Fitzpatrick's Dermatology in General Medicine.* Vol. 1. 7th Ed. New York, NY: McGraw-Hill; 2008:219–225.

■■ Diagnosis Synopsis

Infantile seborrheic dermatitis is an inflammatory disease of the scalp, face, postauricular, presternal, and intertriginous areas ("seborrheic areas") of infants. Characteristically, the rash begins within the first month of life and gradually resolves by 4 months of age. It is hypothesized that increased activity of the sebaceous glands in response to elevated infantile hormones plays an important role in its pathogenesis.

◉ Look For

Well-defined, erythematous macules and plaques with varying degrees of greasy, yellow scale (Figs. 4-150–4-153). The scale adheres to the skin and may be confluent. Common sites of involvement include the scalp, face, skin folds, postauricular, presternal, and intertriginous areas. Scalp disease tends to be minimally inflamed, whereas the skin folds often display significant erythema and maceration. In darkly pigmented infants, the rash may be associated with postinflammatory hypopigmentation.

●● Diagnostic Pearls

- Maceration and erosions in the diaper area often signify *Candida albicans* superinfection.
- If acutely weeping with superficial erosions, consider secondary infection with group A streptococcus species.
- Severe or generalized seborrheic dermatitis requires consideration of immunodeficiency.

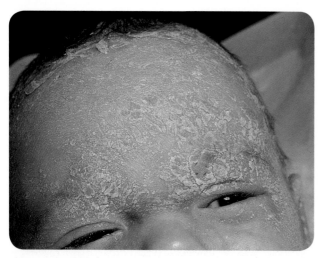

Figure 4-150 Seborrheic dermatitis with thick, waxy, yellow scale and underlying erythema.

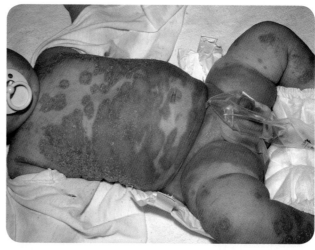

Figure 4-151 Seborrheic dermatitis with greasy scale and involvement of the diaper area, skin folds, and torso.

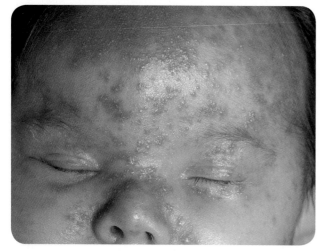

Figure 4-152 Seborrheic dermatitis on the scalp, forehead, and nasolabial fold, typical locations in adults as well.

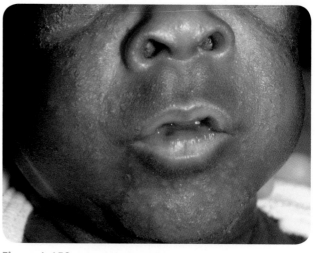

Figure 4-153 Seborrheic dermatitis with prominent slightly edematous facial involvement.

?? Differential Diagnosis and Pitfalls

- The most difficult diagnoses to separate from infantile seborrheic dermatitis are psoriasis and atopic dermatitis. Both psoriasis and atopic dermatitis, however, have dry rather than greasy scale. Additionally, psoriasis more commonly affects the lower abdomen and umbilicus than seborrheic dermatitis, and atopic dermatitis more commonly affects the shins and forearms than seborrheic dermatitis. Occasionally, it is impossible to distinguish between these diagnoses, and one must follow the patient clinically for more specific signs to develop.
- "Cradle cap" may be caused by seborrheic dermatitis or atopic dermatitis. Atopic dermatitis is much more pruritic, and the scale of atopic dermatitis is dry rather than waxy.
- When localized in the diaper area, dermatoses to consider include the following:

Diaper-induced or Exacerbated Dermatoses

- Candidiasis
- Psoriasis
- Irritant diaper dermatitis
- Allergic contact dermatitis

Dermatoses Unrelated to the Presence of a Diaper

- Acrodermatitis enteropathica
- Cystic fibrosis
- Langerhans cell histiocytosis
- Lichen sclerosus
- Kawasaki disease
- Perianal streptococcal dermatitis
- Congenital syphilis

✓ Best Tests

This is usually a clinical diagnosis. A skin biopsy can be suggestive but not diagnostic of the disease.

▲▲ Management Pearls

- Lesions of seborrheic dermatitis on the body should respond within 2 weeks of starting therapy, and one should consider alternative diagnoses if lesions are persistent.
- Avoid salicylic acid preparations, as they may cause salicylism or irritation.

Therapy

Scalp

For mild disease, wash the scalp with a mild shampoo ("no tears" shampoo) daily. If not responsive, wash daily with a selenium sulfide shampoo.

For thick scale, massage mineral or baby oil onto the scalp daily prior to bathing.

For inflammatory lesions, apply a mild topical steroid daily (Derma-Smoothe/FS oil, hydrocortisone 2.5% ointment).

Body

Mild Class 6 or 7 topical steroid creams or ointments (desonide or hydrocortisone 2.5% twice daily) are usually sufficient.

Topical antiyeast creams (i.e., ketoconazole 2% cream) may also be applied once to twice daily to increase efficacy.

Suggested Readings

Gupta AK, Batra R, Bluhm R, et al. Skin diseases associated with Malassezia species. *J Am Acad Dermatol.* 2004;51(5):785–798.

Gupta AK, Bluhm R, Cooper EA, et al. Seborrheic dermatitis. *Dermatol Clin.* 2003;21(3):401–412.

Henderson CA, Taylor J, Cunliffe WJ. Sebum excretion rates in mothers and neonates. *Br J Dermatol.* 2000;142(1):110–111.

Plewig G, Jansen T. Seborrheic dermatitis. In: Wolff K, Goldsmith LA, Katz SI, Gilchrest BA, Paller AS, Leffell DJ, eds. *Fitzpatrick's Dermatology in General Medicine.* Vol. 1. 7th Ed. New York: McGraw-Hill; 2008:219–225.

■■ Diagnosis Synopsis

Epidermal nevi (nevi verrucosus) affect 0.1% of the population and are usually recognized at birth, but may not appear until childhood when they are seen as a linear array of smooth, hyperpigmented, thin plaques or rough skin-colored papules and plaques. Epidermal nevi are hamartomas of ectodermal origin; the term encompasses a variety of lesions with various histologic and clinical patterns. The most typical presentation is as a linear verrucous epidermal nevus. Most develop sporadically, although familial cases have been reported.

Occasionally, epidermal nevi may be associated with other cutaneous, CNS, skeletal, and ocular abnormalities previously known as epidermal nevus syndrome. This entity is now thought to include many distinct genetic diseases, all sharing a phenotype reflecting genetic mosaicism.

◉ Look For

Linear, verrucous, thin plaques that gradually enlarge and become warty in appearance (Figs. 4-154–4-156). The lesions tend to be oriented along the lines of Blaschko (Fig. 4-157). The pattern is linear and whorled with a midline demarcation.

●● Diagnostic Pearls

There is a tendency for epidermal nevi to assume a more verrucous appearance with age, particularly at puberty.

?? Differential Diagnosis and Pitfalls

- Verruca vulgaris—verrucous papules and plaques, however, do not tend to assume a whorled pattern and do not respect the midline.
- Epidermal nevi may reflect a somatic mosaicism for K1/K10 mutations as seen in epidermolytic hyperkeratosis (EHK). If these patients have gonadal mosaicism, the offspring may have full-blown EHK. Mosaicism for ATP2A2 mutations can cause segmental Darier disease. As in EHK, if these patients have gonadal mosaicism, the offspring may have full-blown Darier disease.
- Nevus sebaceus—papillomatous, yellow-orange, linear plaque on the scalp or face.
- Psoriasis—may present in a segmental fashion (nevoid psoriasis) but responds to topical steroids.
- Inflammatory linear verrucous epidermal nevus—congenital pruritic, linear, psoriasiform plaque.
- Lichen striatus—presents in childhood as asymptomatic linearly arranged, small, flat-topped, pink to skin-colored papules within the lines of Blaschko, usually on an extremity. These lesions spontaneously resolve over months to a few years.
- Mosaic EHK—skin biopsy reveals reticulate degeneration of the epidermis.
- Mosaic Darier disease—skin biopsy reveals acantholytic dyskeratosis.

✓ Best Tests

Skin biopsy reveals hyperkeratosis, papillomatosis, and acanthosis.

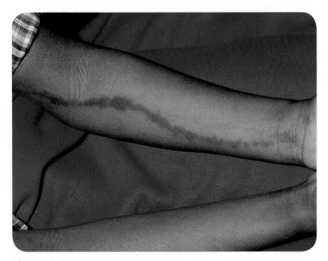

Figure 4-154 Epidermal nevus in a long, linear distribution. Lesions are usually slightly papular and wartlike.

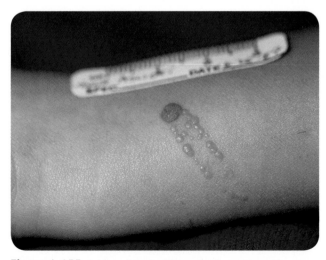

Figure 4-155 Epidermal nevi with a smooth papular and a verrucous component.

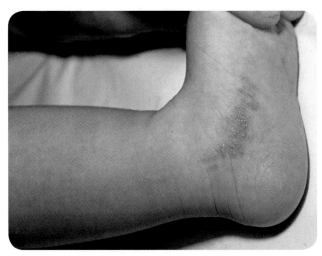

Figure 4-156 Epidermal nevi may involve the palms, soles, or the nail bed.

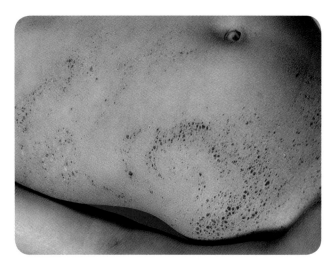

Figure 4-157 Epidermal nevi may have a complex configuration related to development; whorllike structure follow the lines of Blaschko.

▲▲ Management Pearls

- Epidermal nevi are benign. Biopsy should be considered to rule out mosaic EHK. Those patients bearing epidermal nevi with histopathologic features of EHK should receive genetic counseling for possible mutations in sperm or egg leading to a child with generalized EHK.
- Symptom-directed screening should be performed in patients with widespread epidermal nevi, and an interdisciplinary team of neurologists, orthopedists, cardiologists, ophthalmologists, oncologists, and rehabilitation specialists should be employed as indicated.

Therapy

Epidermal nevi can be a cosmetic problem. Excisional surgery can be used for small lesions. However, this results in scarring, and extension can still occur even after excision. Carbon dioxide laser has been used to ablate lesions with variable success, but also results in scarring.

Suggested Readings

Bolognia JL, Jorizzo JL, Rapini RP, eds. *Dermatology*. Vol. 2. 2nd Ed. St Louis, MO: Mosby; 2008:1671–1672.

Boyce S, Alster TS. CO_2 laser treatment of epidermal nevi: Long-term success. *Dermatol Surg.* 2002;28(7):611–614.

Cohen BA, ed. *Pediatric Dermatology*. 3rd Ed. St Louis, MO: Mosby; 2005:55.

James WD, Berger TG, Elston DM, eds. *Andrews' Diseases of the Skin*. 10th Ed. Philadelphia, PA: WB Saunders; 2006:633–635.

Paller AS, Syder AJ, Chan YM, et al. Genetic and clinical mosaicism in a type of epidermal nevus. *N Engl J Med.* 1994;331(21):1408–1415.

Spitz JL. *Genodermatoses. A Clinical Guide to Genetic Skin Disorders.* 2nd Ed. Philadelphia, PA: Lippincott Williams & Wilkins; 2004:44–47.

■ Diagnosis Synopsis

Ichthyosis vulgaris is a common heritable condition of abnormal cornification, resulting in dry scaly skin. It is often seen in association with atopic dermatitis. Extreme dryness of the skin presents as fine, fishlike scale. The condition is more prominent in winter and in climates with low relative humidity. Ichthyosis vulgaris usually begins in childhood between 3 and 12 months of age and follows a favorable course in which the scaling alleviates in intensity by adulthood.

◉ Look For

Dry, fine, scaling skin forming a network of fish skinlike scale (Figs. 4-158–4-161). Usually, most apparent on the extensor extremities.

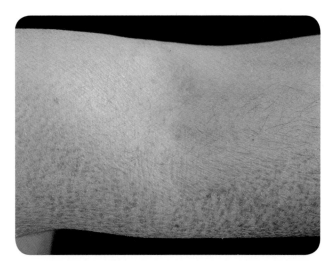

Figure 4-158 Ichthyosis vulgaris with antecubital sparing is characteristic.

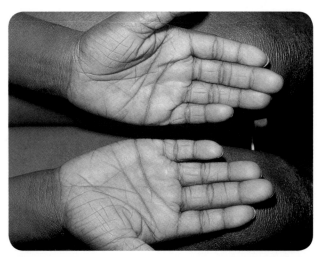

Figure 4-159 Ichthyosis vulgaris with accentuated palmar markings.

●● Diagnostic Pearls

- Look for accentuated palmar creases and scaly palms.
- Flexural sparing, extensor accentuation.
- Frequently associated with atopic dermatitis and keratosis pilaris.

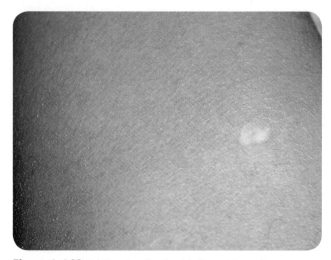

Figure 4-160 Ichthyosis vulgaris with fine, white scale.

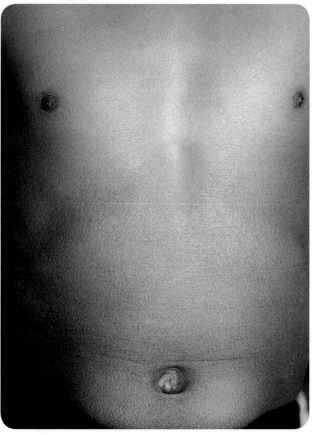

Figure 4-161 Ichthyosis vulgaris with very fine body scale.

?? Differential Diagnosis and Pitfalls

Consider X-linked ichthyosis in males, which has a darker scale and involves a wider distribution, including lateral neck, and usually starts before the age of 1 year.

✓ Best Tests

Skin biopsy showing an absent or very thinned granular layer, though the diagnosis is usually made on clinical grounds. Most patients have a mutation in the filaggrin gene, but precise gene testing is usually not indicated.

▲▲▲ Management Pearls

Emollients are the mainstay of therapy. Creams applied after bathing help the epidermis retain water. Use nondrying soaps (e.g., Dove) or nonsoap cleansers (e.g., Cetaphil or similar).

Therapy

A moisturizing cream/ointment applied directly to wet skin after bathing. For more scaling or hyperkeratotic areas, an alpha hydroxy acid or urea-based lotion or cream applied to wet skin with an additional application of an emollient may improve the condition. Use mild-potency topical steroids (Classes 6 and 7) on thinner skin and on the face, or use topical calcineurin inhibitors (pimecrolimus or tacrolimus) when dermatitis is coexistent. Use steroid ointments that have fewer preservatives in them if there seems to be flaring with multiple topical medications.

Propylene glycol (20% to 60%) in water applied under occlusion can be used as an effective keratolytic.

Suggested Readings

Goldsmith LA, Baden HP. Management and treatment of ichthyosis. *N Engl J Med.* 1972;286(15):821–823.

Oji V, Traupe H. Ichthyoses: Differential diagnosis and molecular genetics. *Eur J Dermatol.* 2006;16(4):349–359.

Shwayder T. Disorders of keratinization: Diagnosis and management. *Am J Clin Dermatol.* 2004;5:17–29.

Diagnosis Synopsis

X-linked ichthyosis is a genetic disorder of abnormal corni-fication caused by a deficiency in steroid sulfatase (STS), which is involved in normal desquamation of the stratum corneum. It is classically characterized by dirty-appearing scale on the sides of the neck ("dirty neck") and the peri-umbilical area. The remainder of the trunk and extremities are also involved, with classic sparing of the face, palms, and soles, as well as the popliteal and antecubital fossae. This con-dition is almost exclusive to males, with exaggerated neonatal desquamation along the flanks of neonates being a common presentation. However, the disease phenotype ranges from absent to marked and diffuse scaling.

The placenta is of fetal origin and is also deficient in ste-roid sulfatase. For this reason, mothers with affected children experience prolonged labor, possibly requiring cesarean sec-tion or vacuum-assisted delivery.

Look For

Fine, white or thick, dark brown scale symmetrically affecting the torso, extensor surfaces of the extremities, posterior and lateral neck, scalp, and lateral face (Figs. 4-162–4-165). The palms, soles, antecubital, and popliteal fossae are charac-teristically spared. Scaling may present within the first weeks of life, develop within several years, or never develop at all.

Parents should be asked about abnormal eye examina-tions, as asymptomatic corneal opacities are present in 10% to 50% of patients and female carriers after the first decade of life.

Diagnostic Pearls

The scale characteristically improves during the more humid summer months.

Differential Diagnosis and Pitfalls

- Lamellar ichthyosis—may begin as a collodion membrane and involves the face, palms, soles, and flexural surfaces (i.e., antecubital and popliteal fossae)
- Ichthyosis vulgaris—hyperlinear palms and soles, often associated with atopy

Best Tests

- This diagnosis is generally made clinically. A skin biopsy may show hyperkeratosis and a normal or thickened stra-tum granulosum. However, changes are subtle and can be difficult to differentiate from lamellar ichthyosis and normal skin. Fluorescent in situ hybridization will reveal absence of the STS gene in 90% of affected individuals.

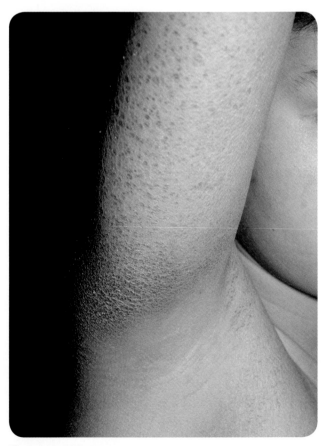

Figure 4-163 X-linked ichthyosis. Axillae and antecubital and popliteal fossae may be spared.

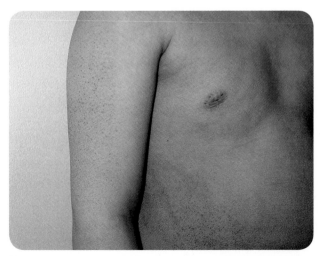

Figure 4-162 X-linked ichthyosis with small, dark brown scale.

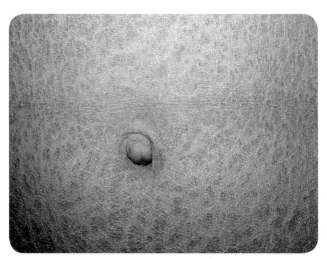

Figure 4-164 X-linked ichthyosis with typical dark polygonal scales.

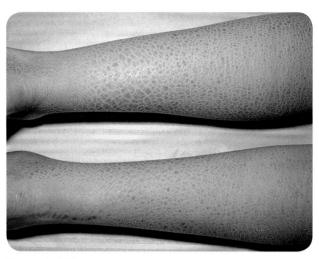

Figure 4-165 X-linked ichthyosis typically has large discrete scales compared with ichthyosis vulgaris.

- Other less commonly employed tests include the following: lipoprotein electrophoresis (increased mobility of the low-density lipoprotein fraction); steroid sulfatase assay on serum, leukocytes, or fibroblasts; Southern blot analysis; and blood cholesterol sulfate level (elevated).

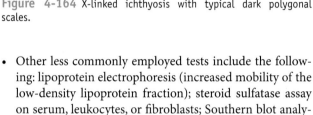 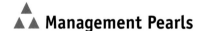

Management Pearls

Up to 25% of infants with X-linked ichthyosis will have concurrent deletions of adjacent genes on the X-chromosome leading to associated syndromes (contiguous gene syndromes). Therefore, infants should receive a complete physical examination and regular developmental evaluations to monitor for early signs of potentially associated syndromes (Kallmann syndrome, idiopathic familial short stature, X-linked recessive chondrodysplasia punctata, X-linked mental retardation, and ocular albinism).

Therapy

The mainstay of therapy for the skin involves frequent and liberal use of moisturizers, emollients, and humectants. Topical retinoids and keratolytics may be used in localized areas, but patients may find them irritating. Oral retinoids have been used but are associated with possible systemic side effects, especially if used long term. Topical amino acids and α-hydroxy acids have also been reported to be helpful in some cases.

Special Considerations in Infants

X-linked ichthyosis is most commonly diagnosed prenatally due to a low estriol on a maternal triple screen and confirmed by fluorescent in situ hybridization. The first signs of disease in infants are most often fine scaling on the scalp and flanks and abnormal testicular descent, which occur in up to 28% of infants.

Suggested Readings

Fleck CA. Managing ichthyosis: A case study. *Ostomy Wound Manage.* 2006;52(4):82–86, 88, 90, passim.

Shwayder T. Disorders of keratinization: Diagnosis and management. *Am J Clin Dermatol.* 2004;5(1):17–29.

Williams ML, Bruckner A, Nopper A. Generalized disorders of cornification (the ichthyoses) In: Harper J, Oranje A, Prose NS, eds. *Textbook of Pediatric Dermatology.* 2nd Ed. Hoboken, NJ: Wiley-Blackwell; 2006:1304–1358.

Juvenile Plantar Dermatosis

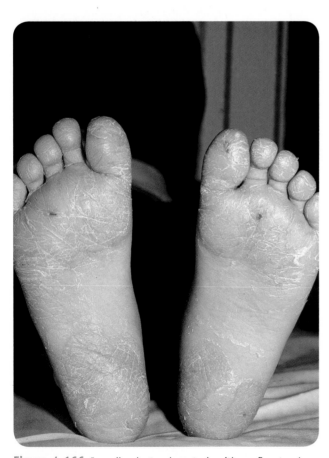

Diagnosis Synopsis

Juvenile plantar dermatosis is a localized scaling and fissuring dermatitis of the plantar surface seen in prepubertal and early teenage children. The condition is more frequently encountered in atopic children. It is thought to be caused by repeated maceration followed by drying, inducing impairment of the superficial epidermis.

Look For

Taut, shiny-appearing plantar skin with accentuation of the skin folds (Figs. 4-166–168). Fissures can be prominent (Fig. 4-169). Although sweating can be marked, the skin feels dry and scaly. Flares are episodic and last 1 to 2 weeks.

Diagnostic Pearls

The great toe, ball of the foot, and heel are most often involved. Interdigital and arch areas are usually spared. Patients often pick at the scale and cause painful wounds.

?? Differential Diagnosis and Pitfalls

- Allergic contact dermatitis to shoes more commonly involves the dorsal surface of the foot.
- Tinea pedis may present similarly but can be easily differentiated by demonstrating fungal elements using a KOH preparation from scale.
- Keratoderma often involves the palms as well, and patients may report a family history of similar findings.
- Psoriasis can also affect the bilateral soles. Additional pertinent skin and nail findings can help make this diagnosis.

✓ Best Tests

This is a clinical diagnosis. Rule out dermatophytosis with a KOH examination of the scale.

▲▲ Management Pearls

Encourage patients to use a different pair of shoes on alternating days to allow the shoes to dry out.

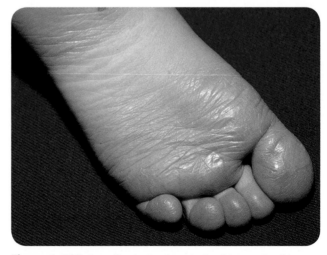

Figure 4-166 Juvenile plantar dermatosis with confluent redness and scaling on pressure areas. Note sparing on the proximal portions of the second, third, fourth, and fifth toes.

Figure 4-167 Juvenile plantar dermatosis with smooth, shiny erythema.

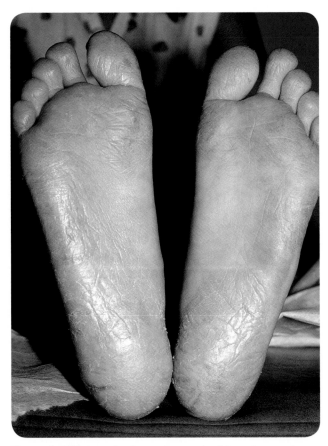

Figure 4-168 Juvenile plantar dermatosis with erythema and sparing on the instep of the foot.

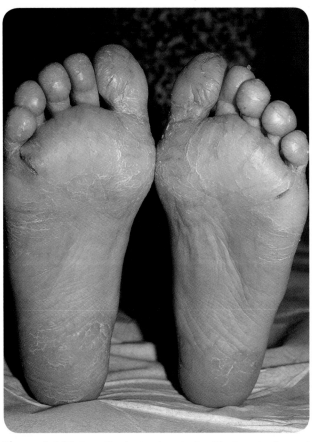

Figure 4-169 Juvenile plantar dermatosis with sharp borders and prominent fissures.

Therapy

Avoid excessive moisture and maceration followed by complete drying. Encourage use of foot powders, thick absorbent or moisture-wicking socks, and absorbent insoles. White petrolatum or urea-containing preparations (Carmol) may be helpful to repair barrier function of the epidermis.

Suggested Readings

Bolognia JL, Jorizzo JL, Rapini RP, eds. *Dermatology*. Vol. 1. 2nd Ed. St Louis, MO: Mosby; 2008:224–225.

Cohen BA, ed. *Pediatric Dermatology*. 3rd Ed. St Louis, MO: Mosby; 2005:85.

James WD, Berger TG, Elston DM, eds. *Andrews' Diseases of the Skin*. 10th Ed. Philadelphia, PA: WB Saunders; 2006:81.

Diagnosis Synopsis

Lichen planus is a pruritic papulosquamous eruption of unknown etiology. Cell-mediated autoimmune reactions, possibly mediated by a drug or virus, may be important in the pathogenesis.

Drugs causing lichen planus-like eruptions (lichenoid drug reactions) include antihypertensives (ACE inhibitors: captopril and enalapril; β-blockers: propranolol and labetalol), thiazide diuretics, antimalarials (quinidine and hydroxychloroquine), penicillamine, NSAIDs, gold, griseofulvin, tetracycline, antiepileptics, and many other drugs. Childhood lichen planus has been described after hepatitis C infection and hepatitis B vaccination.

Lichen planus usually affects the glabrous skin and sometimes the mucosa, scalp, and nails. The frequency of childhood lichen planus varies from 2.1% to 11.2% of all cases of lichen planus.

The majority of children who develop lichen planus develop the classical form. Other variants include actinic, hypertrophic, linear, eruptive, follicular, atrophic, and bullous lesions.

Lichen planus lesions may resolve spontaneously over several months. However, the disease generally has a chronic course with frequent remissions and exacerbations.

Look For

Classical lichen planus—small, flat-topped, polygonal violaceous papules and plaques on the flexural surface of the wrists, legs, and lower back (bilaterally symmetrical) (Figs. 4-170–4-172). The surface of the lesions shows the characteristic fine, linear white lines known as Wickham striae. Koebnerization, linear in a linear configuration, from scratching or trauma, is uncommon.

Actinic lichen planus—annular plaques with central hyperpigmentation and a raised, well-defined hypopigmented border. Sites include the forehead and extensor forearms and dorsa of hands.

Annular lichen planus—cluster of flat-topped, polygonal violaceous papules in a ringlike pattern with clear or atrophic center. Sites include the lower abdomen, back, and penis.

Lichen planus hypertrophicus—markedly thickened verrucous plaques.

Eruptive (guttate) lichen planus—this is an acute widespread form including numerous classical lichen planus papules on the trunk and extremities.

Lichenoid drug reactions—psoriasiform, eczematous, or a more inflammatory type of lesions, predominantly on the photoexposed areas, which heal with deep residual hyperpigmentation. Skin biopsy shows parakeratosis, and the cellular infiltrate consists of eosinophils and plasma cells.

Mucosal lichen planus is seen in 30% to 39% of children with lichen planus. The typical mucosal lesions are asymptomatic reticulate white papules arranged in a lacelike pattern on the inner cheeks. On the lips, the papules are arranged in an annular pattern. Other types of lesions are plaques, bullous, or ulcerative forms.

Nail changes are seen in up to 15% of the pediatric lichen planus patients, and these include thinning or ridging of the nail plate. The typical nail change of pterygium is sometimes seen.

Follicular lichen planus or lichen planopilaris is primarily a variant of lichen planus involving the hair follicles. Scalp involvement causes scarring alopecia.

Diagnostic Pearls

- Wickham striae, the grayish white streaks on the surface of the lesion, are highly diagnostic of lichen planus.

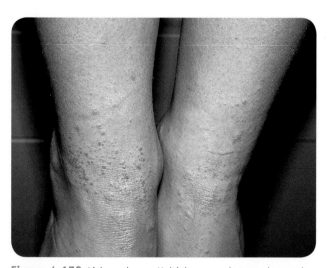

Figure 4-170 Lichen planus. Multiple, somewhat purple papules; the linear group of lesions on the left leg are characteristic.

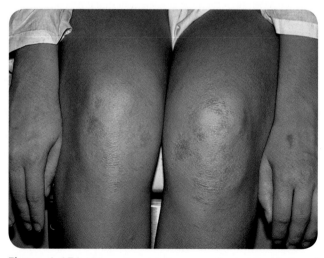

Figure 4-171 Lichen planus lesions are often symmetrical, and lesions may be grouped.

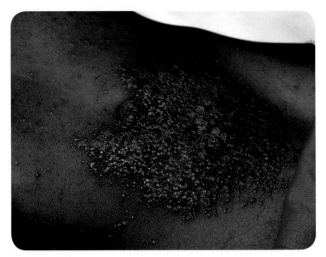

Figure 4-172 Lichen planus with discrete papules at the periphery of a large hyperpigmented group of lesions resembling nickel dermatitis.

- Linear lesions may be present as a result of trauma (Koebner phenomenon) (Fig. 4-173).
- Children with trachyonychia or 20-nail dystrophy may have lichen planus. Nail matrix biopsy is needed to confirm the diagnosis, especially in the absence of skin lesions.
- If you suspect lichen planus on the glabrous skin or nails, carefully examine the oral mucosa for reticular, lacy network papules or plaques.

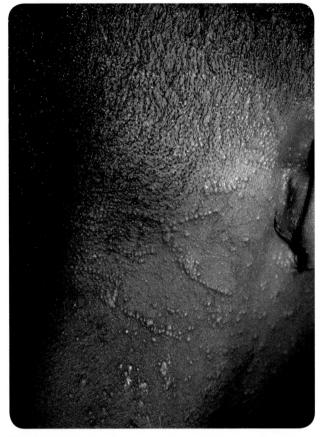

Figure 4-173 Lichen planus with several linear and curvilinear characteristic groups of lesions.

?? Differential Diagnosis and Pitfalls

- Psoriasis—erythematous papules and plaques (on trauma-prone areas such as knees, elbows, and scalp) covered with silvery scale.
- Lichen nitidus—small pinpoint (1 mm) sized (monomorphic), flesh-colored, round or dome-shaped papules in clusters. Common sites include the forearms, trunk, abdomen, and genitalia.
- Lichen striatus—linear arrangement of hypopigmented or hyperpigmented inflammatory lichenoid to eczematous papules on the extremities. No Wickham striae or violaceous hue. Much less pruritus than lichen planus.
- Pityriasis lichenoides chronica—small, oval, pink-brown papules covered with thin scale and crust that resolve with hypopigmentation.
- Granuloma annulare—skin-colored beaded papules in an annular pattern (hands and feet). No surface changes.
- Sarcoidosis—erythematous to violaceous edematous papuloplaques (face, extremities). No surface changes. Associated lymphadenopathy, uveitis, and chest symptoms.

✓ Best Tests

- Skin biopsy will confirm the diagnosis.
- If there are any signs of liver dysfunction, order LFTs and consider a hepatitis antibody panel. In some parts of the world, there is a frequent association of oral and also severe lichen planus with viral hepatitis.

▲▲ Management Pearls

- Children with erosive/ulcerative (skin and mucosal) lichen planus should follow up periodically. In adults, the lesions may evolve into squamous cell carcinoma. No such association is known in children.
- In adults, urolithiasis and diabetes are known to occur in association with lichen planus.
- The scalp should be examined in all children with follicular lichen planus. This may cause irreversible scarring alopecia.

Therapy

For Focal Lesions
- Use high-potency topical steroids
- Fluocinonide 0.05% (Lidex)
- Clobetasol ointment

For Hypertrophic Lesions
- Use Class 1 potent topical steroids (clobetasol propionate 0.05%, halobetasol propionate 0.05%) under occlusion.

Or

- Intralesional triamcinolone: 5 to 10 mg/mL

For Widespread Lesions
- Consider a short course of systemic steroids.
- Prednisolone: 1 mg/kg/day

Other Therapies for Treatment of Lichen Planus
- Topical tacrolimus
- Dapsone, griseofulvin, metronidazole, thalidomide, cyclosporine, PUVA, or narrow band ultraviolet B.

Treatment of Oral Lichen Planus
- Topical steroids (triamcinolone acetonide [0.1%] paste)

Or

- Topical tacrolimus or topical cyclosporine

Or

- Systemic steroids

Suggested Readings

Handa S, Sahoo B. Childhood lichen planus: A study of 87 cases. *Int J Dermatol.* 2002;41(7):423–427.

Luis-Montoya P, Domínguez-Soto L, Vega-Memije E. Lichen planus in 24 children with review of the literature. *Pediatr Dermatol.* 2005;22(4):295–298.

Malhotra AK, Khaitan BK, Sethuraman G, et al. Betamethasone oral minipulse therapy compared with topical triamcinolone acetonide (0.1%) paste in oral lichen planus: A randomized comparative study. *J Am Acad Dermatol.* 2008;58(4):596–602.

Sandhu K, Handa S, Kanwar AJ. Familial lichen planus. *Pediatr Dermatol.* 2003;20(2):186.

Sharma R, Maheshwari V. Childhood lichen planus: A report of fifty cases. *Pediatr Dermatol.* 1999;16(5): 345–348.

Diagnosis Synopsis

Lichen striatus is an uncommon, self-limited skin disorder in younger children of unknown etiology. It has been reported in children as young as 3 months. It presents with linear bands of slightly scaly, pinpoint, and lichenoid papules that follow the lines of Blaschko. Lesions are usually on an extremity; however, lichen striatus can occur anywhere. Lichen striatus is typically asymptomatic.

Look For

Uniform, red, pink, or skin-colored, slightly scaly, pinpoint, flat-topped papules in a curvilinear configuration distributed along the lines of Blaschko (Figs. 4-174–4-177). It is most commonly seen on the extremities, though involvement of the trunk and face may occur. The band of involvement may be one continuous band, or it may be interrupted. Papules and plaques are linear and can involve the entire length of an extremity, including the nail. Involvement of the nail can occur without any other cutaneous involvement. The lesions are often subtle and resolve leaving hypopigmentation or hyperpigmentation.

Diagnostic Pearls

The onset is usually fairly rapid and may reach maximal involvement within a few days to weeks.

?? Differential Diagnosis and Pitfalls

- Linear epidermal nevus
- Linear porokeratosis
- Incontinentia pigmenti
- Linear lichen planus

✓ Best Tests

This is generally a clinical diagnosis. A punch biopsy may be helpful if the diagnosis is in question.

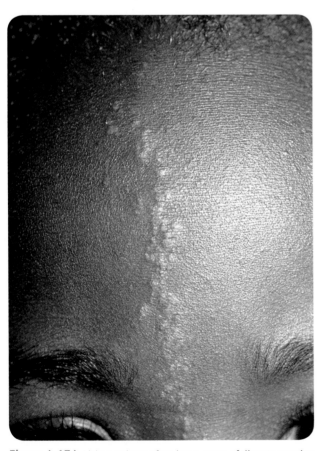

Figure 4-174 Lichen striatus often has a group of discrete papules.

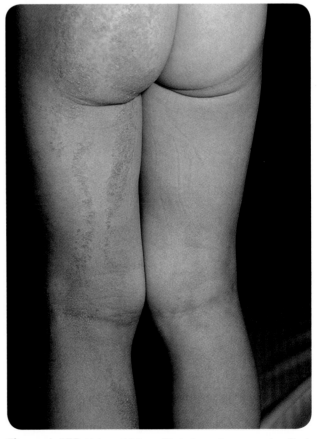

Figure 4-175 Lichen striatus with lesions along an extremity is common.

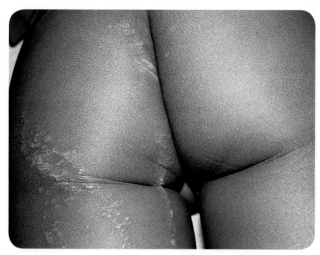

Figure 4-176 Lichen striatus has completely normal skin between the sets of linear lesions.

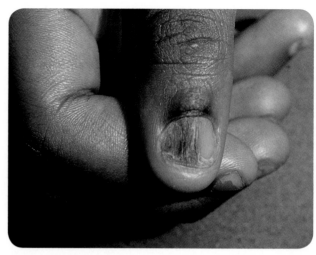

Figure 4-177 Lichen striatus may involve the nail fold and matrix, impairing the growth of the nail plate.

▲▲▲ Management Pearls

The disease is self-limited, so aggressive treatment is not indicated. It typically resolves spontaneously within 1 to 2 years.

Therapy

Midstrength topical corticosteroids may hasten resolution and can be helpful if pruritus is present.

Suggested Readings

Tilly JJ, Drolet BA, Esterly NB. Lichenoid eruptions in children. *J Am Acad Dermatol.* 2004;51(4):606–624.

■ Diagnosis Synopsis

Neonatal lupus erythematosus is an autoimmune disorder of the newborn caused by maternal autoantibodies. Anti-SSA/Ro, anti-SSB/La, and anti-U1RNP antibodies can be found in both the fetal and maternal circulation. The main concern in patients with neonatal lupus is congenital heart block, which is irreversible in almost all cases. Elevated liver enzymes, thrombocytopenia, anemia, and neutropenia may also be seen. These will resolve as the maternal antibodies are cleared, usually between the ages of 6 and 8 months.

◉ Look For

At birth of shortly thereafter, erythematous scaly plaques in a periorbital or forehead distribution, though they may appear anywhere (Figs. 4-178–4-181). These lesions are present at birth in two thirds of the patients; the remainder of the time they appear by the age of 5 months. Lesions generally heal within a year and may be associated with telangiectasia and atrophy.

Diagnostic Pearls

Look for periorbital plaques that seem to worsen with the infant's first sun exposure.

?? Differential Diagnosis and Pitfalls

- Seborrheic dermatitis
- Bloom syndrome
- Rothmund–Thompson syndrome
- Congenital rubella
- Congenital syphilis

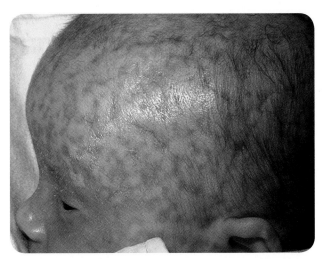

Figure 4-178 Neonatal lupus erythematosus with multiple areas of atrophy on the scalp.

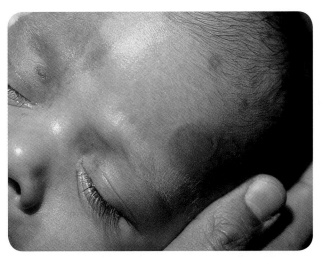

Figure 4-179 Neonatal lupus erythematosus with multiple scaly plaques.

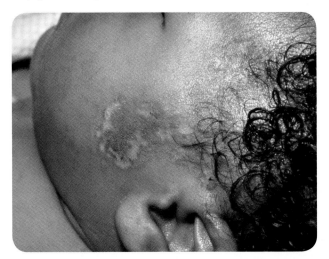

Figure 4-180 Neonatal lupus erythematosus with polyarcuate borders and hyperpigmentation.

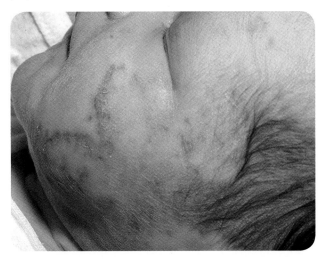

Figure 4-181 Neonatal lupus erythematosus with large arcuate areas and erosions.

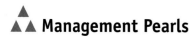

Best Tests

- Maternal and patient serum should be checked for ANA, anti-SSA/Ro, anti-SSB/La, and anti-U1RNP antibodies.
- A complete blood count with differential and liver function tests should be checked. An electrocardiogram and echocardiogram should also be checked on the patient.
- Skin biopsy is usually unnecessary but will demonstrate histologic features of lupus.

▲▲▲ Management Pearls

Pediatric cardiology should be consulted as soon as neonatal lupus is suspected. Congenital heart block can occur in approximately 20% of siblings born subsequent to a patient with congenital heart block.

Therapy

Avoid sun exposure and use sunscreen if exposed. Midpotency topical corticosteroids may be helpful for the skin rash. No other treatment is required, as the skin lesions will resolve by the age of 6 to 8 months.

Suggested Readings

Izmirly PM, Rivera TL, Buyon JP. Neonatal lupus syndromes. *Rheum Dis Clin North Am.* 2007;33(2):267–285, vi.

◼◼ Diagnosis Synopsis

Pityriasis lichenoides et varioliformis acuta (PLEVA), or Mucha–Habermann disease, is an idiopathic cutaneous disease within the spectrum of diseases known as pityriasis lichenoides. It is clinically characterized by recurrent crops of papules that become necrotic and then heal with pigmentary change or minor scarring. Febrile ulceronecrotic Mucha–Habermann disease and pityriasis lichenoides chronica are the other entities within the pityriasis lichenoides group. They are characterized by large coalescent, ulcerative lesions with systemic symptoms or an indolent course with lesions that resolve without necrosis, respectively. PLEVA has a peak onset at ages 5 and 10 years and may last weeks to years before spontaneously resolving. Although generally considered a benign disease, rare case reports have documented possible transformation to T-cell lymphomas.

◉ Look For

Crops of 2 to 10 mm macules that rapidly evolve into scaly papules (Figs. 4-182–4-185). The centers of the papules become vesicular, pustular, and then necrotic with an overlying red-to-brown hemorrhagic crust. Due to successive crops, lesions are in different stages of evolution, usually localized to the trunk, proximal extremities, and flexural surfaces. Lesions may be asymptomatic or mildly pruritic. Fever and malaise are rarely present.

●● Diagnostic Pearls

In darker-skinned individuals, look for numerous regularly sized, oval, hypopigmented macules of postinflammatory hypopigmentation.

?? Differential Diagnosis and Pitfalls

- Nodules, plaques, tumors, severe pain, and severe systemic symptoms do not occur in PLEVA, and their presence should strongly suggest alternate diagnoses.
- Guttate psoriasis presents as widespread, monomorphic, well-defined erythematous plaques with overlying silvery scale. A preceding history of streptococcal infection is frequently elicited.
- Lymphomatoid papulosis may be difficult to distinguish clinically. The presence of CD30+ cells within the inflammatory infiltrate helps establish this diagnosis.
- Cutaneous T-cell lymphoma is rare in children and tends to present with larger atrophic patches and plaques.
- Cutaneous small vessel vasculitis presents with palpable purpura, most frequently on the lower extremities.
- History as well as viral culture and/or Varicella Zoster Virus PCR may be necessary to exclude the possibility of varicella.
- Insect bites most frequently present as pruritic papules involving the ankles and distal lower extremities.
- Gianotti–Crosti syndrome presents as symmetrically distributed monomorphous, pink-brown, flat-topped papules or papulovesicles on the face, extensor limbs, and buttocks.

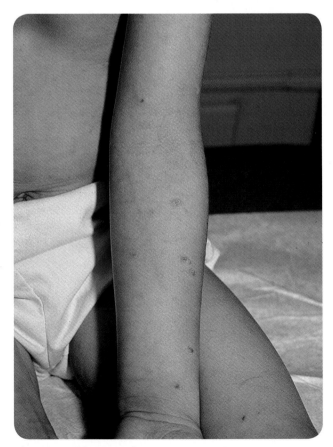

Figure 4-182 Pityriasis lichenoides et varioliformis acuta with characteristic scattered lesions.

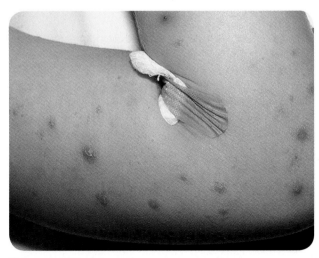

Figure 4-183 Pityriasis lichenoides et varioliformis acuta with red papules and some pustules.

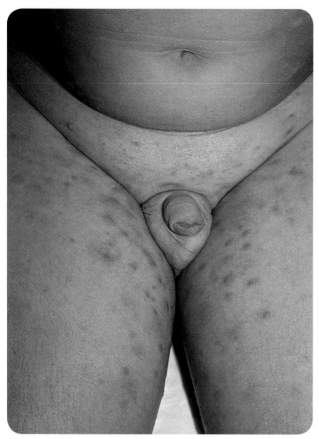

Figure 4-184 Pityriasis lichenoides et varioliformis acuta with inflammatory papules and vesicles in several stages of development.

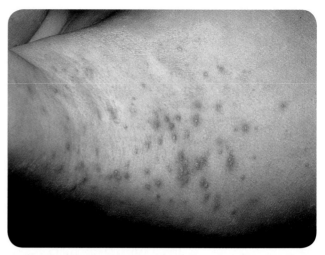

Figure 4-185 Pityriasis lichenoides et varioliformis acuta with many pustules on an inflammatory base.

▲▲ Management Pearls

- The condition is often self-limited and often resolves over a period of weeks to months.
- Phototherapy will improve the postinflammatory hypopigmentation.

Therapy

Unfortunately, treatment options are based on small case series, case reports, or anecdotal evidence. For persistent cases, treatment options include the following:

– Azithromycin 10 mg/kg up to 500 mg on day 1, then 5 mg/kg up to 250 mg daily to complete a 5-day course, given bimonthly until resolution.
– Erythromycin 40 mg/kg/day until resolution.
– Tetracycline 500 mg has been reported to be of value. However, its restriction to children aged 8 and older is a significant limitation.
– Narrowband UVB, two to three times per week until resolution.
– Prednisone 1 mg/kg/day may be considered for severe disease.

- A careful history is helpful in differentiating PLEVA from a drug eruption.
- The primary lesion observed in cases of folliculitis is a pustule. The pathogenic organism can be cultured from lesions.
- Erythema multiforme presents with predominantly acrally located target lesions. Patients often show evidence of coexisting herpes orolabialis.
- Patients with dermatitis herpetiformis may also present with crusted erythematous papules and vesicles. Areas of greatest involvement include the extensor forearms, elbows, knees, and buttocks. Histopathology and immunofluorescence are helpful in establishing this diagnosis.

✓ Best Tests

Skin biopsy reveals a lymphocytic infiltrate with disruption of the dermoepidermal junction and epidermal changes. Atypical cells and vasculitic changes are rare to absent.

Suggested Readings

Bolognia JL, Jorizzo JL, Rapini RP, eds. *Dermatology*. Vol. 1. 2nd Ed. St Louis, MO: Mosby; 2008:323, 1206.

Bowers S, Warshaw EM. Pityriasis lichenoides and its subtypes. *J Am Acad Dermatol*. 2006;55(4):557–572.

Cohen BA, ed. *Pediatric Dermatology*. 3rd Ed. St Louis, MO: Mosby; 2005:88–89.

James WD, Berger TG, Elston DM, eds. *Andrews' Diseases of the Skin*. 10th Ed. Philadelphia, PA: WB Saunders; 2006:736–737.

Pityriasis Rosea

■ Diagnosis Synopsis

Pityriasis rosea (PR) is a common, mildly inflammatory, papulosquamous eruption that mostly affects the trunk and proximal extremities. While human herpes virus types 6 and 7 have been implicated, the etiology remains unknown. The eruption is self-limited, typically lasting 4 to 16 weeks, and is often nonpruritic. PR is most common in adolescents, occurring most frequently during the spring and autumn months.

● Look For

Macules in an oval or circular pattern with an associated fine, central scale (Figs. 4-186–4-189). The condition usually begins with one larger truncal plaque (herald patch) and then new patches and plaques form in a "Christmas-tree"

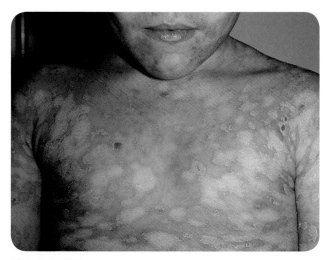

Figure 4-186 PR with polycyclic discrete and confluent scaling on trunk and face.

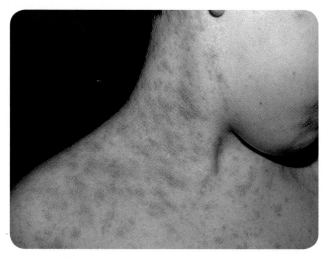

Figure 4-187 PR with salmon-colored papules on chest and neck.

distribution (i.e., following the skin cleavage lines) on the trunk. Although lesions almost never occur on the face, hands, or feet in adults, facial lesions—particularly on the forehead—are not infrequent in children. Oral buccal erosions may occur, and the scalp may be involved during early childhood. Rarely, lesions may be concentrated in the axillae and groin (the inverse form of PR).

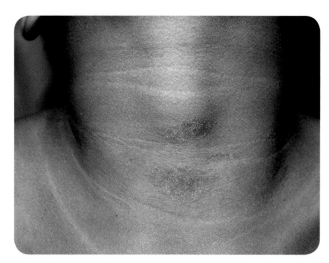

Figure 4-188 PR with oval hyperpigmented lesions roughly following skin tension lines.

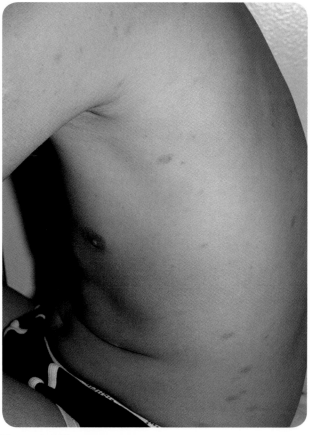

Figure 4-189 PR with small oval truncal lesions.

Other variants include vesicular, papular, pustular, and urticarial forms.

Significant postinflammatory hyperpigmentation can occur in pigmented skin.

Diagnostic Pearls

Patients will usually give a history of an asymptomatic macule that appeared before the rest of the lesions (the herald patch).

Differential Diagnosis and Pitfalls

- Tinea corporis
- Tinea versicolor
- Psoriasis
- Parapsoriasis
- Secondary syphilis

Best Tests

Diagnosis is usually made on clinical grounds. A biopsy is rarely indicated. A KOH should be performed to rule out tinea.

Management Pearls

Pityriasis is self-limited, and patient education is important because the eruption often results in a general health concern due to the widespread nature of the process.

Therapy

No treatment is necessary as the condition is self-limited. If pruritus is present, topical corticosteroids and oral antihistamines may be used.

Other treatments that have been successful in some reports include a 2-week course of oral macrolides or narrowband UVB.

Suggested Reading

Stulberg DL, Wolfrey J. Pityriasis rosea. *Am Fam Physician*. 2004;69(1): 87–91.

Psoriasis

■■ Diagnosis Synopsis

Psoriasis is a chronic skin disease marked by hyperproliferation of epidermal cells and inflammation that results in thickened, scaly, erythematous plaques. The cause of psoriasis is incompletely understood and appears to be multifactorial, with genetic and environmental components. Psoriasis is fairly common in childhood but rare in infancy. Several clinical patterns exist, and multiple forms may be observed in a single patient. Typical plaque-type psoriasis (psoriasis vulgaris) is discussed here; other forms include guttate psoriasis (which often follows streptococcal pharyngitis), palmar–plantar psoriasis, erythrodermic psoriasis, and pustular psoriasis. Psoriasis can also be strictly limited to the fingernails or to body areas such as the genitals, scalp, feet, or even a solitary fingertip. Psoriasis lesions usually develop slowly but may have a sudden onset. The condition is common and is estimated to affect 1% to 2% of the population, with 20% of cases presenting before 20 years of age. Distribution is worldwide.

Approximately 8% of patients develop psoriatic arthritis. Those with nail involvement seem to be at increased risk for developing this erosive seronegative arthritis that can be a source of considerable morbidity.

◉ Look For

Symmetrically distributed erythematous plaques with overlying silvery (micaceous) scale (Figs. 4-190–4-193). Areas of greatest involvement include the elbows, knees, umbilicus, and scalp. Characteristic nail findings include pitting, oil spots (yellowish-brown discoloration), and distal onycholysis.

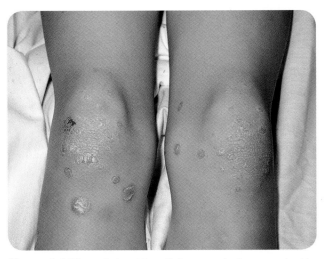

Figure 4-190 Psoriasis with well-demarcated plaques and white scales in a typical location.

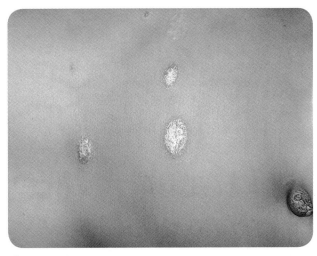

Figure 4-191 Psoriasis with scattered silvery-scaled plaques.

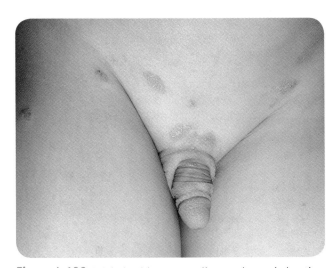

Figure 4-192 Psoriasis with sparse scaling on plaques in locations of skin folds.

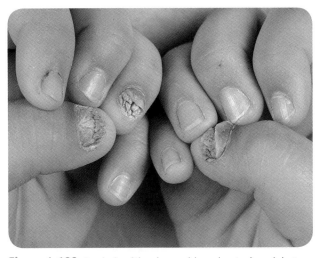

Figure 4-193 Psoriasis with subungual hyperkeratosis and destruction of nail plates.

Diagnostic Pearls

- Removal of scale will result in pinpoint bleeding (Auspitz sign), suggesting the diagnosis. Trauma may induce local plaques of psoriasis (the isomorphic response or Koebnerization). Patients may interpret these lesions as "slow-healing wounds."
- Certain drugs, such as lithium, β-blockers, antimalarials, interferon, and rapid taper of corticosteroids, are known to induce psoriasis.

?? Differential Diagnosis and Pitfalls

- Pityriasis rosea may easily be confused with guttate psoriasis. The presence of a larger herald patch and the orientation of plaques along skin tension lines are a helpful clue to the diagnosis.
- Pityriasis rubra pilaris presents as large coalescing orange-red plaques with prominent foci of uninvolved skin (islands of sparing).
- Mycosis fungoides is rare in children and tends to present with atrophic scaly patches involving sun-protected sites.
- Lichen planus presents with pruritic violaceous papules with overlying white reticulated markings (Wickham striae), most often involving the wrists and ankles.
- While psoriasis usually involves the extensor surfaces of knees and elbows, the lichenified pruritic plaques of chronic atopic dermatitis typically involve the flexor surfaces of the extremities.
- Seborrheic dermatitis is yellowish and greasier, as opposed to the silvery, dry scale of psoriasis. Lesions are also ill-defined, unlike the well-defined plaques of psoriasis.
- Tinea corporis can be easily differentiated from psoriasis by the demonstration of hyphal elements on KOH preparation.

✓ Best Tests

The diagnosis is a clinical one. If in doubt, however, a skin biopsy can be helpful.

Management Pearls

- Psoriasis may be triggered by streptococcal infection in susceptible individuals.
- Ultraviolet light is one of the best therapies to treat extensive or widespread disease. Consider UVB three times weekly or recommend natural sun exposure if possible. As excess UV exposure can result in sunburn and potentially elicit an isomorphic response, patients must be carefully counseled if this treatment is recommended.

Therapy

Topical corticosteroids remain the mainstay in the treatment of psoriasis. Patients should be counseled on their proper use and followed for signs of skin atrophy and striae formation.

Localized Disease (Topical Treatments)
Midpotency topical corticosteroids (Classes 3 and 4) need supervision with scheduled follow-up to observe for steroid atrophy.

- Triamcinolone, ointment (Kenalog, Aristocort)—apply twice daily (15, 30, 60, 120, and 240 g)
- Mometasone, ointment (Elocon)—apply twice daily (15 and 45 g)
- Fluocinolone, ointment (Synalar)—apply twice daily (15, 30, and 60 g)

High-potency topical corticosteroids (Class 2) should be limited to the thickest plaques and used for short periods of time.

- Fluocinonide, ointment (Lidex)—apply twice daily (15, 30, 60, and 120 g)
- Desoximetasone, ointment (Topicort) 0.25%—apply twice daily (15, 60, and 120 g)
- Halcinonide, ointment (Halog)—apply twice daily (15, 60, and 240 g)
- Amcinonide, ointment (Cyclocort)—apply twice daily (15, 30, and 60 g)

Vitamin D Analog
- Calcipotriol (Dovonex) cream—apply twice daily to affected areas (30, 60, and 100 g tubes) (60 mL scalp solution)

Patients can use these preparations as steroid-sparing agents by rotating therapy with steroid treatment. For example, a patient may use a vitamin D analog twice daily on weekdays and topical steroid ointment on weekends.

Intertriginous and Facial
Use low-potency topical steroids on thinner-skin areas of the face and intertriginous areas.

- Desonide (DesOwen) or Aclovate ointment or cream—twice daily 30 g
- Tacrolimus ointment 0.03% and 0.1% twice daily
- Pimecrolimus 1% cream twice daily

Tar-based Therapy
- 10% liquor carbonis detergens in Aquaphor ointment—apply daily, compound 440 g jar of Aquaphor

- Anthralin (Drithocreme) 0.1%, 0.25%, and 0.5% creams—begin with lowest strength and apply short contact (e.g., 10 min); advance as tolerated
- Tar bath oils, Balnetar 2.5% coal tar, (240 mL), Zetar (180 mL), and Doak oil (240 mL)

Scalp Therapy

Thick, scaly plaques within the scalp can be a difficult management problem. Consider loosening scale with an oil-based treatment such as Baker P&S applied nightly (120 mL) or treating with Derma-Smoothe F/S applied nightly (fluocinolone in peanut oil) supplied 120 mL. Have patient shampoo with tar-based shampoos such as Neutrogena T/Gel.

Tazarotene gel (0.05% or 0.1%) applied to lesions nightly may be better tolerated when used with a topical corticosteroid.

Systemic Therapy

Phototherapy can be an excellent treatment option for patients with extensive cutaneous involvement. Narrowband UVB (311 to 313 nm) is now considered the most optimal form of phototherapy for these patients.

Methotrexate, cyclosporin, acitretin, and newer biologic agents such as etanercept, alefacept, infliximab, and adalimumab are effective treatment options for patients with severe extensive disease. As these agents have multiple, acute, chronic, and potentially severe side effects such as lymphoma, referral to a dermatologist or other provider skilled in the use of these agents is indicated for management with these systemic agents.

Suggested Readings

Bolognia JL, Jorizzo JL, Rapini RP, eds. *Dermatology*. Vol. 1. 2nd Ed. St Louis, MO: Mosby; 2008:115–135.

Cohen BA, ed. *Pediatric Dermatology*. 3rd Ed. St Louis, MO: Mosby; 2005:67–70.

James WD, Berger TG, Elston DM, eds. *Andrews' Diseases of the Skin*. 10th Ed. Philadelphia, PA: WB Saunders; 2006:193–202.

Paller AS, Siegried EC, Langley RG, et al. Etanercept treatment for children and adolescents with plaque psoriasis. *N Engl J Med*. 2008;358(3):241–251.

Psoriasis, Guttate

Diagnosis Synopsis

Guttate psoriasis is a particular variant of psoriasis that typically follows an acute streptococcal infection. It is characterized by an abrupt papulosquamous eruption arising in children and young adults. The prognosis in children is typically better than in adults, with many children spontaneously clearing within several weeks to months. Nevertheless, most patients will go on to develop chronic psoriatic disease several years later.

Look For

Hundreds of small (2 mm to 1 cm), droplike (guttate), scaly papules and plaques concentrated on the trunk (Figs. 4-194–4-197).

Diagnostic Pearls

Streptococcal pharyngitis is the most common preceding infection in the older child. In young children, consider perianal streptococcal infection as a potential trigger.

?? Differential Diagnosis and Pitfalls

- Patients with pityriasis rosea also present with multiple truncal scaly plaques, often with a history of preceding respiratory illness. Plaques in patients with pityriasis rosea, however, are typically thinner and oriented along skin tension lines.
- Dermatophytosis may be easily distinguished from guttate psoriasis by demonstrating hyphal elements on a KOH preparation.

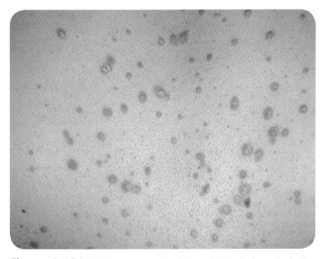

Figure 4-194 Guttate psoriasis with multiple lesions including many small drop-size lesions.

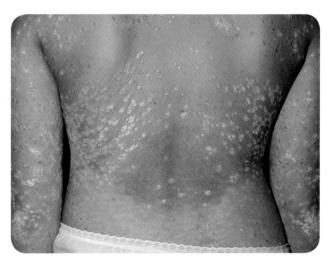

Figure 4-195 Guttate psoriasis with some small lesions and larger plaques.

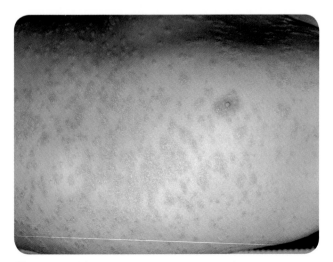

Figure 4-196 Guttate psoriasis with multiple lesions with little scale.

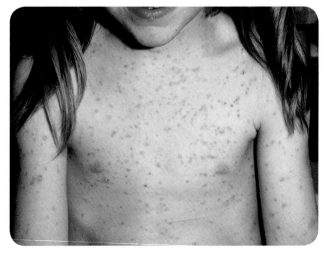

Figure 4-197 Guttate psoriasis with multiple small lesions in the same stage of development.

- The plaques of atopic dermatitis are pruritic, lichenified, and typically distributed over the popliteal fossae, antecubital fossae, and posterior neck.
- Pityriasis lichenoides et varioliformis acuta presents with recurrent crops of crusted, vesicular, or pustular lesions.
- The erythema in plaques of small plaque parapsoriasis is typically less intense than that of guttate psoriasis. This condition is more frequently encountered in adults.

✓ Best Tests

- The diagnosis is typically a clinical one. A skin biopsy may be performed if the diagnosis is in question.
- Throat culture, perianal culture, and ASO titer may be performed to document streptococcal infection.

▲▲ Management Pearls

Early treatment of cutaneous lesions can lessen the severity of each episode. In some cases, treatment of the underlying infection results in clearing of the psoriasis. This observation has prompted many clinicians to empirically treat for potential underlying streptococcal infection in patients presenting with guttate psoriasis. Long-term therapy with antibiotics has not been shown to improve chronic psoriasis.

Therapy

If cultures are positive, treat the underlying streptococcal infection with penicillin, cephalosporin, or erythromycin for at least 10 days.

Limited disease can be treated with topical midpotency corticosteroids (Classes 3 and 4):

- Triamcinolone cream, ointment (Kenalog, Aristocort)—apply twice daily (15, 30, 60, 120, and 240 g)

- Mometasone cream, ointment (Elocon)—apply twice daily (15 and 45 g)
- Fluocinolone ointment, (Synalar)—apply twice daily (15, 30, and 60 g)

Use low-potency topical steroids on the face and intertriginous areas:

- Desonide (DesOwen) or Aclovate ointment or cream 30 g twice daily

Treatment with topical steroids in patients with guttate psoriasis is often impractical due to the extent of cutaneous involvement. Narrowband UVB is an excellent option if the patient has easy local access to this treatment.

Use of systemic agents such as methotrexate, acitretin, cyclosporin, or newer biologic agents should be reserved for patients with severe, treatment-resistant disease under the care of a dermatologist familiar with their use.

Suggested Readings

Bolognia JL, Jorizzo JL, Rapini RP, eds. *Dermatology*. Vol. 1. 2nd Ed. St Louis, MO: Mosby; 2008:118–119.

Cohen BA, ed. *Pediatric Dermatology*. 3rd Ed. St Louis, MO: Mosby; 2005:67–70.

James WD, Berger TG, Elston DM, eds. *Andrews' Diseases of the Skin*. 10th Ed. Philadelphia, PA: WB Saunders; 2006:194.

Nanda A, Kaur S, Kaur I, et al. Childhood psoriasis: An epidemiologic survey of 112 patients. *Pediatr Dermatol*. 1990;7(1):19–21.

Wilson JK, Al-Suwaidan SN, Krowchuk D, et al. Treatment of psoriasis in children: Is there a role for antibiotic therapy and tonsillectomy? *Pediatr Dermatol*. 2003;20:11–15.

■ Diagnosis Synopsis

Psoriasis is a chronic inflammatory skin disease that is seen in <1% of infants by 1 year of age and 2% of infants by age 2. Infantile psoriasis resembles adult psoriasis with discrete oval, erythematous plaques with white scale often involving the trunk, extremities, and face. There is usually less white scale on the plaques in infants as compared to adults. Lesions may be pruritic. The disease process results in hyperproliferation of epidermal cells causing thickened, often scaly skin. Lesions usually develop slowly but may have a sudden onset. Psoriasis in infancy typically involves the diaper area and face. Nail findings of pitting, onycholysis, oil spots, and subungual hyperkeratosis are present in 10% of affected infants.

◉ Look For

Red, or salmon-red, plaques often with silvery-white or grayish-white scale (Figs. 4-198–4-201). The plaques are usually symmetrical and well demarcated. In infants, the diaper area will often have bright red plaques with no scale. The scalp, palms, and soles may have diffuse erythema and scale.

●● Diagnostic Pearls

- Areas of increased friction in diaper area (e.g., under elastic bands) is involved first with subsequent spread to the face, trunk, and body folds. Infantile psoriasis is rarely generalized.
- There is often a strong family history of psoriasis.
- Infantile psoriasis is rarely pruritic.

?? Differential Diagnosis and Pitfalls

- Occasionally, it is impossible to distinguish between alternative diagnoses, and one must follow the patient clinically for more specific signs to develop.
- Seborrheic dermatitis—favors intertriginous areas and has a greasy rather than dry, flaky scale.
- Atopic dermatitis—usually spares the diaper area and more commonly affects the shins and forearms.
- Cutaneous candidiasis—responds to antifungal therapy, has satellite pustules, and pseudohyphae using KOH preparation.
- Acrodermatitis enteropathica—initially vesicular or bullous; periorificial and acral preference; often associated with diarrhea, alopecia, and failure to thrive.
- Irritant diaper dermatitis—spares skin folds and limited to diaper area.

✔ Best Tests

A skin biopsy may help to differentiate psoriasis from seborrheic dermatitis, but because the treatment is similar, empiric therapy is reasonable before biopsy. KOH preparation may help distinguish from *Candida*.

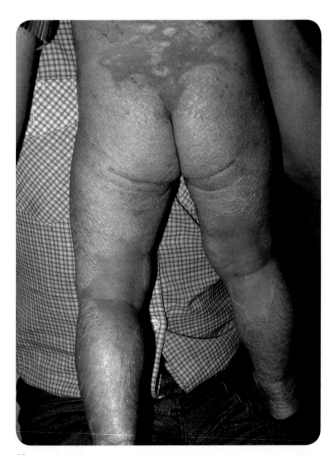

Figure 4-198 Infantile psoriasis in an 18 month old with confluent affected areas.

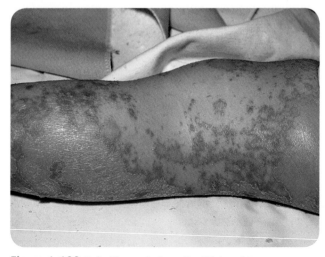

Figure 4-199 Infantile psoriasis on the thigh and leg.

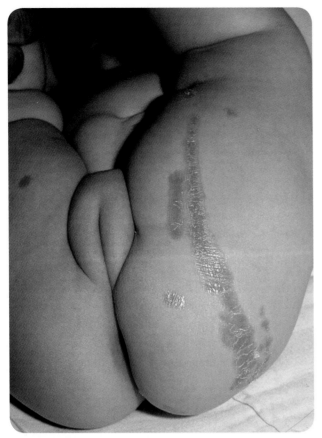

Figure 4-200 Infantile psoriasis with linear buttock lesions.

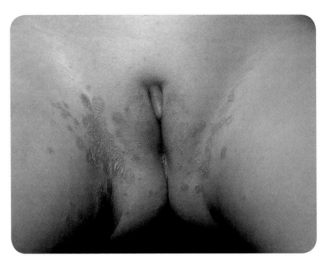

Figure 4-201 Infantile psoriasis with plaques with some white scale.

▲▲ Management Pearls

Barrier creams such as zinc oxide ointment may be used in the diaper area to reduce irritation and Koebnerization. Infantile psoriasis usually responds well to minimal topical therapy.

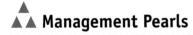

Diaper Area

Low-potency topical corticosteroids (Class 6 or 7) and emollient creams are often effective in this site. Careful monitoring for signs of cutaneous atrophy is imperative.

While useful in older patients, the topical calcineurin inhibitors tacrolimus and pimecrolimus are not approved for use in patients aged younger than 2 years.

Topical Treatment for Body Plaque Psoriasis

Applying low- to mid-potency topical steroids (Classes 4 to 6) twice daily to involved areas is usually sufficient treatment.

Scalp Therapy

Thick, scaly plaques within the scalp can be a difficult management problem. Consider loosening scale with an oil-based treatment, such as Baker P&S applied nightly (120 mL), or mineral oil. Have parents shampoo the child with selenium-based shampoos such as Selsun or Sebulex.

Suggested Readings

Bolognia JL, Jorizzo JL, Rapini RP, eds. *Dermatology*. Vol. 1. 2nd Ed. St Louis, MO: Mosby; 2008:115–135.

Cohen BA, ed. *Pediatric Dermatology*. 3rd Ed. St Louis, MO: Mosby; 2005:67–70.

James WD, Berger TG, Elston DM, eds. *Andrews' Diseases of the Skin*. 10th Ed. Philadelphia, PA: WB Saunders; 2006:193–202.

▉▉ Diagnosis Synopsis

Scabies is an ectoparasitic infestation caused by the mite *Sarcoptes scabiei* variety *hominis*. Scabies is most common in young children, and the highest prevalence is seen in children aged younger than 2 years. Scabies is transmitted by direct skin-to-skin contact and very rarely by indirect route through infected bedding, clothing, or other fomites. The average number of adult female mites in an infested individual is 10 to 15.

Scabies affects all ethnic groups and socioeconomic levels. Frequent outbreaks are common in kindergarten schools, nursing homes, and orphanages. The predisposing factors are overcrowding, poverty, poor nutrition, poor hygiene, and homelessness.

Symptoms typically develop approximately 3 weeks after primary infestation. The primary symptom of scabies is pruritus. Pruritus is a hallmark of scabies, and a variety of primary and secondary skin lesions occur. Scabies infection may be complicated by id reactions and secondary bacterial infections with both *Streptococcus* and *Staphylococcus*.

◉ Look For

Specific Skin Lesion

- Burrows—Seen in the superficial epidermis, the lesions consist of short, linear, whitish lesions with a tiny black dot at one end, which represents the location of the mite. Common locations include the web spaces of the hands, flexor aspect of the wrists, axillae, umbilicus, nipples, buttocks, and penis.
- Scabies nodules—Severe pruritic, reddish-brown nodules 2 to 20 mm in size, seen in the axillae, male genitalia, buttock, and groin (Fig. 4-202). These lesions represent delayed hypersensitivity reaction to the mites.

Other Nonspecific Primary Lesions

Papules, vesicles, and pustules in the finger web spaces, wrists, elbows, axillae, groin, and genitalia (Figs. 4-203–4-205).

Nonspecific Secondary Lesions

Excoriation, eczematization, and impetiginization.

●● Diagnostic Pearls

- Burrows, nodules, and vesiculopustules in the typical location associated with severe nocturnal itching.
- Similar skin lesions and/or itching in the family or contacts.

?? Differential Diagnosis and Pitfalls

- Papular urticaria—A hypersensitivity reaction to a variety of bites, such as mosquitoes, fleas, bedbugs, and mites.

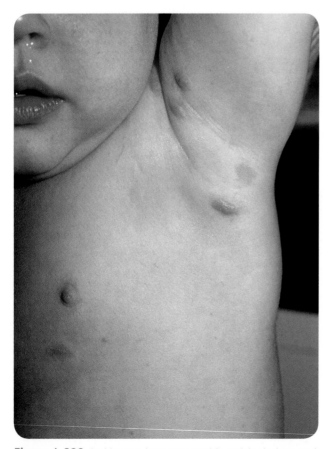

Figure 4-202 Scabies can have very pruritic nodular lesions, such as the one in the axilla.

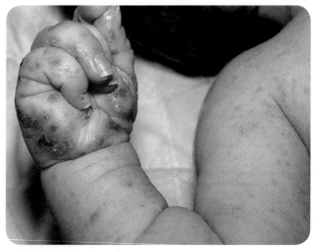

Figure 4-203 Scabies may have pus-filled lesions like those at the base of the thumb.

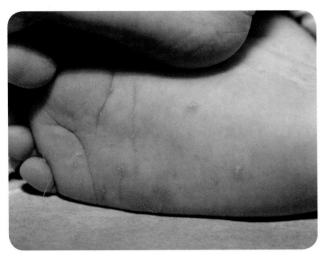

Figure 4-204 Scabies frequently has lesions on the soles and palms.

There may be a seasonal occurrence. Recurrent episodes of excoriated papular and urticarial lesions on the exposed parts of the extremities (extensor aspect) are the cardinal features. Absence of burrows and family history of itching differentiate this from scabies.

- Atopic dermatitis—Eczematous lesions with oozing on the face and flexural areas (cubital and popliteal fossa). Lichenification is seen in chronic dermatitis. Burrows are absent, and lesions are not seen in the web spaces.
- Impetigo—Erythematous vesiculopustular lesions that rupture, forming the pathognomonic honey-colored crust. Lesions may involve the face, neck, and extremities.
- Other differential diagnoses include Langerhans cell histiocytosis, insect bites, tinea corporis, dermatitis herpetiformis, eczema herpeticum, pityriasis rosea, and viral exanthems.

✓ Best Tests

- Skin scraping—Apply a drop of mineral oil to the lesion, preferably at the terminal black end of the burrow, and using a no. 15 blade, scrape through the lesion. Smear the contents of the scrapping on a glass slide, apply mineral oil on the smear, and place a cover slip. Look for mites, eggs (ova), and feces (scybala).
- Dermatoscopy may also identify the mite at the end of a burrow.

▲▲ Management Pearls

- Treat the entire family and close contacts even if they are asymptomatic. Clothing and bedding should be

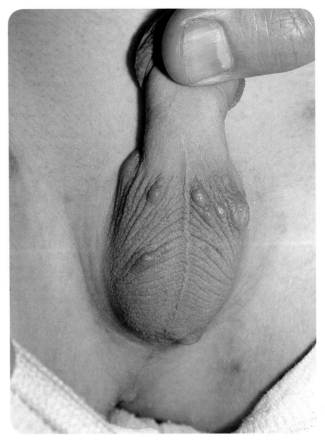

Figure 4-205 Scabies with papulonodular lesions on genitals is not uncommon.

washed in hot water, dry cleaned, or not used for a week.
- Treat the secondary infection.

Therapy

- Permethrin 5% cream is the treatment of choice. Apply to entire body at night, except around the mouth and eyes, and rinse off in the morning. Reapply in 7 days.
- Ivermectin 200 µg/kg, two doses given 1 to 2 weeks apart.
- Lindane 1% cream or lotion—apply from the neck down and rinse off after 8 h.
- Crotamiton 10% cream—apply from neck down for 2 consecutive days and rinse off 48 h after last application.
- Other medications include benzyl benzoate, allethrin, and precipitated sulfur.
- Scabies nodules resolve spontaneously over weeks to months but may be treated with topical or intralesional steroids to speed resolution.
- Antihistamine to relieve pruritus.

Special Considerations in Infants

Scabies is transmitted to the newborn or infant via direct skin-to-skin contact and rarely by fomites. In young infants who have not developed a coordinated itch response, pruritus may manifest as rubbing the head against a caregiver, irritability, insomnia, or poor feeding. In neonates and infants, scabies usually affects the head, face, axillae, diaper area, palms, and soles. The characteristic lesions are erythematous papules, vesiculopustules, and nodules. Burrows are uncommon, owing to secondary impetiginization or eczematization. Scabies should be considered in infants with vesiculopustules on the face, axillae, palms, and soles. Permethrin 5% cream is the treatment of choice. It has been approved for use in infants aged 2 months or older. For infants aged younger than 2 months, apply 6% sulfur ointment for 3 consecutive days. Rinse off 24 h after last application.

Suggested Readings

Chosidow O. Clinical practice. Scabies. *N Engl J Med*. 2006;354(16): 1718–1727.

Hengge UR, Currie BJ, Jäger G, et al. Scabies: A ubiquitous neglected skin disease. *Lancet Infect Dis*. 2006;6(12):769–779.

Malhotra AK, Sethuraman G, Das AK, et al. Scleredema following scabies infestation. *Pediatr Dermatol*. 2008;25:136–138.

Wagner A. Distinguishing vesicular and pustular disorders in the neonate. *Curr Opin Pediatr*. 1997;9(4):396–405.

Tinea Corporis

Diagnosis Synopsis

Tinea corporis is a localized inflammatory skin condition due to fungal colonization of the superficial epidermis. The most commonly implicated species is *Trichophyton*. Fungal organisms are transmitted to children by direct contact with those infected or through fomites. Majocchi granuloma is caused by organisms invading the hair follicle or shaft on nonscalp skin.

Look For

Circular or annular, red, scaly plaques anywhere on the body (Figs. 4-206–4-209). The entire advancing edge of the plaque usually has prominent scale with associated fungal hyphae. Vesicles may also be seen at the periphery of the plaque. The central clearing leads to the appearance of annular shape and thus, the description "ringworm."

Diagnostic Pearls

- Tinea corporis should be within the differential in any patient who presents with a pruritic, scaly plaque. The plaques may be very large.
- If the patient has been treated with a topical steroid, scale and inflammation may be absent (tinea incognito).
- The centers of the lesions are hyperpigmented more often than other dermatoses (pityriasis rosea and nummular dermatitis).

Differential Diagnosis and Pitfalls

- Psoriasis
- Granuloma annulare
- Nummular dermatitis
- Pityriasis rosea
- Erythema annulare centrifugum

Best Tests

A KOH should be performed in all patients in whom tinea is suspected. If Majocchi granuloma is suspected, a biopsy may be necessary.

Management Pearls

Topical steroids should be avoided because they have the potential to worsen the infection.

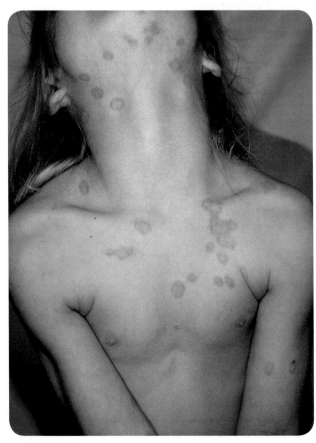

Figure 4-206 Tinea corporis with multiple scaly annular plaques.

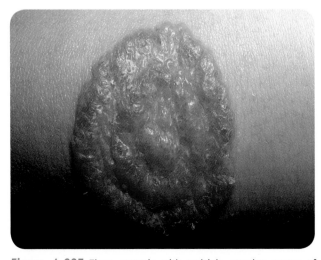

Figure 4-207 Tinea corporis with multiple annular groups of pustules.

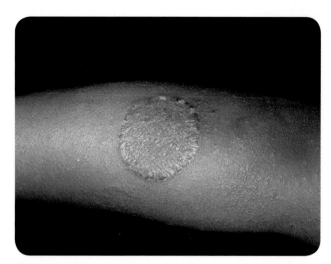

Figure 4-208 Tinea corporis with prominent border with multiple scaly papules.

Therapy

Most cases can be treated with topical antifungal creams. Twice daily application for 2 to 4 weeks is usually sufficient. Patients should be instructed to apply the cream to the lesion as well as a 2 cm area surrounding it for 1 to 2 weeks after clinical resolution.

For more extensive involvement or Majocchi granuloma, oral griseofulvin or terbinafine can be used. Griseofulvin is dosed at 20 mg/kg/day for 4 to 6 weeks; terbinafine is dosed at 6 mg/kg/day for 2 weeks.

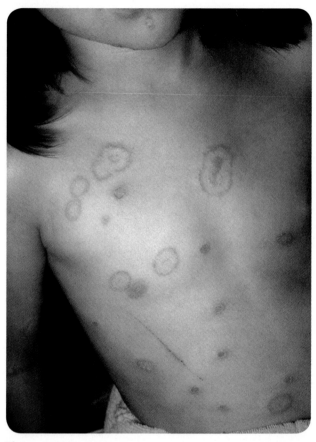

Figure 4-209 Tinea corporis with multiple lesions with red annular rims.

Suggested Readings

Gilaberte Y, Rezusta A, Gil J, et al. Tinea capitis in infants in their first year of life. *Br J Dermatol*. 2004;151(4):886–890.

Möhrenschlager M, Seidl HP, Ring J, et al. Pediatric tinea capitis: Recognition and management. *Am J Clin Dermatol*. 2005;6(4):203–213.

Sethi A, Antaya R. Systemic antifungal therapy for cutaneous infections in children. *Pediatr Infect Dis J*. 2006;25(7):643–644.

Tinea Pedis (Athlete's Foot)

◼◼ Diagnosis Synopsis

Tinea pedis (athlete's foot) is a localized inflammatory condition due to a fungal infection. It is more common in adolescents than in younger children. The infection causes dry scale on the feet, maceration between the toes, and, in some cases, destruction of the nail plate (onychomycosis). Factors leading to this infection include high levels of humidity; occlusive footwear; and the use of communal pools, showers, or baths (locker rooms).

◉ Look For

Four types of tinea pedis have been described: chronic intertriginous, chronic hyperkeratotic (Figs. 4-210 and 4-211), vesiculobullous (Fig. 4-212), and acute ulcerative. Chronic intertriginous is the most common type and presents with erythema and scale of the web spaces. Bacterial coinfection can lead to maceration (Fig. 4-213). The hyperkeratotic form involves erythema and scale on the plantar surface; the dorsum of the foot is not involved. Involvement of one hand may also be seen with this form, leading to two feet-one hand syndrome.

Acute ulcerative and vesiculobullous types are rarely seen in children.

●● Diagnostic Pearls

- Intertriginous tinea pedis often involves the third and fourth web spaces of the foot, unlike atopic dermatitis, which favors the first and second web spaces.
- Evaluation of toenails may reveal coexistent onychomycosis with thickening, whitening, or onycholysis.
- Tinea pedis is especially common among athletes. Pruritus may be severe.

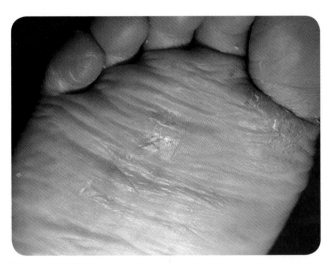

Figure 4-210 Tinea pedis in a 9 year old with scaly plaques on sole.

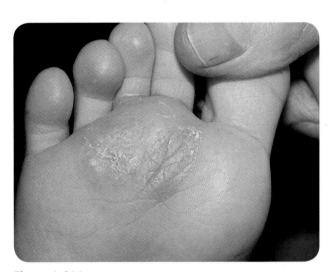

Figure 4-211 Tinea pedis in a 2 year old.

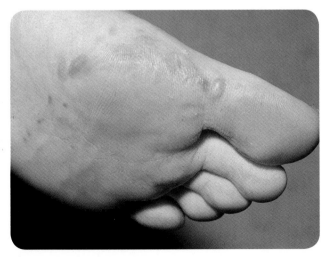

Figure 4-212 Tinea pedis with a deep vesicle.

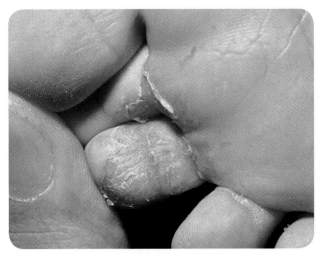

Figure 4-213 Tinea pedis with scaling and erythema.

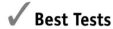

Differential Diagnosis and Pitfalls

- Granuloma annulare
- Contact dermatitis
- Psoriasis
- Juvenile plantar dermatosis
- Keratoderma (hereditary)

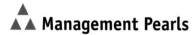

Best Tests

A KOH test should be performed in any patient in whom tinea pedis is suspected. If bacterial coinfection is suspected (pustules, crust, or significant inflammation), a bacterial culture should also be sent.

▲▲▲ Management Pearls

Small, localized lesions can be treated topically. With extensive disease, systemic antifungals may be required (griseofulvin 4 to 6 weeks, dosage as below). Check for nail involvement, which will require prolonged therapy (12 weeks of oral therapy) to prevent recurrence.

Therapy

Topical antifungals are generally sufficient. A treatment course can last anywhere from 1 to 6 weeks depending on the extent of involvement. Patients should be instructed to limit the use of occlusive footwear in order to keep their feet dry. Drying powders may also be used.

Oral antifungals are usually not necessary but may be used if there is extensive involvement or if topical treatment is not successful. Terbinafine at 6 mg/kg/day may be used for 2 weeks. Griseofulvin may also be used at a dose of 20 mg/kg/day for 4 weeks.

Topical antibacterials may be necessary if bacterial coinfection is present. Oral antibiotics are rarely necessary.

Suggested Readings

Wolff K, Goldsmith LA, Katz SI, et al., eds. *Fitzpatrick's Dermatology in General Medicine.* Vol. 1. 7th Ed. New York: McGraw-Hill; 2008:1815–1819.

Tinea Versicolor

■■ Diagnosis Synopsis

Tinea versicolor is also known as pityriasis versicolor. It is a superficial fungal infection resulting from infection with *Malassezia furfur*. The yeast phase of this organism, *Pityrosporum orbiculare*, is part of the normal skin flora. Skin lesions arise when the hyphal form predominates. It is a condition more likely to occur in adolescents than in younger children. It is seen with frequency in tropical areas with high humidity and temperatures. In most patients, the condition is nonpruritic, and the primary concern is over its appearance.

◉ Look For

Hyperpigmented or hypopigmented scaly macules and patches on the upper trunk and arms (Figs. 4-214–4-217). Facial involvement can occur and is more frequent in infants. The eruption favors oily areas of skin (seborrheic areas). Occasionally, erythematous lesions may arise.

●● Diagnostic Pearls

Stretching of the involved skin will accentuate the fine scale of tinea versicolor.

?? Differential Diagnosis and Pitfalls

- Confluent and reticulated papillomatosis of Gougerot–Carteaud presents with lesions in similar locations on the upper trunk but has a negative skin scraping.
- Pityriasis rosea may mimic tinea versicolor. Lesions in pityriasis are often not limited to seborrheic areas, and skin scrapings are negative.

- Seborrheic dermatitis may be difficult to clinically distinguish from tinea versicolor. Skin scraping with KOH examination is a helpful test.
- Atopic dermatitis presents with lichenified plaques and is more pruritic.
- Erythrasma.
- Tinea corporis is typically not as widespread in distribution. KOH test results reveal long, branching hyphae and no yeast.
- Psoriasis presents with thicker erythematous plaques with silvery, KOH-negative scale.
- Cutaneous candidiasis has a predilection for skin folds and typically presents with erythematous papules and pustules. Pseudohyphae can be seen on KOH preparation.
- Vitiligo presents with depigmented macules and patches that lack scale. Woods lamp examination is helpful to distinguish it from the hypopigmented lesions seen in tinea versicolor.

✓ Best Tests

Lightly scrape scale within the skin lesions onto a glass slide. Add a small drop of 10% KOH. Heat over an open flame for 1 to 3 s. Look for short, nonbranching hyphae and yeast cells.

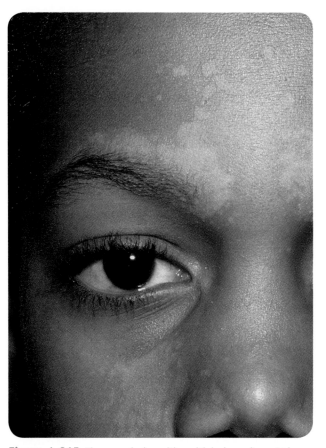

Figure 4-215 Tinea versicolor with multiple hypopigmented papules on the face.

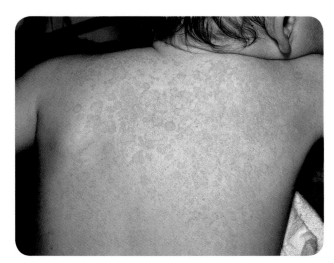

Figure 4-214 Tinea versicolor with multiple light brown papules on the trunk.

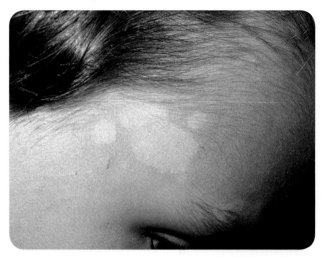

Figure 4-216 Tinea versicolor with less apparent scale until scraped.

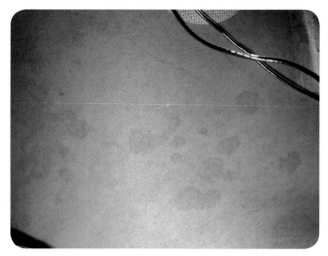

Figure 4-217 Tinea versicolor. Multiple discrete and confluent reddish-brown papules.

▲▲ Management Pearls

Parents should be informed that pigmentary changes take several months to resolve after proper therapy.

Therapy

The condition typically responds to short courses of topical or oral antifungals. Prophylactic treatments are usually necessary to prevent relapse.

Selenium sulfide 2.5% lotion applied for 10 min daily for 7 days is a cost-effective treatment. Once clear, weekly to monthly use can be an effective prophylactic measure.

Zinc pyrithione 2% soap or shampoo may also be used in a similar fashion.

Other topical agents reported to be effective include imidazoles, triazoles, ciclopirox olamine, sulfur preparations, propylene glycol, salicylic acid preparations, and benzoyl peroxide.

Ketoconazole 400 mg orally at monthly intervals is an effective treatment and prophylactic measure.

Similar results have been reported with oral itraconazole and fluconazole.

Suggested Readings

Bolognia JL, Jorizzo JL, Rapini RP, eds. *Dermatology.* Vol. 1. 2nd Ed. St Louis, MO: Mosby; 2008:1136–1137.

Cohen BA, ed. *Pediatric Dermatology.* 3rd Ed. St Louis, MO: Mosby; 2005:95–96.

James WD, Berger TG, Elston DM, eds. *Andrews' Diseases of the Skin.* 10th Ed. Philadelphia, PA: WB Saunders; 2006:313.

Diagnosis Synopsis

Common warts, also known as verruca vulgaris, are caused by the human papillomavirus (HPV), most frequently HPV types 1, 2, and 4. Infection is usually at sites prone to frequent trauma, such as fingers, hands, knees, and elbows, but can occur on virtually any epidermal surface as well as mucosal surfaces. Warts may be pruritic, and scratching can produce a linear array of lesions via autoinoculation. Widespread, persistent lesions may be a clue to underlying inherited or acquired immunodeficiency.

Look For

Hyperkeratotic, exophytic papules or nodules on the dorsal hands, fingers, elbows, or knees (Figs. 4-218–4-221). Confluent verrucous plaques may form in sites of longstanding lesions. Scratching often leads to a linear array of papules due to autoinoculation.

Diagnostic Pearls

Look for tiny blackish-red dots within the wart. These are thrombosed capillaries and foci of capillary hemorrhage.

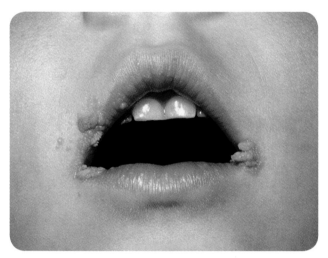

Figure 4-218 Common warts are frequently seen on the lips in children.

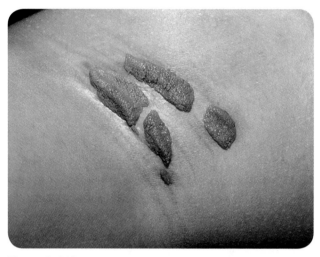

Figure 4-219 Common warts as large sessile nodules in the axilla.

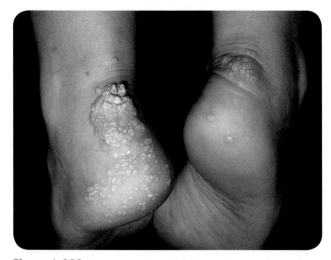

Figure 4-220 Common wart over Achilles tendon may be confluent with plantar warts.

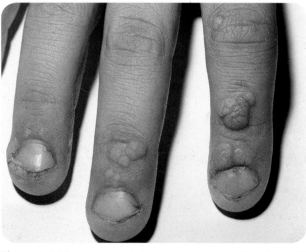

Figure 4-221 Common warts in a very common location. The fourth finger has a periungual wart that is often a treatment challenge.

Also look for interruption in the normal skin lines (dermato-glyphs).

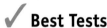 ## Differential Diagnosis and Pitfalls

- Corns and calluses typically arise of the plantar surfaces of the feet and between toes. These lesions lack the punctate black dots seen in warts. Paring of a wart often better illustrates this feature.
- Molluscum contagiosum presents as domed, shiny papules, often with a central dell.
- Prurigo nodularis presents as a pruritic lichenified hyperpigmented papule or nodule.

✓ Best Tests

This is usually a clinical diagnosis.

▲▲ Management Pearls

A multitude of treatments are available, and the list of therapies below is by no means exhaustive. Treatment is aimed at lesion destruction and/or elicitation of an effective host immune response. No treatment is successful in all patients. Additionally, it has been reported that 60% of warts will resolve spontaneously within 2 years. This underscores the importance of choosing treatments that limit potential scarring and are age/location appropriate.

Therapy

Paring of hyperkeratotic debris, followed by application of liquid nitrogen, either via cotton swab or use of a spray canister, is an effective treatment. Three to four treatments, spaced 3 to 4 weeks apart, are often curative. Pain is a limiting factor in some patients.

Multiple over-the-counter salicylic acid-containing products are available for home use in the form of liquid that can be painted onto lesions or impregnated adhesive plaster. Soaking of lesions followed by paring in between daily applications improves response. Increased effectiveness is seen when combined with cryotherapy.

Topical 5-fluorouracil 5% cream applied one to two times daily until resolution has been described more recently as an effective treatment option. This treatment may also be combined with in-office cryotherapy.

Pulsed dye laser is another treatment option for recalcitrant warts.

Non-FDA-approved therapies include intralesional candida antigen and treatment with contact sensitizers. Intralesional candida antigen is often successful in eliciting a host immune response directed at the wart. One to ten lesions are injected with 0.1 mL each of *Candida albicans* skin test antigen. Avoid treatment of lesions on the digits as a painful compartment syndrome-like response has been reported with its use at these sites.

Contact immunotherapy with squaric acid dibutyl ester has been used with good results in patients with lesions resistant to other treatments. This treatment requires access to a compounding pharmacy and is best prescribed by a dermatologist familiar with its use.

Suggested Readings

Bolognia JL, Jorizzo JL, Rapini RP, eds. *Dermatology*. Vol. 1. 2nd Ed. St Louis, MO: Mosby; 2008:1183–1198.

Cohen BA, ed. *Pediatric Dermatology*. 3rd Ed. St Louis, MO: Mosby; 2005:121–126.

James WD, Berger TG, Elston DM, eds. *Andrews' Diseases of the Skin*. 10th Ed. Philadelphia, PA: WB Saunders; 2006:404–406.

Diagnosis Synopsis

Plantar warts, also called verruca plantaris, are caused by the human papillomavirus (HPV), most frequently HPV types 1, 2, and 4. The warts favor pressure points of the ball of the foot and under the metatarsal heads, but they may develop anywhere else on the sole. Multiple adjacent warts frequently fuse to form one large plaque, called a mosaic wart. Due to an endophytic growth pattern and position over areas of pressure, these lesions are often painful.

Look For

Well-demarcated callus-like plaques on the sole of the foot with scattered, central black dots **(Figs. 4-222–4-225)**. Normal dermatoglyphics are disrupted. Usually, there are several lesions on one foot that can merge and form one large mosaic wart.

Diagnostic Pearls

Look for tiny punctate, blackish-red dots within the wart (thrombosed capillaries), which are best visualized by paring the surface of the wart with a no. 15 surgical blade.

?? Differential Diagnosis and Pitfalls

- Differentiate from hard corns and calluses by looking for the characteristic thrombosed capillaries.
- Acquired digital fibrokeratoma presents as a skin-colored papule with a rim of raised skin, most commonly on a finger. Lesions on the sole of the foot have been described.

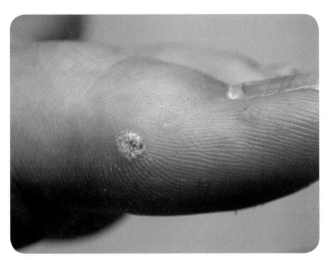

Figure 4-222 Plantar wart with characteristic black dots from thrombosed capillaries.

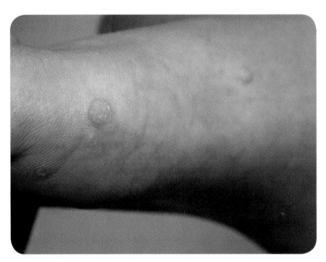

Figure 4-223 Plantar warts in a common location, over the great toe.

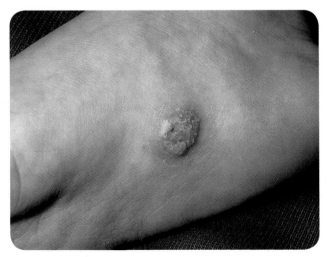

Figure 4-224 Plantar wart with one hemorrhagic site.

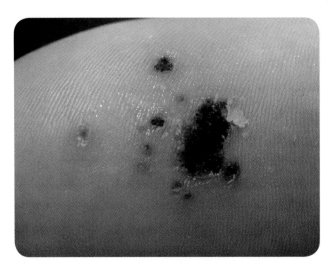

Figure 4-225 Plantar warts. Multiple lesions are common.

- In nonresponding lesions, consider verrucous carcinoma, a form of squamous cell carcinoma, that can appear warty. These uncommon tumors are typically found in elderly men and are extremely rare in children.

 Best Tests

This is usually a clinical diagnosis. If necessary, a skin biopsy should reveal characteristic histopathological findings.

 Management Pearls

If treatment is pursued, combination therapy is usually necessary to eradicate it.

Therapy

As warts in young children may resolve spontaneously, reassurance alone is an option for asymptomatic warts. Plantar warts are typically more refractory to treatment than common warts.

For symptomatic warts, aggressive home therapy is required with 40% salicylic acid plaster (Mediplast) applied daily and taped on with strong tape (e.g., duct tape). Have the parent soak, and then pare down the wart between applications of each patch. Diligent treatment is necessary, as larger lesions will often take up to 16 weeks to resolve.

Destructive therapies should be reserved for patients able to tolerate associated pain. These therapies include cryosurgery (liquid nitrogen), laser therapy, or treatment with acids such as bi- or trichloroacetic acid. Make sure to pare the wart down before cryosurgery or application of any topical therapy to improve the chance of treatment success. These treatments, spaced 3 to 4 weeks apart, can be combined with home application of salicylic acid to speed resolution.

Suggested Readings

Bolognia JL, Jorizzo JL, Rapini RP, eds. *Dermatology*. Vol. 1. 2nd Ed. St Louis, MO: Mosby; 2008:1183–1198.

James WD, Berger TG, Elston DM, eds. *Andrews' Diseases of the Skin*. 10th Ed. Philadelphia, PA: WB Saunders; 2006:405.

■■ Diagnosis Synopsis

Acropustulosis of infancy (AI) is a recurrent, self-limited, pruritic vesiculopustular eruption of the hands and feet, typically beginning during the first few weeks to months of life.

Characteristically, lesions appear as recurrent crops every couple of weeks to months, anywhere on hands and feet but more extensively on the palms and soles. Frequently, the condition is initiated by a scabies infestation.

◉ Look For

The classic lesions of AI are recurrent crops of tense 2 to 4 mm well-defined pustules on the palms and soles of an infant that last approximately 1 week (Figs. 4-226–4-229). However, lesions may appear on any surface of the hands and feet, with additional lesions elsewhere on the body; they may be in any stage at presentation. Early lesions are erythematous pinpoint macules or papules. Late lesions may be 2 to 4 mm hyperpigmented macules (postinflammatory hyperpigmentation). Infants are usually irritable, and sleep is deprived due to the pruritus; they are otherwise well.

●● Diagnostic Pearls

Palmar and plantar accentuations are the most important clues to this diagnosis. AI should be diagnosed only after a thorough evaluation of the patient and family members excludes scabies.

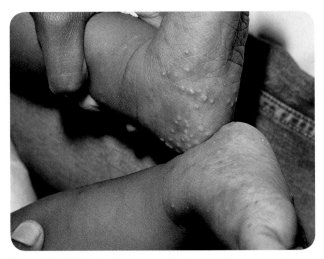

Figure 4-226 Infantile acropustulosis with discrete pustules concentrated on the insteps of the feet.

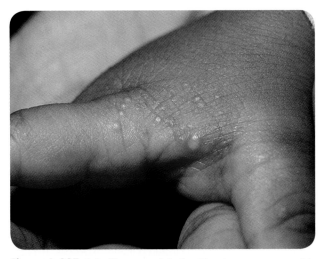

Figure 4-227 Infantile acropustulosis with a larger opaque vesicle on proximal phalanx.

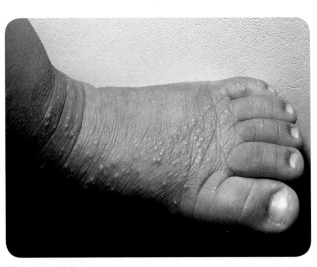

Figure 4-228 Infantile acropustulosis with multiple discrete vesicles and pustules.

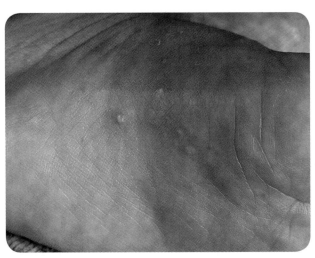

Figure 4-229 Infantile acropustulosis on typical location on sole with discrete vesicles and surrounding erythema.

?? Differential Diagnosis and Pitfalls

- A history of recurrent crops of pustules on the hands and feet is highly suggestive of AI; in the absence of a characteristic history, other diagnoses should be considered.
- Scabies infestation in infants may present identically to AI and may precipitate the disease. Often, burrows will be obscured by vesiculation; careful examination of the entire infant for a typical burrow or vesicular or nodular lesions on the torso is necessary. Family members should also be questioned and examined for pruritus and burrows.
- Eosinophilic folliculitis occurs mainly on the scalp rather than the hands and feet but may cycle concurrently with AI.
- Congenital cutaneous candidiasis, erythema toxicum neonatorum, and transient neonatal pustular melanosis are less pruritic and usually more widespread than AI.
- Hand-foot-and-mouth disease usually affects children after 1 year of age and is associated with constitutional symptoms and oral lesions. The palmar and plantar vesicles are nonpruritic, more oval shaped, and oriented along dermatoglyphics.
- The pustules of pustular psoriasis, bacterial pustulosis, and pustular tinea pedis are less well defined and often coalescent, as opposed to the well-defined 2 to 4 mm pustules of AI.

✓ Best Tests

- Skin scrapings for scabies should be performed on any lesion that resembles a burrow.
- Gram stain, Tzanck smear, and potassium hydroxide preparations will rule out bacterial, herpes virus (multinucleated giant cells), or fungal infections, respectively.

▲▲ Management Pearls

- Unless the diagnosis of AI is obvious, all infants should be treated empirically for scabies on initial presentation, even if skin scrapings are negative for scabies.
- Parents should be instructed that AI is a self-limited disease and that treatment is aimed at controlling the symptoms rather than curing the disease.

Therapy

In children older than 1 year of age, antihistamines in sleep-inducing doses (diphenhydramine 1 to 1.25 mg/kg every 6 h or hydroxyzine 0.5 mg/kg twice daily and 1 mg/kg every night) relieve pruritus but do not alter the course of disease.

High-potency topical glucocorticosteroids such as clobetasol propionate (0.05%) or betamethasone dipropionate (0.05%) ointment twice daily may help relieve flares.

Suggested Readings

Jennings JL, Burrows WM. Infantile acropustulosis. *J Am Acad Dermatol.* 1983;9(5):733–738.

Mancini AJ, Frieden IJ, Paller AS. Infantile acropustulosis revisited: History of scabies and response to topical corticosteroids. *Pediatr Dermatol.* 1998;15(5):337–341.

Van Praag MC, Van Rooij RW, Folkers E, et al. Diagnosis and treatment of pustular disorders in the neonate. *Pediatr Dermatol.* 1997;14(2): 131–143.

Wagner A. Distinguishing vesicular and pustular disorders in the neonate. *Curr Opin Pediatr.* 1997;9(4):396–405.

▪▪ Diagnosis Synopsis

Congenital cutaneous candidiasis (CCC) is an in utero-acquired infection with *Candida* sp. Neonates present within the first 24h of life with either isolated cutaneous or simultaneous cutaneous and systemic disease. In term infants, the infection is almost uniformly limited to the skin and resolves uneventfully with topical antifungals alone. However, preterm infants, especially those <26 weeks' gestation or extremely low birth weight (<1,000 g), are at high risk for systemic disease and death despite appropriate therapy. Risk factors for CCC include prolonged rupture of membranes and the presence of an intrauterine foreign body (i.e., cervical cerclage or intrauterine device).

Look For

Characteristically, it begins as a morbilliform eruption that may be completely macular or consist of some combination of 2 to 4 mm erythematous macules, papulovesicles, and pustules on an erythematous base (Figs. 4-230–4-233). The borders are often well-demarcated. Over days, the eruption becomes more papular, vesicular, and, occasionally, bullous. Lesions coexist in different stages of evolution and cover the face, trunk, buttocks, and extremities, favoring the skin folds. The palms, soles, and nails are often affected whereas the diaper area and oral mucosa are usually spared. In term infants, the rash generally resolves with desquamation within 2 weeks, persisting longest on the palms and soles.

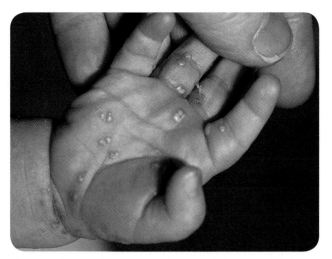

Figure 4-230 Neonatal candidiasis with numerous opaque palmar pustules, both grouped and scattered, on palm.

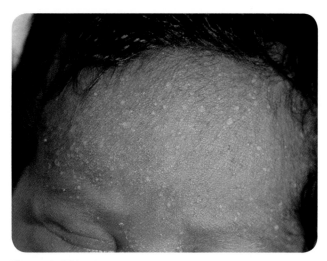

Figure 4-231 Neonatal candidiasis with numerous opaque pustules on forehead.

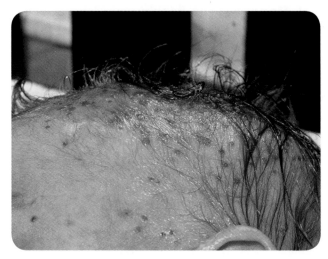

Figure 4-232 Neonatal candidiasis with multiple eroded, scattered lesions. Differentiate from herpes simplex infection.

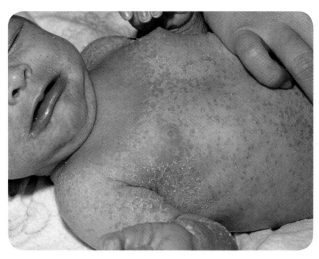

Figure 4-233 Neonatal candidiasis with multiple confluent erosions and scattered pustules.

In premature infants, it tends to be more severe, being more widespread and progressing more rapidly to vesicles and bullae. Patients sometimes present with diffuse, erythematous, burnlike areas that rapidly become eroded or are already denuded at birth.

Systemically infected neonates may show signs of sepsis, including lethargy, poor perfusion, hypotonia, temperature instability, development of or worsening respiratory distress, an elevated white blood count with a left shift, thrombocytopenia, persistent hyperglycemia, or glycosuria. The clinical signs of sepsis may be very subtle, and one should maintain a high index of suspicion in high-risk infants (preterm, very low birth weight, prolonged treatment with broad-spectrum antibiotics, prolonged endotracheal intubation, central intravascular catheters, widespread cutaneous involvement, or major congenital malformations).

 ## Diagnostic Pearls

- Unlike erythema toxicum neonatorum, the palms and soles are often involved, and the eruption is present at birth.
- Examination of the placenta and umbilical cord often reveals chorioamnionitis and/or funisitis. These lesions appear on the umbilical cord as focal granulomatous lesions and well-defined, round, yellow, 2 mm or smaller macules and papules in clusters along the cord. The placenta may be diffusely inflamed, and often there is a yellow exudate covering the fetal surface of the extraplacental membranes.

?? Differential Diagnosis and Pitfalls

Vesiculopustular rashes in the neonate may be divided into infectious, transient, or persistent dermatoses. The first goal in the diagnosis of all vesiculopustular eruptions in the neonate is to rule out infectious etiologies.

Infectious Vesiculopustular Dermatoses

Superficial staphylococcal infection
Listeria monocytogenes
Haemophilus influenza
Group A streptococcal infection
Pseudomonas
Cytomegalovirus
Aspergillus
Herpes simplex infection
Neonatal varicella
Scabies

Transient Noninfectious Vesiculopustular Dermatoses

Erythema toxicum neonatorum
Neonatal pustular melanosis
Miliaria crystallina and rubra
Neonatal acne
Acropustulosis of infancy
Pustular eruption in Down syndrome

Persistent Noninfectious Vesiculopustular Dermatoses

Incontinentia pigmenti
Eosinophilic pustular folliculitis
Langerhans cell histiocytosis
Hyperimmunoglobulin E syndrome
Pustular psoriasis

 ## Best Tests

- Even when the diagnosis is clinically obvious, confirmation by KOH test is rapidly and easily performed.
- Other studies may include smears (Wright stain, Gram stain, direct fluorescent antibodies, and Tzanck prep), and cultures (bacterial, viral, and fungal) of vesicular contents should be performed for all infants with vesiculopustular eruptions to both narrow the differential diagnosis and rule out the infection.
- In neonatal candidiasis, the potassium hydroxide prep would reveal yeast and pseudohyphae, the fungal culture would grow *Candida* sp., and the Wright stain would reveal inflammatory cells; all other tests would be negative.
- Biopsies are rarely indicated.

 ## Management Pearls

All preterm infants with CCC, even when otherwise asymptomatic, should have a complete workup for systemic disease, including cultures from the blood, urine, and cerebrospinal fluid. Because term infants almost uniformly recover uneventfully, only those with systemic signs require more thorough evaluation.

Therapy

Topical imidazole antifungal creams, including ketoconazole or itraconazole, are sufficient for term infants without systemic signs. All preterm neonates and term infants with systemic signs require parenteral antifungal therapy (amphotericin B, flucytosine, and fluconazole).

Suggested Readings

Bendel CM. Candidiasis. In: Remington JS, Klein J, Baker C, Wilson C, eds. *Infectious Diseases of the Fetus and Newborn Infant*. 6th Ed. Philadelphia, PA: Elsevier Saunders; 2005:1107–1128.

Darmstadt GL, Dinulos JG, Miller Z. Congenital cutaneous candidiasis: Clinical presentation, pathogenesis, and management guidelines. *Pediatrics*. 2000;105(2):438–444.

Roqué H, Abdelhak Y, Young BK. Intra amniotic candidiasis. Case report and meta-analysis of 54 cases. *J Perinat Med*. 1999;27(4):253–262.

Wagner A. Distinguishing vesicular and pustular disorders in the neonate. *Curr Opin Pediatr*. 1997;9(4):396–405.

◼◼ Diagnosis Synopsis

Poison ivy, poison oak, or poison sumac dermatitis (contact dermatitis to urushiol) is a type IV delayed hypersensitivity immune reaction that occurs in previously sensitized children. Patients typically present with pruritic papules and vesicles. Pruritus can be intense, and secondary bacterial infection can result from excoriations. Scratching does not spread lesions; the lesions with most antigens appear first and then, as the immune response increases, lesions with less antigens begin to erupt. Skin lesions usually begin to appear after 48 h of initial exposure and will persist 3 to 4 weeks if not treated.

◉ Look For

Asymmetric, linear, and red and brown-red plaques and vesicles, crusted plaques, vesicles, and bullae (Figs. 4-234–4-237). Vesicles quickly rupture, leaking plasma and forming a surface crust. A "black dot variant" has been described (as the oil from the plant leaves a black resin on the skin). Extreme facial edema may be seen if there is significant exposure to the face.

◼◼ Diagnostic Pearls

Distribution is more important than appearance. A linear configuration of pruritic dermatitis on exposed extremities suggests the diagnosis. The family pet may get antigen on its fur and then play with a child, possibly causing an asymmetric multiplicity of lesions.

?? Differential Diagnosis and Pitfalls

- Other diseases with an external environmental exposure may mimic this disorder (e.g., disorders with a light-related causation) as well as contact dermatitis from other plants; however, their distribution and shape are usually not linear on an exposed extremity.
- Scabies can also have vesicles and be extremely pruritic, but it is usually symmetric and involves areas protected by clothing.
- Facial cellulitis—when significant inflammation and edema are present on the face, especially periorbitally; however, patients will not have fever or leukocytosis.
- Herpes simplex virus infection—lesions often coalesce on a red base, usually periorificial; there is often a prodrome of pain and burning. HSV may be associated with fever, malaise, and tender lymphadenopathy. Viral PCR or other viral specific studies will reveal the virus.
- Herpes zoster—localized to dermatomes, grouped vesicles and bullae on a red base with a history of varicella. Viral PCR or other viral specific studies will reveal the virus.
- Impetigo—very fragile vesicles associated with a yellow crust, usually arranged as coalescing plaques with peripheral satellite lesions.

✓ Best Tests

- This is a clinical diagnosis.
- Biopsy is rarely needed and will reveal a nonspecific dermal infiltrate of lymphocytes and eosinophils and intercellular edema or vesiculation of the epidermis.
- Cultures should be obtained if bacterial superinfection is suspected.

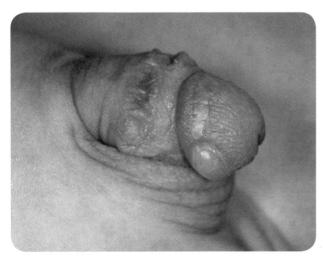

Figure 4-234 Rhus dermatitis with bullae on the penis from urinating in the bushes.

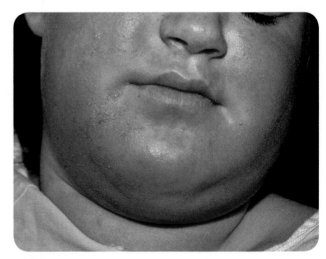

Figure 4-235 Rhus dermatitis may be relatively diffuse depending on the exposure.

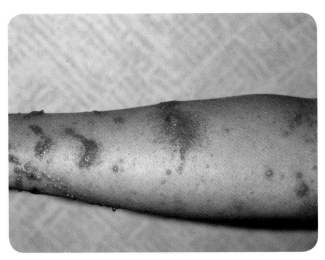

Figure 4-236 Rhus dermatitis with characteristic linear vesicular lesions.

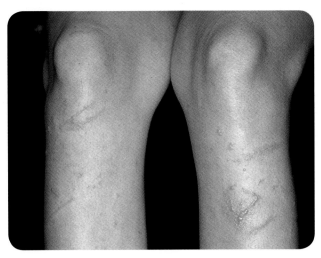

Figure 4-237 Rhus dermatitis with linear lesions from rubbing against plants.

▲▲ Management Pearls

Educate patients to avoid poison ivy, poison oak, and poison sumac, which often have oak-shaped leaves held in threes ("Leaves three, leave it be.").

Therapy

In most patients, this can be managed with Class 1 or 2 topical corticosteroids. Systemic corticosteroids (prednisone 1 to 2 mg/kg/day) may be used in patients with widespread involvement; the length of treatment should be at least 2 weeks to avoid rebound flares.

Oral antihistamines can help with the pruritus but are more useful for their sedating properties, especially when used at night.

Washing exposed skin is helpful to remove the antigen, but this is only helpful within the first 20 to 30 min after exposure. There are barrier creams available commercially that are designed to help prevent the dermatitis if there is expected exposure to the allergen. There are also commercially available cloths designed to remove the antigen after exposure if soap and water are not available.

Suggested Readings

Bolognia JL, Jorizzo JL, Rapini RP, eds. *Dermatology.* Vol. 1. 2nd Ed. St Louis, MO: Mosby; 2008:252–253.

Weston WL. Contact dermatitis in children. *Curr Opin Pediatr.* 1997; 9(4):372–376.

Diagnosis Synopsis

Epidermolysis bullosa (EB) refers to a group of genetic diseases characterized by blistering in response to minor trauma. It is divided into four major categories based on the depth of skin blistering: (i) EB simplex (intraepidermal skin separation), (ii) junctional EB (skin separation at the lamina lucida), (iii) hemidesmosomal EB (skin separation at the hemidesmosomal level), and (iv) dystrophic EB (sublamina densa skin separation).

EB simplex is the most common form of EB. It is caused by defects in keratins 5 and 14, with the vast majority being autosomal dominantly transmitted. Based on the clinical course, EB simplex is divided into three main subtypes: (i) EB simplex Weber–Cockayne (EBS-WC; it is the mildest form with disease limited to the hands and feet), (ii) EB simplex Koebner (EBS-K; it is the intermediate form with generalized blistering), and (iii) EB simplex Dowling–Meara (EBS-DM; it is the most severe form with widespread blistering, possible internal organ involvement, and potential death in the neonatal period).

In milder cases of EB simplex, significant friction or trauma is required to produce blisters, and the first signs may not develop until the patient begins to walk or crawl. In the more severe cases of EB simplex, blistering occurs in response to minimal trauma, and large bullae and erosions are present at birth or within the first few days of life. All forms of EB simplex worsen in hot, humid environments and improve with age.

Look For

When evaluating the patient with EB, it is important to realize that strict clinical criteria for individual subtypes of EB are not defined, and patients may possess characteristics of more than one subtype. On initial evaluation, all children should have a full physical examination with special emphasis on the eyes (photophobia or redness), gastrointestinal tract (polyhydramnios, feeding intolerance, and oral erosions), genitourinary system (gross hematuria or obstruction), and respiratory tract (hoarse voice or stridor).

In all subtypes of EB simplex, vesicles and bullae are tense and painful. The vesicle contents may be dark (hemorrhagic) or clear (serous). Unless punctured and drained, intravesicular hydrostatic pressure tends to cause the vesicles to gradually expand. Lesions tend to heal without scarring or atrophy. Recurrent palmar and plantar vesiculation may lead to callouslike epidermal thickening and lichenification (keratoderma).

EBS-WC: This subtype is usually diagnosed when the child begins to walk. Tense, small vesicles and bullae (<2 cm in diameter) form on the dorsal, palmar, and plantar hands and feet (Fig. 4-238). Individual vesicles are characteristically surrounded by an erythematous halo. Other body sites, the nails, and mouth are almost never affected.

EBS-K: Large bullae and erosions initially develop at birth secondary to trauma during delivery and handling in the nursery (Figs. 4-239 and 4-240). Thereafter, smaller vesicles tend to form only in areas of continual friction, such as the diaper area. Oral lesions tend to be minor and do not interfere with feeding. Children may develop mild thickening of the soles. Nails are almost never affected.

EBS-DM: Large bullae and erosions initially develop at birth secondary to trauma during delivery and handling in the nursery (Fig. 4-241). Later in the neonatal period, bullae tend to favor the hands and feet but may develop anywhere and may appear to develop spontaneously. Vesicles and bullae are often significantly inflamed with surrounding erythema and hemorrhagic vesicular contents. Transient milia may form in healing erosions. With age, vesicles tend to become smaller and grouped but maintain their erythematous, inflammatory base (herpetiform). Mucosal involvement

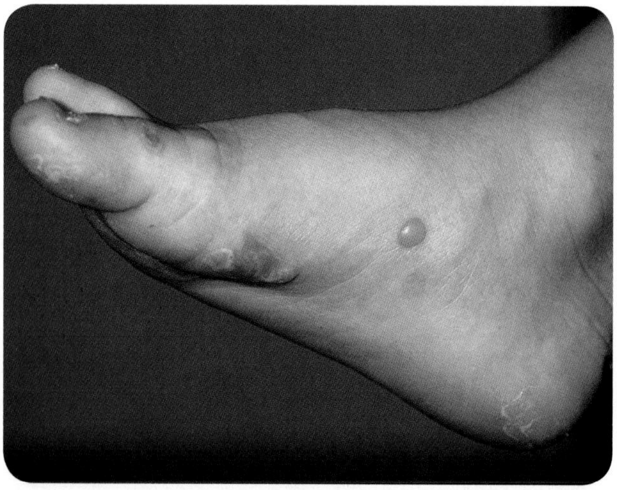

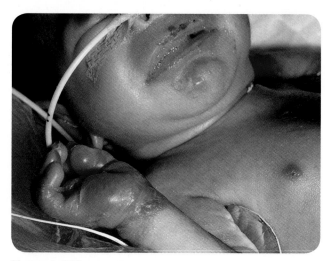

Figure 4-238 EB simplex. Typical blisters of the Weber–Cockayne variant; hyperkeratosis occurs in the areas of recurrent blistering.

Figure 4-239 EB simplex with lesions around the lips, hands, and torso.

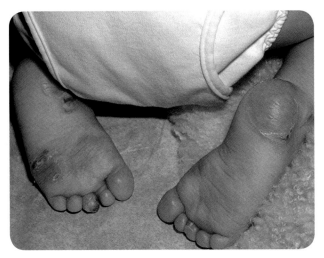

Figure 4-240 EB simplex has blisters commonly on heel and toe, as well as on the knees with crawling.

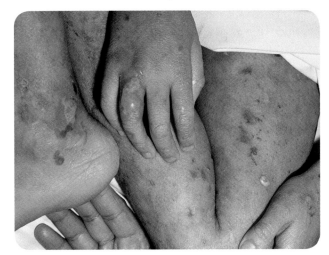

Figure 4-241 EB simplex bullae tend to favor the hands and feet but may occur anywhere in severe forms.

may be significant with interference of feeding (secondary to pain), a hoarse voice and weak cry (secondary to laryngeal involvement), and marked gastroesophageal reflux. Patients often develop significant thickening of the palms, soles, and nails. Nails are often significantly thickened in the neonate.

Diagnostic Pearls

- Parents, siblings, and relatives should also be questioned and examined, as milder forms of EB simplex (i.e., EBS-WC and EBS-K) are almost universally autosomal dominantly inherited.
- Families with EBS-WC may not consider their children to have a medical problem, only an increased tendency to blister, and children may not present until adolescence or adulthood when blistering interferes with strenuous activities such as sports.

Differential Diagnosis and Pitfalls

Traumatic/Idiopathic

Friction blister
Dyshidrotic eczema
Child abuse
Burns

Genetic

Dystrophic EB
Junctional EB
Palmar–plantar keratodermas
Porphyrias

Immune mediated

Chronic bullous dermatosis of childhood (linear IgA disease)
Bullous pemphigoid
Pemphigus vulgaris
Paraneoplastic pemphigus

Toxin/Infectious

Bullous impetigo
Staphylococcal scalded skin syndrome (SSSS)
Toxic epidermal necrolysis
Hand-foot-and-mouth disease

Best Tests

- Skin biopsies from the edge of a freshly induced blister should be sent for (i) routine histology to rule out alternative diagnoses and (ii) immunofluorescence studies and/or electron microscopy to confirm the diagnosis and establish the subtype.
- In new sporadic cases without a family history, genotyping is often indicated for more serious forms of the disorder.

Management Pearls

- Patients with milder forms of EB simplex (EBS-WC and EBS-K) often have long family histories of the disease, and caregivers will be well aware of provoking factors, avoidance strategies, and blister care. The primary role of the health professional is to ensure that patients are properly informed in skin care, treated for secondary infections, and provided with assistance in securing necessary skin care products.

- The Dystrophic Epidermolysis Bullosa Research Association of America, Inc. (DebRA) at www.debra.org provides an excellent Web-based resource, providing extensive information, assistance, and support to families and health professionals caring for children with severe forms of EB.

Therapy

Skin care involves prevention of blisters, blister care, and pain control. One must be more diligent in severe forms (EBS-DM) versus milder forms (EBS-WC and EBS-K), in which therapy is directed more toward foot care in older infants and children.

Prevention of blisters:

- Avoid over heating by providing a cool environment and not over dressing.
- Avoid applying tape, Band-Aids, or adhesives to the skin.
- Dress in loose-fitting clothes (elastic leg bands may be cut from disposable diapers to prevent friction).
- Ideal shoes have soft and permeable leather, ample toe room, and few seams.
- Absorbent powders (e.g., Zeasorb) may be applied inside of socks to prevent friction.
- Ideal socks are cotton, superabsorbent sport socks.
- Avoid friction by patting moist areas dry rather than rubbing and lubricating the skin with Aquaphor or Vaseline.

Blister care:

- Drain blisters that are larger than a dime or that appear tense. Use a sterile needle or lancet to pierce the blister roof, drain the contents, and leave the remaining blister roof intact.
- Apply topical antibiotic ointment (e.g., Bacitracin or Polysporin) to erosions and drained blisters.
- Cover open areas with nonadherent dressings (e.g., Mepitel, Telfa, or Vaseline gauze) and change daily.
- Watch for signs of infection (e.g., yellow crust, foul-smelling exudate, purulence, induration, increased erythema, and severe pain), and culture and treat with systemic antibiotics (e.g., cephalexin or clindamycin).

Pain control with dressing changes:

- Acetaminophen 15 mg/kg orally every 4 to 6 h.
- Ibuprofen 10 mg/kg orally every 6 to 8 h (in infants older than 6 months).
- Opiates may be necessary for more severe pain but can affect feeding/stooling activities of young infants.

Special Considerations in Infants

The differential diagnosis of bullae and erosions in the neonate is broad. When perinatal bullae predominate the clinical picture, the most similar and common alternative diagnoses include sucking blisters, bullous impetigo, SSSS, and other forms of EB. When perinatal erosions and ulcerations predominate the clinical picture, the most similar and common alternative diagnoses include erosions secondary to trauma (scalp electrodes, adhesives, etc.), aplasia cutis, congenital or acquired herpes infection, and other forms of EB. Unlike EB simplex, the bullae of bullous impetigo and SSSS tend to be flaccid, are centrally located (face and trunk), erode quickly, and are associated with significant underlying erythema. Sucking blisters, aplasia cutis, and traumatic ulcerations are isolated and self-limited, unlike EB simplex, which is generalized and chronic.

It is important to realize that once the diagnosis of EB has been established, all categories of EB (dystrophic, junctional, and simplex) may present identically in the neonatal period, and clinical distinction is often not possible until later in infancy or childhood. Therefore, in the newborn period, genetic counseling and anticipatory guidance should be limited until the exact diagnosis is confirmed by immunofluorescence studies and/or electron microscopy.

Suggested Readings

Bello YM, Falabella AF, Schachner LA. Management of epidermolysis bullosa in infants and children. *Clin Dermatol*. 2003;21(4):278–282.

Fine JD. The classification of inherited epidermolysis bullosa (EB): Report of the Third International Consensus Meeting on Diagnosis and Classification of EB. *J Am Acad Dermatol*. 2008;58(6):931–950.

Pessar A, Verdicchio JF, Caldwell D. Epidermolysis bullosa: The pediatric dermatological management and therapeutic update. *Adv Dermatol*. 1988;3:99–120.

Pfender EG, Sadowski SG, Uitto J. Epidermolysis bullosa simplex: Recurrent and de novo mutations in the KRT5 and KRT14 genes, phenotype/genotype correlations, and implications for genetic counseling and prenatal diagnosis. *J Invest Dermatol*. 2005;125:239–243.

Rugg EL, Horn HM, Smith FJ, et al. Epidermolysis bullosa simplex in Scotland caused by a spectrum of keratin mutations. *J Invest Dermatol*. 2007;127(3):574–580.

Yiasemides E, Walton J, Marr P, et al. A comparative study between transmission electron microscopy and immunofluorescence mapping in the diagnosis of epidermolysis bullosa. *Am J Dermatopathol*. 2006;28(5):387–394.

Diagnosis Synopsis

Orofacial herpes (cold sores or fever blisters) is most commonly caused by herpes simplex virus (HSV) type 1 but may be caused by HSV type 2 as well. The condition is highly contagious and is spread by direct contact with a noncrusted lesion. Infection with HSV can present in a variety of ways. In some cases, it is preceded by a prodrome, which may consist of pain, tenderness, or burning; in others, infection is asymptomatic. After the primary infection, the virus remains dormant and may be reactivated by various stimuli, including illness, stress, immunosuppression, or ultraviolet light.

Look For

Grouped vesicles on an erythematous base; some may appear umbilicated (Figs. 4-242–4-245). Gingivostomatitis (involvement of the gingival and buccal mucosa as well as the hard and soft palate) is a common presentation in children.

Diagnostic Pearls

- Herpes infection should be in the differential any time a patient presents complaining of a painful rash.
- Lesions may be pustular or crusted by the time a patient is seen in an office setting.
- The pustular phase is often misdiagnosed as impetigo.

?? Differential Diagnosis and Pitfalls

- Impetigo vesicles and pustules are not as tightly grouped. The individual lesions of impetigo are of varying sizes and stages.

- Herpes zoster presents as a painful vesicular rash as well. Look for a dermatomal distribution.
- Molluscum contagiosum lesions can be pustular and crusted when inflamed.
- Erythema multiforme.

✓ Best Tests

- A Tzanck smear is the fastest and easiest test to help make the diagnosis. An intact vesicle should be unroofed, and a scraping taken from the base should be stained. Once pustular or crusted, the value of a Tzanck decreases significantly.
- Polymerase chain reaction can be used when HSV is suspected clinically and the Tzanck smear is negative.
- A punch biopsy may be performed but is not usually necessary.
- Viral cultures are rarely performed.

▲▲ Management Pearls

- Oral therapy is more effective than topical therapy. Dosing regimens vary depending on whether the infection is primary or recurrent (see below).

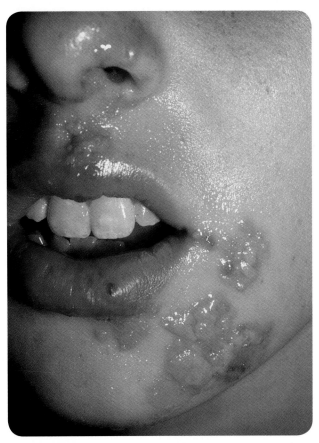

Figure 4-243 Orofacial HSV with moderate lip swelling.

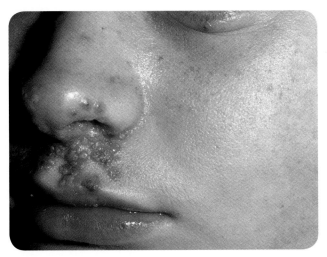

Figure 4-242 Orofacial HSV in a common location with grouped vesicles, pustules, and crust.

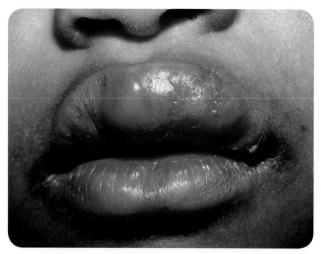

Figure 4-244 Orofacial HSV with severe lip swelling and an opaque vesicle on the upper lip.

- Individual lesions are contagious until they are completely crusted over. Patients should be advised to avoid contact with other children or pregnant women until all lesions are crusted.

Therapy

Acyclovir is approved for use in children. The first episode should be treated at a dose of 20 mg/kg/day divided into five doses for a total of 7 days. Dosing recommendations vary for recurrent episodes. For patients who suffer from frequent recurrences, daily dosing may be necessary.

Valacyclovir is approved for use in children over the age of 12 years. Famciclovir is not approved for use in children. If secondary bacterial infection is suspected, a culture should be taken and the choice of oral antibiotic should be based on the results.

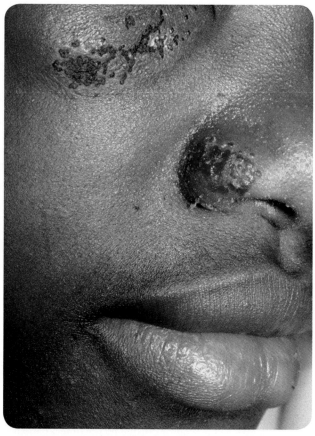

Figure 4-245 Orofacial herpes simplex lesions in two sites innervated by the maxillary branch of the trigeminal nerve.

Suggested Readings

Bolognia JL, Jorizzo JL, Rapini RP. *Dermatology*. Vol. 1. 2nd Ed. St Louis, MO: Mosby; 2008:1199–1204.

Kesson AM. Management of neonatal herpes simplex virus infection. *Paediatr Drugs*. 2001;3(2):81–90.

■■ Diagnosis Synopsis

Bullous impetigo is a localized form of staphylococcal scalded skin syndrome caused by exfoliative toxins (A and B) released by (phage group II) *Staphylococcus aureus*. These toxins cleave desmoglein 1, resulting in superficial blisters locally at the site of infection. It is primarily seen in children and only rarely occurs in teenagers or young adults. Constitutional symptoms and fever are rare and mild, if they occur.

Outbreaks tend to occur during the summer months and in humid climates.

◉ Look For

Superficial flaccid vesicles that progress to large bullae with sharp margins and no surrounding erythema (Figs. 4-246–4-249). These vesicles/bullae rupture easily to form superficial moist, red erosions, which are surrounded by a peripheral collarette of blister roof.

Bullous impetigo affects the moist intertriginous areas such as the axillae, neck, and diaper area.

●● Diagnostic Pearls

- Flaccid bullae and erythematous moist erosions with collarette of blister roof in the intertriginous areas.
- Consider concurrent second dermatoses as the antecedent to impetigo. Scabies, poison ivy, bites, or trauma can lead to impetigo. Primary varicella can present as bullous varicella due to coinfection with *S. aureus*.
- When the lesions are widespread and confluent, consider the diagnosis of SSSS.

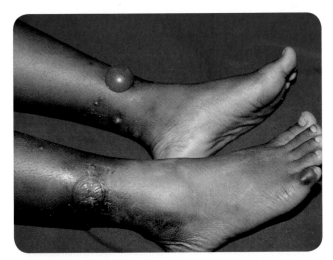

Figure 4-246 Bullous impetigo may have very large intact bullae resembling an arthropod bite.

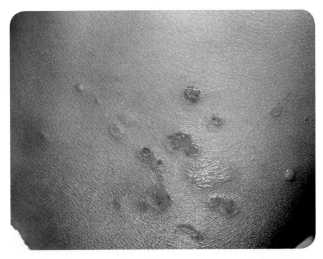

Figure 4-247 Bullous impetigo with small opaque bullae and erosions with a shiny base and rim of scale.

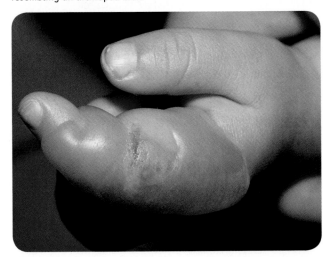

Figure 4-248 Blistering dactylitis with confluent, large bullae on index finger; streptococcal infection is often confused with bullous impetigo.

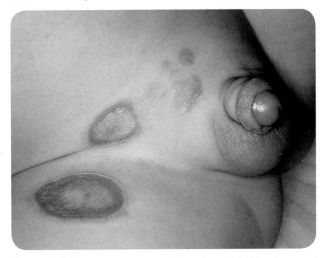

Figure 4-249 Bullous impetigo with erosions with shiny bases and peripheral scale.

?? Differential Diagnosis and Pitfalls

- Varicella—Typical polymorphic lesions in various stages: macules, vesicles, pustules, and crusting. Face, trunk, and proximal extremities are involved. Tzanck smear from a vesicle reveals multinucleated giant cells.
- Stevens–Johnson syndrome—Characteristic target lesions (necrotic center surrounded by erythema and edema [pallor]) along with hemorrhagic crusting of the lips and conjunctiva. There may be associated systemic symptoms.
- Bullous fixed drug eruption—Well-demarcated, circular or oval, erythematous patches that recur in the same site (usually lips, glans penis, and trunk) each time the offending drug is administered. Lesions characteristically heal with hyperpigmentation.
- Herpes simplex virus infection—Tiny, grouped vesicles on an erythematous base that rupture to form polycyclic erosions. Prodromal symptoms are usually present. The skin of the face and hands is commonly affected.
- Bullous insect bite reactions—Linear, irregular streaks of dermatitis with vesiculation at the site of bite, often with a "kissing pattern."
- Scabies—Pruritic erythematous papules and vesiculopustules on the intertriginous areas, face, genitalia, and palms and soles. Burrows may be present in the finger web spaces, flexor aspect of the wrist, axilla, umbilicus, nipples, buttocks, and penis.
- Cutaneous candidiasis affects the intertriginous areas, especially the groin or neck, in the form of confluent erythematous patches with multiple small satellite pustules. KOH test from a pustular lesion reveals budding spores and pseudohyphae that confirm *Candida* infection.
- Chronic bullous dermatosis of childhood—Tense (subepidermal) blisters in the groin, lower abdomen, back, and perioral region. The characteristic rosette-like vesicles resembling a cluster of pearls surrounding a central healing bulla.

✓ Best Tests

Gram stain of blister fluid demonstrating Gram-positive cocci. Culture and sensitivity.

▲▲ Management Pearls

- *S. aureus* readily spreads from person to person and contaminates the environment. Hence, appropriate infection-control measures should be taken, which involves identifying the infected patients, isolating them from other noninfected patients, cleaning of the environment, and, most importantly, proper hand hygiene. Alcoholic antiseptic hand rubs offer an alternative to antiseptic hand washes and increase the compliance.

- In cases of severe bullous impetigo, such as rapidly progressing lesions or recalcitrant disease, community-acquired MRSA infection should be considered. In the setting of a nursery or intensive care unit, nosocomial MRSA infection should be suspected. Skin swab for the bacterial culture and sensitivity should be performed.
- In cases of recurrent impetigo or in the setting of an epidemic outbreak, treat the nasal or perineum carriage of *S. aureus* with topical mupirocin (0.5 g into each nostril twice daily for 5 days).

Therapy

For limited disease, either topical mupirocin or fusidic acid (not available in the United States) is used (both three times daily until clear).

For widespread infections or those with systemic symptoms, use systemic antibiotics.

First-line Therapy
- Cloxacillin/dicloxacillin 50 to 100 mg/kg/day four times daily for 10 days (suspension is poorly tolerated due to taste)
- Cephalexin 25 to 50 mg/kg/day three to four times daily for 10 days

Second-line Therapy
- Amoxicillin/clavulanate and other cephalosporins (cefadroxil and cefprozil)
- Erythromycin, azithromycin, clarithromycin, and loracarbef

Treatment of MRSA
Clindamycin, trimethoprim/sulfamethoxazole, or vancomycin

Treatment of Multidrug-resistant *S. aureus*
Linezolid and quinupristin/dalfopristin

Special Considerations in Infants

Impetigo can present in the first 2 weeks of life. In neonates, the infection is commonly centered on the umbilicus or circumcision sites. Neonates with bullous impetigo can appear well.

Suggested Readings

Ladhani S, Garbash M. Staphylococcal skin infections in children: Rational drug therapy recommendations. *Paediatr Drugs*. 2005;7(2):77–102.

Sandhu K, Kanwar AJ. Generalized bullous impetigo in a neonate. *Pediatr Dermatol*. 2004;21(6):667–669.

Stanley JR, Amagai M. Pemphigus, bullous impetigo, and the staphylococcal scalded-skin syndrome. *N Engl J Med*. 2006;355(17):1800–1810.

Miliaria Crystallina

▪▪ Diagnosis Synopsis

Miliaria crystallina, or sudamina, is a common transient vesicular eruption resulting from superficial blockage of eccrine sweat ducts. Typically, high fever and sweating in association with occlusion of the skin lead to miliaria crystallina. It is most likely to be seen in those who have recently moved to a tropical climate from a more temperate one. It also follows excessive sweating, sunbathing, warming in a hot tub, high fever, or occlusion of the skin from dressings, immobility in a hospital bed, or clothing.

◉ Look For

Crops or widespread areas of tiny, fragile, clear fluid vesicles resembling water droplets (Figs. 4-250–4-253). The lesions often involve the forehead, upper trunk, and volar aspects of the arms. They appear within days to weeks of exposure to warm, humid weather and resolve within hours to days.

●● Diagnostic Pearls

- Gently rubbing the vesicles will cause them to rupture and disappear.
- Lesions are usually in the same stage of development and are most prominent in areas with occlusion.

?? Differential Diagnosis and Pitfalls

- The diagnosis is usually self-evident. However, occasional cases become more inflammatory or pustular and need to be distinguished from other vesiculopustular rashes of the neonate.
- Vesicular drug eruptions—larger tense vesicles.
- Varicella—larger vesicles on an erythematous base.
- Eosinophilic pustular folliculitis—tense pustule on an erythematous base.
- AGEP (acute generalized exanthematous pustulosis)—pustules are opaque, not clear as in miliaria.
- Superficial staphylococcal infection—tense pustule on an erythematous base.
- Scabies.

✓ Best Tests

- Skin biopsy will confirm but is not necessary.
- Smears and stains of vesicular contents are usually acellular.

▲▲ Management Pearls

- Miliaria rarely becomes secondarily infected, and cultures and antibiotics should be started when lesions become pustular and develop surrounding inflammation.

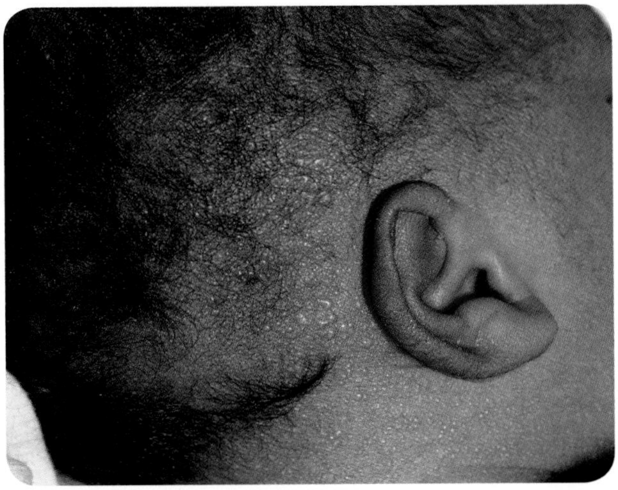

Figure 4-250 Miliaria crystallina with multiple closely-grouped, clear vesicles on the scalp.

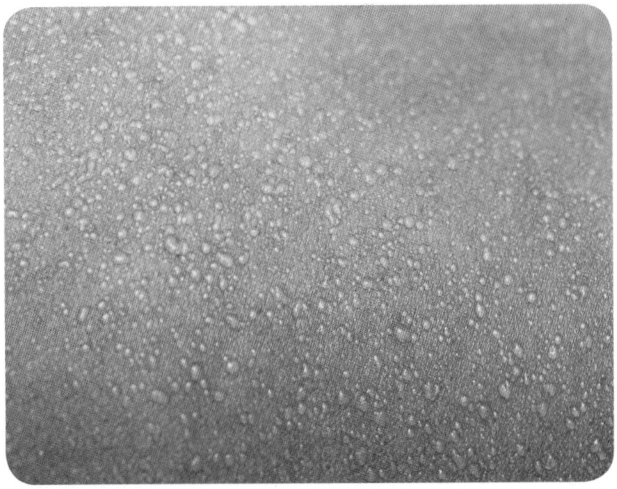

Figure 4-251 Miliaria crystallina. Multiple tiny-walled, clear vesicles of varying sizes.

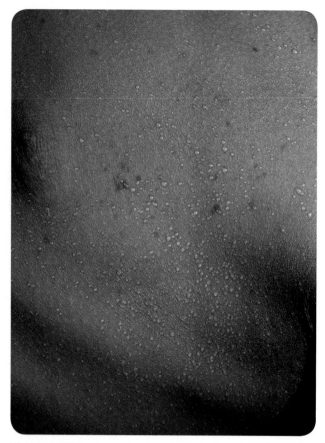

Figure 4-252 Miliaria crystallina with multiple vesicles in a nonfollicular distribution.

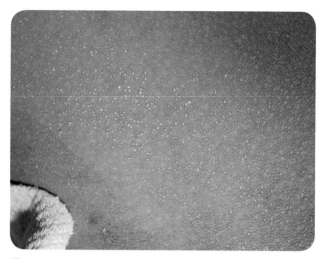

Figure 4-253 Miliaria crystallina with clear vesicles.

Special Considerations in Infants

In infants, miliaria crystallina usually occurs toward the end of the first week of life. The differential diagnosis of persistent or pustular eruptions in neonates and infants should include the following:

- Congenital cutaneous candidiasis
- Neonatal varicella
- Erythema toxicum neonatorum
- Neonatal pustular melanosis
- Miliaria rubra
- Neonatal acne
- Acropustulosis of infancy
- Incontinentia pigmenti

- Treat underlying fever and prevent occlusion of sweat ducts. Keep patient in a cool environment. Overdressing of young children is a common cause of this condition; recommend less clothes if this etiology seems likely.

Therapy

Miliaria will rapidly resolve by treating fever and reducing environmental heat (e.g., less clothing, cool bathing, and air conditioning). If an incubator is necessary, reducing humidity is helpful.

Suggested Readings

Bolognia JL, Jorizzo JL, Rapini RP, eds. *Dermatology*. Vol. 1. 2nd Ed. St Louis, MO: Mosby; 2008:540–541.

Schachner L, Press S. Vesicular, bullous and pustular disorders in infancy and childhood. *Pediatr Clin North Am*. 1983;30:609–629.

■■ Diagnosis Synopsis

Transient neonatal pustular melanosis (TNPM) is an idiopathic pustular disease of term newborns. Lesions begin in utero as pustules that then rupture, leaving behind collarettes of scale and hyperpigmented macules. Depending on the eruption's stage of evolution, infants are born with some combination of pustules, scale, and hyperpigmented macules. The pustules and scale resolve within 2 weeks of birth, leaving behind hyperpigmented macules that persist for several months. New lesions do not form after delivery.

◉ Look For

The eruption presents at birth as some combination of pustules, collarettes of scale, and/or hyperpigmented macules affecting any cutaneous surface, including the palms and soles (Figs. 4-254–4-257). Favored sites include the chin, neck, upper chest, lower back, and buttocks. Typically, all three stages are simultaneously present at birth. Pustules measure 2 to 6 mm in diameter and have no surrounding erythema. The pustules are very fragile and rupture with mild friction, leaving behind superficial collarettes of scale or brown crusts. In darker-skinned infants, lesions resolve with

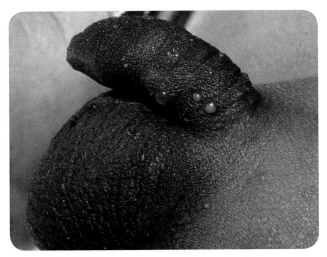

Figure 4-254 Transient neonatal pustular dermatosis. Multiple pustules on the penis. (Same patient as in Fig. 4-257.)

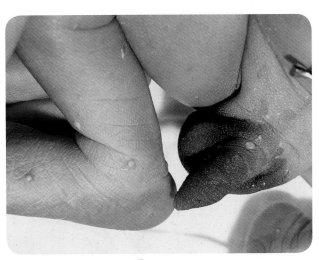

Figure 4-255 Transient neonatal pustular dermatosis. Note the collarettes of scale left behind as the fragile pustules rupture. (Same patient as in Fig. 4-256.)

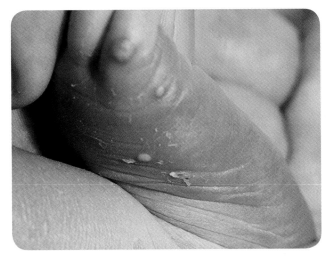

Figure 4-256 Transient neonatal pustular dermatosis with pustules of varying sizes.

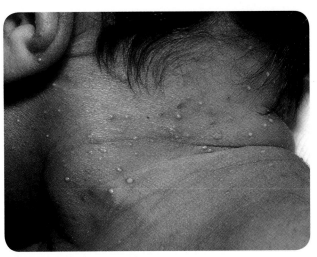

Figure 4-257 Transient neonatal pustular dermatosis with multiple pustules with minimal erythema on the neck.

postinflammatory hyperpigmentation (hyperpigmented macules); however, hyperpigmentation is usually not a feature in white infants.

Diagnostic Pearls

- The pustules of TNPM are very fragile and often ruptured upon removal of the vernix caseosa. Pustules may rupture in utero as well. New lesions do not form after delivery. Therefore, pustules may not be present on examination, leading one to consider the diagnosis of multiple cutaneous lentigines. The hyperpigmented macules of TNPM, however, are less well-defined than lentigines and are often surrounded by collarettes of scale in the first few days of life. Furthermore, even when part of a syndrome (LEOPARD syndrome, Carney syndrome, or Peutz–Jeghers syndrome), lentigines tend to be few at birth and develop progressively thereafter, whereas the hyperpigmented macules of TNPM are numerous at birth and fade over time.
- TNPM may also be confused with erythema toxicum neonatorum, which, unlike TNPM, is almost never present at birth and has significant underlying erythema.

?? Differential Diagnosis and Pitfalls

If mainly consisting of scale

Bullous impetigo
Staphylococcal scalded-skin syndrome
Ichthyosis bullosa of Siemens
Postmaturity desquamation

If mainly consisting of pigmented macules

Multiple lentigines
LEOPARD syndrome
Carney complex
Peutz–Jeghers syndrome
Multiple melanocytic nevi

If there are many pustules: Infectious vesiculopustular dermatoses

Congenital cutaneous candidiasis
Superficial staphylococcal infection
Listeria monocytogenes
Haemophilus influenza
Group A streptococcal infection
Pseudomonas
Cytomegalovirus
Aspergillus

Herpes simplex virus infection
Neonatal varicella
Scabies

Transient noninfectious vesiculopustular dermatoses

Neonatal pustular melanosis
Miliaria crystallina and rubra
Neonatal acne
Acropustulosis of infancy
Pustular eruption in Down syndrome

Persistent noninfectious vesiculopustular dermatoses

Incontinentia pigmenti
Eosinophilic pustular folliculitis
Langerhans cell histiocytosis
Hyperimmunoglobulin E syndrome
Pustular psoriasis

✓ Best Tests

- A Wright stain of pustular fluid shows polymorphonuclear leukocytes with occasional eosinophils.
- A skin biopsy is not necessary because this is a clinical diagnosis; however, if performed, a biopsy will show subcorneal pustules with neutrophils.

Management Pearls

Parents should be reassured that this is a benign, nonscarring, self-limited disease that is not associated with any internal problems.

Therapy

None, as the condition is self-limited.

Suggested Readings

Lucky AW. Transient benign cutaneous lesions in the newborn. In: Eichenfield LF, Frieden IJ, Esterly NB, eds. *Neonatal Dermatology.* 2nd Ed. Philadelphia, PA: Elsevier; 2008:85–97.

Van Praag MC, Van Rooij RW, Folkers E, et al. Diagnosis and treatment of pustular disorders in the neonate. *Pediatr Dermatol.* 1997;14(2):131–143.

Wagner A. Distinguishing vesicular and pustular disorders in the neonate. *Curr Opin Pediatr.* 1997;9(4):396–405.

Varicella (Chickenpox)

Diagnosis Synopsis

Varicella, or chickenpox, is an acute, highly contagious exanthem caused by primary infection with varicella–zoster virus (VZV). The virus is believed to be spread by respiratory droplets and skin vesicles from individuals with varicella or herpes zoster (a dermatomal rash caused by reactivated endogenous VZV) to the respiratory tract of susceptible children. In immunologically normal children, the illness typically begins after an incubation period of 2 to 3 weeks, lasts 3 to 7 days, and resolves without complication. Rare cases, however, are associated with prolonged courses and severe complications, including bacterial superinfection, pneumonia, encephalitis, bleeding disorders, and hepatitis. Adolescents and immunocompromised children (e.g., malignancy, congenital defects in cell-mediated immunity,

organ transplant recipients, or HIV-infected children) are at elevated risk for complications.

Look For

Typical varicella begins with a 1 to 3 day prodrome of fever and malaise followed by a rapidly progressive vesiculopustular eruption. The eruption is characterized by crops of erythematous macules that develop central papules, which progress into 2 to 3 mm diameter vesicles, pustules, and crusts within 12 to 48 h (Figs. 4-258–4-261). Crops of lesions continue to develop over 3 to 4 days before becoming completely crusted over by 6 to 7 days. The pathognomonic picture is that of a centrally focused eruption with lesions in all stages of evolution simultaneously. Lesions may concentrate within areas of inflammation, such as a sunburn or

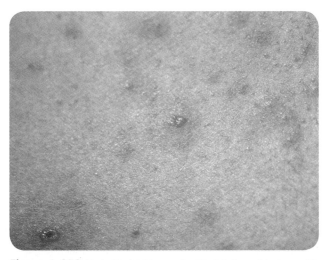

Figure 4-258 Varicella (chickenpox) with faintly red lesions with some umbilicated vesicles.

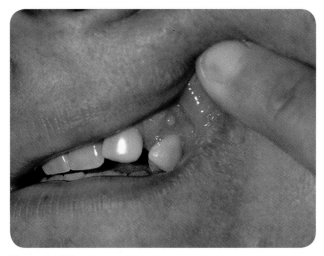

Figure 4-259 Varicella (chickenpox) with vesicular lesion in the mouth.

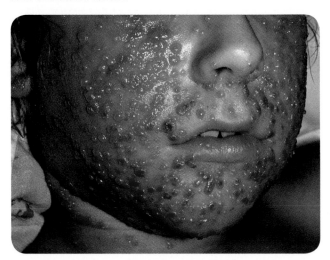

Figure 4-260 Varicella (chickenpox) with multiple vesicles and some with umbilication. Many lesions are in the same stage of development, which brings up the differential diagnosis of smallpox.

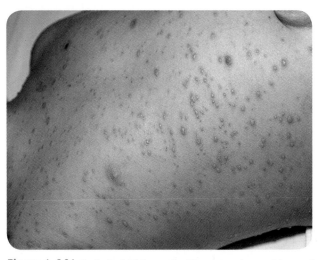

Figure 4-261 Varicella (chickenpox) with red macules, vesicles, and umbilicated vesicles.

169

dermatitis. Mucous membranes may also be involved with 2 to 3 mm shallow ulcerations. Patients typically develop 250 to 500 lesions.

●● Diagnostic Pearls

The vesicle is classically described as a dewdrop on a rose petal. The vesicle is thin-walled and easily broken.

?? Differential Diagnosis and Pitfalls

- Eczema herpeticum—prior history of eczema; lesions favor the extremities, and vesicles are often grouped or confluent.
- Drug eruption—associated with drug exposure.
- Miliaria—no viral symptoms; lesions do not rapidly progress to pustules and crusts.
- Disseminated herpes simplex—concentrated in sites typically infected by HSV (oral mucosa, perioral area, and genitalia) and occurs in patients with depressed immunity or underlying dermatoses.
- Hand-foot-and-mouth disease—favors hands, feet, and oral mucosa.
- Impetigo—gradually progressive, superficial erosions; very fragile bullae; favors exposed sites.
- Insect bite reactions—larger papules and vesicles; lesions do not rapidly progress to pustules and crusts; favor exposed sites.
- Molluscum contagiosum—no viral symptoms; lesions do not rapidly progress to pustules and crusts.
- Variola (smallpox)—all lesions at the same stage; favors extremities.
- PLEVA (pityriasis varioliformis et acuta)—recurrent crops of papulovesicles that crust and resolve with residual hypopigmentation; less pruritus; no mucous membrane involvement.

✓ Best Tests

- The most sensitive and specific method for detection of VZV in clinical specimens is PCR of viral DNA.
- When PCR is not available, direct fluorescent antibody examination may be performed.
- Tzanck preparations can be read quickly revealing multinucleate giant cells and margination of the nucleoplasm, but is not as sensitive or specific as molecular methods or culture.
- Skin biopsy is usually not necessary but will show multinucleated giant cells, intranuclear inclusion bodies, and reticular degeneration of the epidermis.
- Viral culture is highly specific but requires several days to develop.

- Serologic studies of acute and convalescent IgM and IgG are also not useful for early diagnosis.

▲▲ Management Pearls

- Fever that persists beyond one week or recurs after crusting of the lesions may signify a secondary bacterial infection or other complication.
- Children with varicella are contagious from 2 days before the exanthem appears until all vesicles are crusted, typically 3 to 7 days after onset of the exanthem.
- **Note:** The CDC Advisory Committee on Immunization Practices recommends that all health care workers ensure that they are immune to varicella, since nosocomial transmission of varicella is well recognized. If susceptible persons must enter the room of a patient known or suspected to have varicella, they should wear respiratory protection (N95 respirator). Persons immune to varicella need not wear respiratory protection.
- **Precautions:** Standard and airborne (isolate patient in a negative pressure room, wear respiratory protection [N95 mask], and limit patient transport).
- In the United States, varicella is reportable in many states.
- Per the CDC, morbidity or mortality due to varicella is Nationally Notifiable via the National Notifiable Diseases Surveillance System.

Therapy

Symptomatic treatment for varicella includes oral antihistamines (hydroxyzine 2 mg/kg/day divided three times a day), calamine lotion, trimming of fingernails to discourage scratching, and acetaminophen (15 mg/kg four times daily) for fever and pain.

Antiviral therapy is reserved for those with severe varicella or at risk for severe varicella. Adolescents, children receiving intermittent or aerosolized corticosteroids, those on long-term salicylate therapy, and patients with chronic skin or lung disease may be given a closely monitored course of oral acyclovir (20 mg/kg four times daily for 5 days). All severely affected and immunosuppressed patients should be given intravenous acyclovir until no new lesions appear for more than 48 h. Foscarnet may be given to resistant cases.

Passive immunization with varicella–zoster immune globulin (VariZIG) is recommended as postexposure prophylaxis (within 96 h of exposure) for immunocompromised children.

Varicella vaccine may be given to normal children within 5 days of exposure to prevent or ameliorate varicella.

Suggested Readings

American Academy of Pediatrics Committee on Infectious Diseases. The use of oral acyclovir in otherwise healthy children with varicella [published erratum appears in *Pediatrics*. 1993;91(4):858]. *Pediatrics*. 1993;91(3):674–676.

Centers for Disease Control and Prevention (CDC). A new product (VariZIG) for postexposure prophylaxis of varicella available under an investigational new drug application expanded access protocol. *MMWR Morb Mortal Wkly Rep*. 2006;55(8):209–210.

Dahl H, Marcoccia J, Linde A. Antigen detection: The method of choice in comparison with virus isolation and serology for laboratory diagnosis of herpes zoster in human immunodeficiency virus-infected patients. *J Clin Microbiol*. 1997;35(2):347–349.

Gershon AA. Varicella–zoster virus infections. *Pediatr Rev*. 2008;29(1):5–10; quiz 11.

Heininger U, Seward JF. Varicella. *Lancet*. 2006;368(9544):1365–1376.

Myers MG, Seward JF, LaRussa. Varicella-zoster virus. In: Kliegman RM, Behrman RE, Jenson HB, Stanton BF, eds. *Nelson Textbook of Pediatrics*. 18th Ed. Philadelphia, PA: WB Saunders; 2007:1366–1372.

Sauerbrei A, Eichhorn U, Schacke M, et al. Laboratory diagnosis of herpes zoster. *J Clin Virol*. 1999;14(1):31–36.

■■ Diagnosis Synopsis

Neonatal varicella, or neonatal chickenpox, is an infection with varicella–zoster virus (VZV) during the first 4 to 6 weeks of life. Neonates may be infected (i) in utero by transplacental viremia, (ii) at birth by ascending infection, or (iii) after birth by respiratory droplets or direct contact with infectious lesions. The incubation period of VZV is usually between 10 and 14 days; therefore, onset of symptoms within the first 10 days of life is usually caused by intrauterine transmission. Onset of symptoms after 10 days is usually indicative of postnatally acquired infection.

Intrauterine-acquired neonatal varicella is common in infants born to mothers who contract a primary varicella infection during the last 3 weeks of pregnancy. The severity of neonatal disease is dependent on the presence of transplacentally acquired maternal antibodies. Hence, onset of the rash of primary maternal VZV infection between 6 and 21 days prior to delivery allows for maternal antibody production, transplacental transfer to the fetus, and nonfatal neonatal varicella. Conversely, onset of maternal rash between 5 days before and 2 days after delivery does not allow sufficient time for maternal antibody production, and one can expect a fulminant course.

Postnatally acquired VZV infections are usually self-limited in healthy full-term infants. However, severe varicella may result in neonates <28 weeks' gestation or below 1,000 g at birth.

◉ Look For

Typical varicella begins with a 1 to 3 day prodrome of fever and malaise followed by a rapidly progressive vesiculopustular eruption. The eruption is characterized by crops of erythematous macules that develop central papules, which progress into 2 to 3 mm diameter vesicles, pustules, and crusts within 12 to 48 h (Figs. 4-262–4-265). Crops of lesions continue to develop over 3 to 4 days before becoming completely crusted over by 6 to 7 days. The pathognomonic picture is that of a centrally focused eruption with lesions in all stages of evolution simultaneously. Lesions may concentrate within areas of inflammation, such as diaper dermatitis. Mucous membranes may also be involved with 2 to 3 mm shallow ulcerations. Postnatally acquired infection in nonimmune, otherwise healthy neonates is usually limited to the skin with an average of 250 to 500 lesions.

In utero-acquired infection, on the other hand, may be more or less severe than postnatally acquired infection, depending on the presence of maternally acquired antibodies, as discussed in the Diagnosis Synopsis. The day of rash onset is highly predictive of the severity of in utero-acquired infection. Newborns who first develop lesions at age 0 to 4 days may have only a few scattered lesions. However, neonates who first develop the rash at age 5 to 10 days will likely develop hundreds of lesions, pneumonitis, hepatitis, encephalitis, and respiratory distress. Mothers of neonates with in utero-acquired VZV infection may report a history consistent with chickenpox during the last weeks of pregnancy.

●● Diagnostic Pearls

- The early vesicle is classically described as a dewdrop on a rose petal.
- The vesicle is thin-walled and easily broken.
- In utero, acquired neonatal varicella does not occur after uncomplicated maternal herpes zoster.

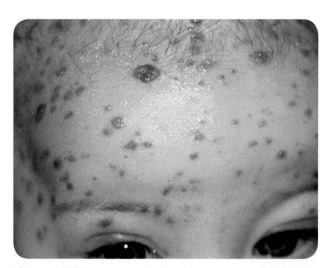

Figure 4-262 Neonatal varicella with lesions becoming impetiginized.

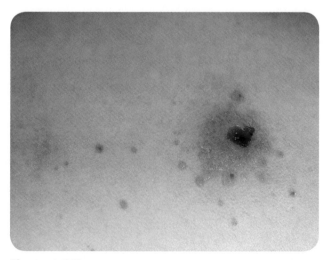

Figure 4-263 Neonatal varicella with larger, eroded lesion and small vesicles.

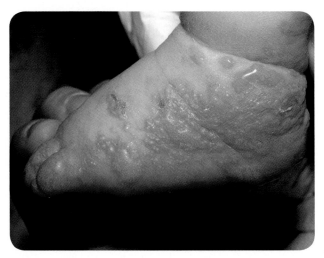

Figure 4-264 Neonatal varicella with bullous lesions on the feet.

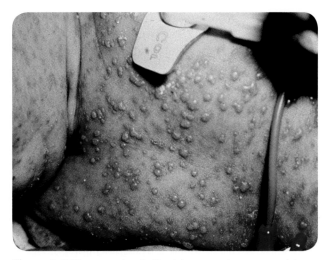

Figure 4-265 Neonatal varicella with very erythematous vesicles on chest and more crusts on face.

Langerhans cell histiocytosis
Hyperimmunoglobulin E syndrome
Pustular psoriasis

Differential Diagnosis and Pitfalls

- Vesiculopustular rashes in the neonate may be divided into infectious, transient, or persistent dermatoses.
- The first goal in all vesiculopustular eruptions in the neonate is to rule out infectious etiologies.

Infectious Vesiculopustular Dermatoses

Superficial staphylococcal infection
Listeria monocytogenes
Haemophilus influenza
Group A streptococcal infection
Pseudomonas
Cytomegalovirus
Aspergillus
Herpes simplex
Congenital cutaneous candidiasis
Scabies

Transient Noninfectious Vesiculopustular Dermatoses

Erythema toxicum neonatorum
Neonatal pustular melanosis
Miliaria crystallina and rubra
Neonatal acne
Acropustulosis of infancy
Pustular eruption in Down syndrome

Persistent Noninfectious Vesiculopustular Dermatoses

Incontinentia pigmenti
Eosinophilic pustular folliculitis

✓ Best Tests

- VZV infection in the neonate can be confirmed by culture, histology, antigen detection, polymerase chain reaction (PCR), or antibody titers.
- The most sensitive and specific method for detection of VZV in clinical specimens is PCR of viral DNA and is the method of choice for rapid detection of VZV in skin swabs or biopsies.
- When PCR is not available, immunofluorescent VZV-specific antigen staining (direct fluorescent antibody [DFA] examination) is preferred.
- Both PCR of VZV DNA and antigen detection yield results within one day.
- Viral culture is highly specific but requires several weeks for cytopathic changes to develop.
- Tzanck preparations can be read within minutes, revealing multinucleate giant cells and margination of the nucleoplasm, but is not as sensitive or specific as molecular methods or culture.
- Skin biopsy is usually not necessary but will show multinucleated giant cells, acidophilic intranuclear inclusion bodies, and reticular degeneration of the epidermis.
- Serologic studies of acute and convalescent IgM and IgG are not useful for early diagnosis.

Management Pearls

- Fever that persists beyond one week or recurs after crusting of the lesions may signify a secondary bacterial infection or other complication.

- All exposed neonates should be closely monitored and placed in isolation for 2 to 3 weeks (one full incubation period) after the onset of rash in the index case.
- All exposed infants who receive varicella–zoster immune globulin (VZIG) should remain in respiratory isolation for 28 days.
- Mothers with varicella at the time of delivery should be isolated from their infants until all lesions have crusted.

Therapy

Therapy is directed at reducing severe complications in at-risk neonates by using a combination of VZIG and acyclovir. The decision to treat is based on maternal history and neonatal health.

Acyclovir (10 to 15 mg/kg every 8 h) for all symptomatic neonates within 48 h of the onset of rash.

VZIG (dosage: 125 units intramuscularly) is given to neonates when

- Mothers develop primary varicella within 5 days before or 2 days after delivery.

- Preterm infants fewer than 1,000 g or 28 weeks' gestation are exposed to VZV (regardless of maternal history).
- Premature infants of mothers with a negative (or unreliable) history of varicella are exposed to VZV.

Infants with neonatal varicella who are born after 28 weeks' gestation to mothers with a positive history of varicella do not require VZIG.

Suggested Readings

Centers for Disease Control and Prevention (CDC). A new product (VariZIG) for postexposure prophylaxis of varicella available under an investigational new drug application expanded access protocol. *MMWR Morb Mortal Wkly Rep*. 2006;55(8):209–210.

Centers for Disease Control and Prevention (CDC). Prevention of varicella: Recommendations of the Advisory Committee on Immunization Practices (ACIP). *MMWR Recomm Rep*. 1996;45(RR-11):1–36.

Dahl H, Marcoccia J, Linde A. Antigen detection: The method of choice in comparison with virus isolation and serology for laboratory diagnosis of herpes zoster in human immunodeficiency virus-infected patients. *J Clin Microbiol*. 1997;35(2):347–349.

Sauerbrei A, Eichhorn U, Schacke M, et al. Laboratory diagnosis of herpes zoster. *J Clin Virol*. 1999;14(1):31–36.

Sauerbrei A, Wutzler P. Neonatal varicella. *J Perinatol*. 2001;21(8):545–549.

Zoster (Shingles)

Diagnosis Synopsis

Zoster, or shingles, is a reactivation of a latent infection with varicella–zoster virus (VZV). Annual incidence is <1/1,000 in children aged younger than 10 years. Maternal varicella infection during pregnancy, infection during the first year of life, and immunocompromised status are risk factors for zoster development in childhood.

Though the onset of cutaneous zoster in adults typically involves a 1 to 3 day prodrome of pain or tingling in the affected dermatome, this is rarely observed in children. Postherpetic neuralgia is also rare in children.

If it occurs, zoster encephalitis usually appears in the first 2 weeks after the onset of lesions and has a 10% to 20% mortality rate. Disseminated zoster occurs 5 to 10 days after the onset of dermatomal disease. It is defined as more than 20 lesions outside the initial dermatome of involvement.

Look For

Grouped vesicles or small bullae on an erythematous base usually confined to one or multiple contiguous dermatomes (Figs. 4-266–4-269). Early lesions may be urticarial. Vesicles may be confluent, sparse, or discrete. Commonly, vesicles become hemorrhagic or pustular within several days. The lesions typically crust over and resolve after a 7 to 14 day course. Scarring is a common sequelae. Regional adenopathy can occur. Pain and/or pruritus may precede or accompany the appearance of rash.

Diagnostic Pearls

- Consider zoster when there is a history of primary varicella infection before the first birthday, or an intrauterine infection.

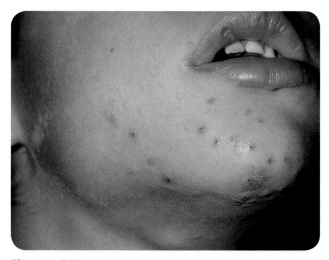

Figure 4-266 Herpes zoster in a mandibular distribution (V3) with an upper lip lesion (V2).

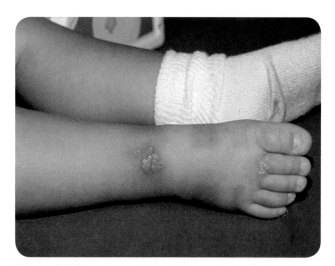

Figure 4-267 Herpes zoster. The mother had varicella at 5 months of gestation.

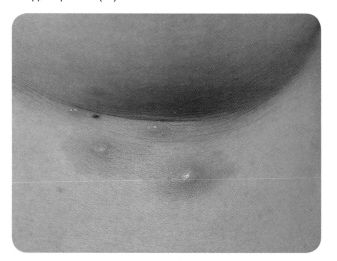

Figure 4-268 Herpes zoster with vesicle on erythematous macule.

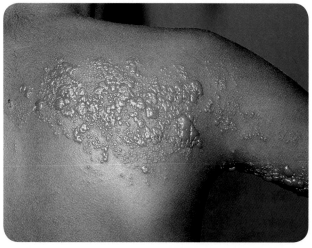

Figure 4-269 Herpes zoster in a dermatomal distribution.

- Patients may not have a definite history of previous varicella infection. In such cases, serologic evaluation should suggest prior exposure.

?? Differential Diagnosis and Pitfalls

- Herpes simplex occurring within a dermatomal distribution is the primary differential diagnosis. Serology, viral culture, or PCR may be necessary to distinguish this diagnosis from zoster.
- Allergic contact dermatitis may present as a well-defined vesicular plaque. A dermatomal distribution suggests zoster.
- Molluscum contagiosum, when inflamed, can be confused with varicella. Cases are typically of longer duration, and VZV PCR studies are negative. The presence of coexisting noninflamed molluscum lesions is a helpful diagnostic clue.

✓ Best Tests

- PCR can be useful in diagnosis, although most disease is diagnosed clinically by typical appearance and distribution of lesions.
- The Tzanck smear is the most rapid and least expensive test. A smear is made of cells scraped from the base of the bullae that are stained and examined under the microscope for multinucleated giant cells. Infection with herpes simplex virus will appear identical.
- Viral culture may also be used.

▲▲ Management Pearls

- Patients with active vesicular lesions can spread the infection to immunocompromised hosts.
- Zoster is much less contagious than varicella.

Therapy

Antiviral therapy (acyclovir and prodrug forms), if administered in the first 48 to 72 h, can shorten the length and severity of the acute episode in adults. Because post zoster neuralgia is rare in children, conservative treatment is also appropriate. Aluminum acetate or Burrow soaks can help to alleviate crusted cutaneous symptoms. Observe for secondary bacterial infection.

Special Considerations in Infants

Herpes zoster in infants is usually due to in utero exposure to varicella. Although not FDA approved for children aged younger than 2 years, many practitioners treat infantile herpes zoster with oral acyclovir at 50 to 100 mg/kg/day for 5 to 7 days.

Suggested Readings

Bolognia JL, Jorizzo JL, Rapini RP, eds. *Dermatology*. Vol. 1. 2nd Ed. St Louis, MO: Mosby; 2008:1204–1208.

James WD, Berger TG, Elston DM, eds. *Andrews' Diseases of the Skin*. 10th Ed. Philadelphia, PA: WB Saunders; 2006:379–385.

Kurlran JG, Connelly BL, Lucky AW. Herpes zoster in the first year of life following postnatal exposure to varicella–zoster virus: Four case reports and a review of infantile herpes zoster. *Arch Dermatol*. 2004;140(10):1268–1272.

Nikkels AF, Nikkels-Tassoudji N, Piérard GE. Revisiting childhood herpes zoster. *Pediatr Dermatol*. 2004;21(1):18–23.

Intertrigo

Diagnosis Synopsis

Intertrigo is inflammation of approximating skin surfaces predominantly found in the perineum and neck creases, though any intertriginous area may be involved. Intertrigo is exacerbated by any condition that increases heat, wetness, and friction of opposing skin surfaces. Intertrigo is often complicated by superficial skin infection with yeast or bacteria. Intertrigo caused by cutaneous infection with streptococcus can be seen at the neck, axillae, inguinal fold, or perianal regions.

Look For

An erythematous lesion with serous discharge is the initial lesion, which may progress to maceration and crusting (Figs. 4-270–4-273). Fissuring may occur following erosion. Pustules or vesicles usually indicate secondary infec-

tion (*Candida*, *Staphylococcus*, or other). Any skin fold may be involved with intertrigo. In infants (or older adolescents/adults) who are obese, inflammation may occur in neck creases, in popliteal or antecubital fossae, as well as in the thigh and groin folds, and less commonly under pendulous breast or abdominal folds.

Diagnostic Pearls

Look at other skin folds of the body for similar lesions.

?? Differential Diagnosis and Pitfalls

- Streptococcal intertrigo of the neck, axillae, or inguinal folds manifests with intense, well-circumscribed erythema with moist erosions. A bacterial cause should be suspected if standard topical treatment is ineffective.

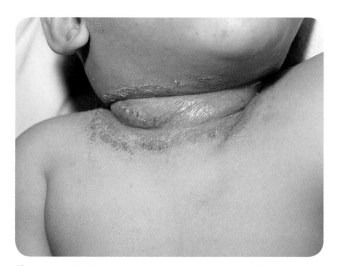

Figure 4-270 Intertrigo with crusting, peripheral scale, and vesicles requiring culture for *Staphylococcus*.

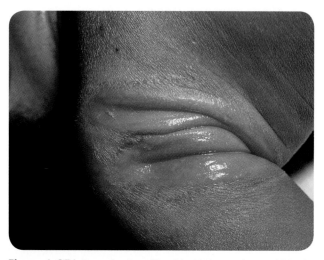

Figure 4-271 Intertrigo in axilla with shining erythema within the skin folds.

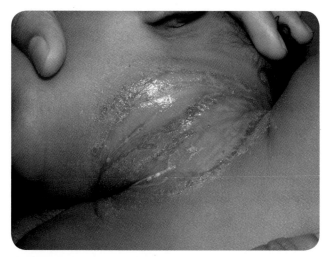

Figure 4-272 Intertrigo in a common location in an infant.

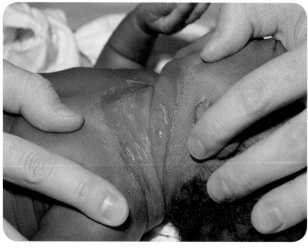

Figure 4-273 Intertrigo without redness beyond the lesion.

- Seborrheic dermatitis is usually seen on the scalp and forehead of infants, but it can be seen in skin folds and the diaper area.
- Candidiasis often involves the diaper area skin folds (whereas an irritant dermatitis will spare the skin folds). Look for satellite lesions.
- Langerhans cell histiocytosis—If involvement is widespread, includes petechiae/purpura, has associated hepatosplenomegaly, and/or standard treatments are not effective.

 Best Tests

- KOH preparation to look for yeast and a bacterial culture should be performed.
- If vesicles are present, a Tzanck smear should also be performed.

 Management Pearls

Be sure to examine all skin folds. If standard treatments are ineffective and cultures are negative, consider a skin biopsy.

Therapy

First-line treatment involves liberal use of barrier creams such as zinc oxide or petroleum jelly. Excessive swaddling leads to increased temperature and should be avoided as well. Antifungals are often helpful, as intertrigo is often colonized with Candida or other fungal organisms. In the case of bacterial superinfection, oral antibiotics are necessary. Low-potency topical steroids may be used for short periods as well as in conjunction with topical antifungals.

Suggested Readings

Honig PJ, Frieden IJ, Kim HJ, et al. Streptococcal intertrigo: An underrecognized condition in children. *Pediatrics*. 2003;112(6 Pt 1):1427–1429.

Nanda S, Reddy BS, Ramji S, et al. Analytical study of pustular eruptions in neonates. *Pediatr Dermatol*. 2002;19(3):210–215.

Diagnosis Synopsis

Pitted keratolysis (keratoma plantare sulcatum, ringed keratolysis) is a noninflammatory bacterial infection of the soles of the feet caused by the corynebacteria *Micrococcus sedentarius*, which produces a proteolytic enzyme that digests the stratum corneum. Those with excessive perspiration involving the feet during periods of hot, humid weather are most susceptible. Previously thought to affect mostly those living in tropical climates, the condition is now known to have a worldwide distribution. The plantar lesions often go unnoticed but are frequently malodorous.

Look For

A few or numerous shallow, rounded depressions or pits on the weight-bearing portions of the soles (Figs. 4-274–4-277). Lesions can coalesce to form furrows, and a background of maceration can be present.

Diagnostic Pearls

Noninflammatory, superficial, "punched-out," small pits are characteristic.

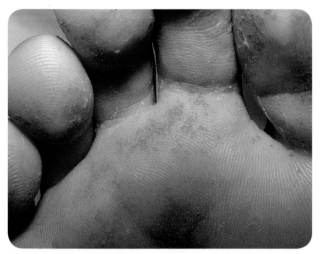

Figure 4-274 Pitted keratolysis with shallow erosions between toes and on weight-bearing skin.

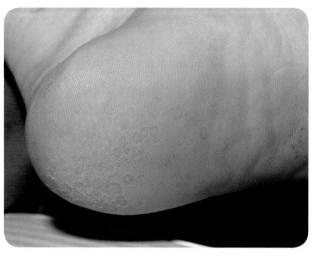

Figure 4-275 Pitted keratolysis on heel with large, superficial eroded islands.

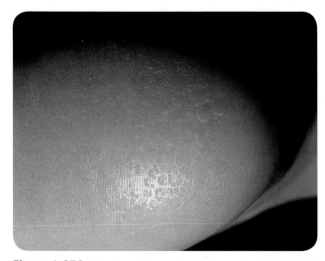

Figure 4-276 Pitted keratolysis with erosions not reflecting light as the intact skin does.

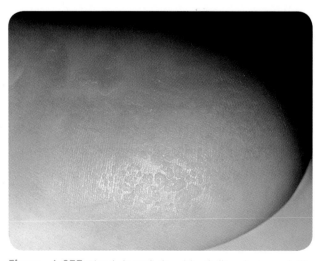

Figure 4-277 Pitted keratolysis with shallow honeycomb-like erosions.

Differential Diagnosis and Pitfalls

- Tinea pedis presents with scaly erythematous plagues. Hyphal elements can be demonstrated using a KOH preparation.
- There are no inflammatory lesions as seen in dyshidrotic eczema.
- Keratolysis exfoliativa is another noninflammatory asymptomatic condition that can affect the soles and presents with scaling in annular or circinate patterns. Some believe that this condition represents a phenotype of different processes (eczema, psoriasis, etc.).

✓ **Best Tests**

- This is a clinical diagnosis. Skin biopsy will reveal organisms in the walls and bases of punched-out defects in the stratum corneum.
- Organisms may be highlighted using methenamine sliver stain.
- Gram stain of stratum corneum shavings may also reveal the organism.

 Management Pearls

Keep the feet dry with frequent sock changes, and prescribe aluminum chloride 20% twice daily to reduce hyperhidrosis.

Therapy

Erythromycin 2% solution, clindamycin 1% solution, or benzoyl peroxide 5% gel twice daily for 2 to 4 weeks are effective treatments.

In those with associated severe hyperhidrosis, injection of botulinum toxin A may be helpful.

Suggested Readings

Bolognia JL, Jorizzo JL, Rapini RP, eds. *Dermatology*. Vol. 1. 2nd Ed. St Louis, MO: Mosby; 2008:1088–1089.

James WD, Berger TG, Elston DM, eds. *Andrews' Diseases of the Skin*. 10th Ed. Philadelphia, PA: WB Saunders; 2006:268–269.

Takama H, Tamada Y, Yano K, et al. Pitted keratolysis: Clinical manifestations in 53 cases. *Br J Dermatol*. 1997;137(2):282–285.

Striae

Diagnosis Synopsis

Striae (stretch marks) are common in all ages and are due to thinning or atrophic defects in the skin. They occur at sites of dermal connective tissue damage, usually when systemic or topical steroids have been used or when the skin stretches excessively. Various physiologic states, including puberty, pregnancy, growth spurts, rapid weight gain, obesity, or cortisol excess are associated with striae formation. In adolescent females, they are seen most frequently on the abdomen, thighs, buttocks, and breasts. Striae occurring in pregnancy are most common on the abdomen and breasts. In adolescent boys, they tend to occur on the thighs and lumbosacral region. While rarely symptomatic and without serious medical consequences, the appearance of striae is frequently distressing to patients.

Look For

Initially, look for thin; raised; red-, pink-, or purplish-hued; linear lesions in a longitudinal configuration, perpendicular to lines of skin tension (Figs. 4-278–4-281). The streaks may be several millimeters to 20 cm or more in length. Over time, the color fades, and linear streaks become more atrophic, finally appearing as a skin-colored or pearly-white wrinkle-like thinning of the skin.

When due to endogenous or exogenous corticosteroid excess, striae can be widespread.

Diagnostic Pearls

- Striae in unusual locations, such as the face or axillae, are likely due to topical application of steroids.
- Striae appear in specific directions depending on the area: hips—transverse, buttocks—oblique, lumbosacral region—transverse, breasts—radiated from the nipple, shoulders—oblique.

?? Differential Diagnosis and Pitfalls

- Anetoderma is caused by focal loss of elastic fibers within the dermis and present as flaccid, well-circumscribed areas of slack skin. Saclike protrusions can occasionally be observed in some lesions.
- Lichen sclerosus presents as flat, yellowish-white plaques surrounded by a red-, purple-, or violet-colored border.
- Linear focal elastosis (elastotic striae) is a rare condition that presents as asymptomatic atrophic yellow lines on the mid or lower back, thighs, arms, or breasts.
- Scars are raised, firm nodules or plaques at sites of previous trauma.

✓ Best Tests

This is a clinical diagnosis.

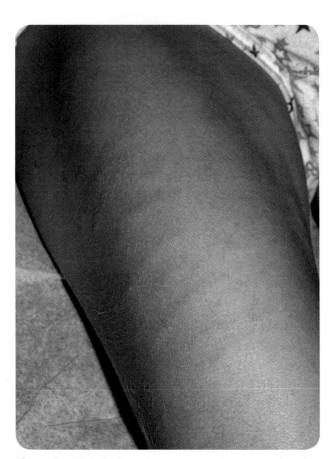

Figure 4-278 Striae in a raised, early stage in a common location.

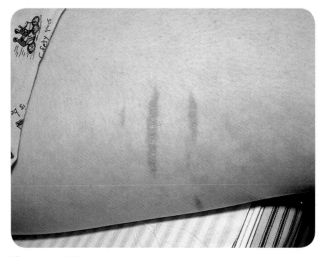

Figure 4-279 Striae in a common location.

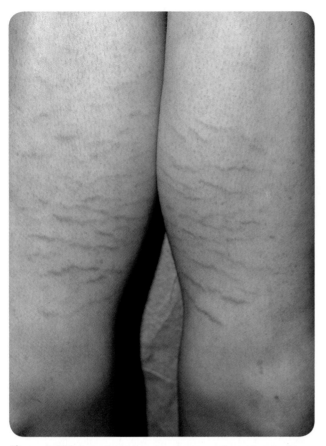

Figure 4-280 Striae in this location may occur after topical steroid use.

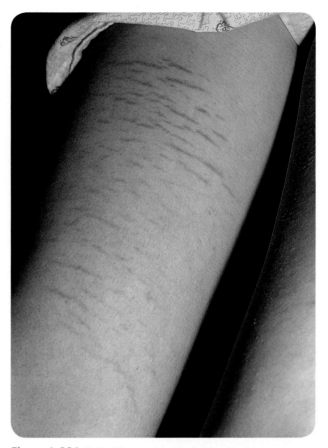

Figure 4-281 Striae. (Same patient as in Fig. 4-280.)

▲▲ Management Pearls

Patients should be informed that striae improve over months to years.

Therapy

Topical tretinoin 0.1% cream may improve appearance and potentially decrease the length and width of lesions if applied in early stages.

Pulsed dye laser has been used effectively to improve associated erythema within striae.

Suggested Readings

Bolognia JL, Jorizzo JL, Rapini RP, eds. *Dermatology*. Vol. 1. 2nd Ed. St Louis, MO: Mosby; 2008:1508–1509.

James WD, Berger TG, Elston DM, eds. *Andrews' Diseases of the Skin*. 10th Ed. Philadelphia, PA: WB Saunders; 2006:516–517.

Cellulitis

▪ Diagnosis Synopsis

Cellulitis is an inflammatory bacterial infection of subcutaneous tissues most often caused by *Streptococcus pyogenes, Staphylococcus aureus,* or *Haemophilus influenzae.* These bacteria invade through small cracks, fissures, or breaks in the skin. The clinical manifestations include rapidly progressive areas of skin edema, redness, heat, and pain with or without associated lymphangitis or adenopathy. Systemic symptoms of fever, malaise, and chills are common. In immunosuppressed individuals, the infection can spread to cause large abscesses, necrosis, and dissemination into blood. Predisposing factors include conditions that compromise the barrier function of the skin or weaken host defenses, such as obesity, trauma, or chronic edema.

Other causes of cellulitis include nongroup A β-hemolytic streptococci, *Pasteurella multocida* (usually acquired from animal bites) or, in the immunocompromised, rarely *Streptococcus pneumoniae, Neisseria meningitidis, Campylobacter jejuni, Bacteroides fragilis, Yersinia enterocolitica,* and *Cryptococcus.*

Although many cases of cellulitis are attributable to streptococci, it is important to be cognizant of the rising prevalence of MRSA. CA-MRSA (Community-associated MRSA) has increasingly been identified as the agent of skin and soft tissue infections in otherwise healthy individuals lacking the traditional risk factors for such infections (participation in contact sports, etc.).

◉ Look For

The initial infection shows mild redness that quickly progresses to tenderness and edema. Look for diffuse erythema, warmth, a tender plaque with peripheral enlargement, and lymphangitic streaking (Figs. 4-282–4-285). Superficial hemorrhage, necrosis, and blisters are common. Trauma or bite sites, such as a cat scratch, are typical predisposing factors. The extremities and the face are common sites.

●● Diagnostic Pearls

Distinguishing cellulitis from necrotizing fasciitis requiring immediate surgical intervention may be challenging. The following clinical features suggest a deep necrotizing infection:

- Constant pain that is often quite severe
- Presence of bullae
- Skin necrosis or ecchymosis that precedes necrosis
- Gas in the soft tissues
- Edema extending beyond areas of erythema
- Systemic toxicity (fever, delirium, renal failure, hypotension, and tachycardia)
- Cutaneous anesthesia
- Rapid spread despite antibiotic therapy

?? Differential Diagnosis and Pitfalls

Some of the most common masqueraders are the following:

- Contact dermatitis
- Insect bite reactions

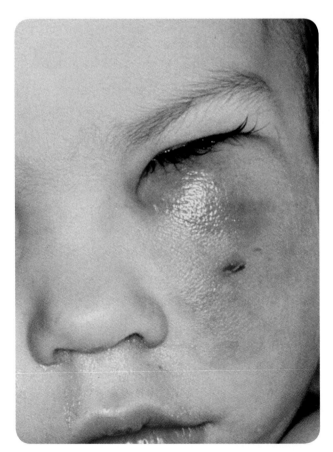

Figure 4-282 Cellulitis due to a human bite with edema and redness.

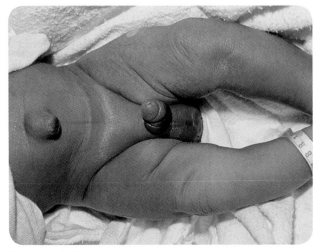

Figure 4-283 Cellulitis in an infant, with involvement of legs, genitals, and lower abdomen.

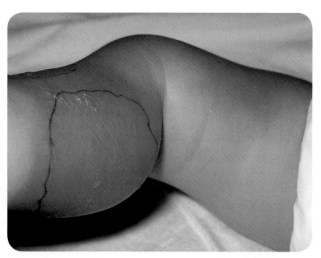

Figure 4-284 Cellulitis is often fairly well demarcated, as in this lesion on the lower leg.

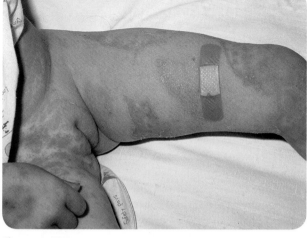

Figure 4-285 Cellulitis in a patient with acute lymphocytic leukemia, thrombocytopenia, and staphylococcal infection.

- Necrotizing fasciitis
- Eosinophilic cellulitis
- Deep venous thrombosis
- Thrombophlebitis
- Panniculitis
- Sweet syndrome
- Erythema nodosum
- Erysipelas

✓ Best Tests

- The diagnosis of cellulitis is made primarily on clinical appearance and history.
- Blood cultures are of little utility in patients lacking signs of systemic toxicity (tachycardia and hypotension). Needle aspiration of lesions and culture of skin biopsy specimens are also unnecessary in straightforward cases. These diagnostic modalities may prove more fruitful in individuals who are slow to respond to initial treatment or those with diabetes, malignancy, immunodeficiency, or obvious nidus of infection.
- Culture any vesicular fluid or pus, if present. Sensitivities should be performed on all *S. aureus* isolates to determine antibiotic resistance. Consider oropharyngeal, nasal, and conjunctival cultures if there is facial involvement. Toe web cultures of patients with lower extremity cellulitis and tinea pedis may yield a causative organism in older children.

▲▲ Management Pearls

- While most cases can be managed on an outpatient basis, severe cases or facial or orbital cellulitis require hospitalization.

- Patients should be instructed to keep the affected area elevated whenever possible. In patients with recurring cellulitis, treatment aims should include aggressive management of any underlying predisposing condition such as tinea pedis or other chronic skin disease. Reports of the efficacy of prophylactic antibiotics in such cases are mixed.
- Given the prevalence of MRSA, maintain a high index of suspicion and make the initial choice of empiric antibiotic therapy accordingly. It is helpful to be aware of patterns of antimicrobial resistance within your community.
- **Precautions:** Standard and contact (isolate patient, wear gloves and a gown, limit patient transport, and avoid sharing patient-care equipment).
- In the United States, infections due to MRSA, Vancomycin resistant *S. aureus* (VRSA), vancomycin-intermediate *S. aureus* (VISA), vancomycin-resistant *Enterococcus* sp., or vancomycin-resistant *S. epidermidis* are reportable in most states.
- Per the CDC, infections due to VISA and VRSA are nationally notifiable via the National Notifiable Diseases Surveillance System (NNDSS).
- In the United States, infections due to invasive Group A *Streptococcus* are reportable in all states **except** AL, CO, MS, MT, ND, OR, and UT.
- Per the CDC, infections due to invasive Group A *Streptococcus* are nationally notifiable via the NNDSS.

Therapy

Mild infections in otherwise healthy patients can be managed initially on an outpatient basis with close follow-up and oral antibiotics.

For *H. influenzae*:

- Cefotaxime 100 to 200 mg/kg/day p.o. divided three times daily for 7 days.
- Ceftriaxone 50 to 100 mg/kg/day IM/IV daily for 7 to 14 days.
- Chloramphenicol 75 to 100 mg/kg/day p.o. divided four times daily for 7 to 14 days.

For *S. aureus*:

- Dicloxacillin or cephalexin 25 mg/kg/day divided three to four times daily for 10 to 14 days.
- Patients should be assessed frequently (every 24 to 72 h) to determine appropriate response to therapy.

For infections in which an organism cannot be identified:

- Cefazolin 50 to 100 mg/kg/day, not to exceed 6 g/day p.o. divided three times daily for 10 days.
- Patients exhibiting signs or symptoms of systemic involvement or with rapidly progressing infections or significant comorbidities (i.e., immunosuppressed) should be hospitalized for observation and parenteral antibiotic administration.

Suggested regimens include the following:
Nafcillin or oxacillin 100 to 150 mg/kg/day IV divided into four doses or cefazolin 50 mg/kg/day IV divided into three doses.

Standard cephalosporins and penicillins are of no benefit in treating MRSA. In recent studies, CA-MRSA has demonstrated a high degree of susceptibility to trimethoprim–sulfamethoxazole and rifampin (100%), clindamycin (95%), and tetracycline (92%). Inducible resistance to clindamycin should be excluded by performing a D-zone disk-diffusion test on any isolates.

Possible antibiotic regimens for MRSA include:

- Clindamycin 25 to 40 mg/kg/day IV in three doses or 10 to 20 mg/kg/day p.o. divided three times daily
- Trimethoprim–sulfamethoxazole 8 to 12 mg/kg/day p.o. divided twice daily

Critically ill patients with MRSA or suspected MRSA should receive vancomycin or linezolid:

- Vancomycin 40 mg/kg/day IV divided into four doses or linezolid 10 mg/kg IV or p.o. every 12 h

Special Considerations in Infants

Neonates (especially preterm) are relatively immunocompromised and are at risk for perinatally transmitted infections. *H. influenzae* may cause plaques of cellulitis on the face in young children, but the incidence of this infection in Western countries has markedly decreased by the Hib vaccine. Look for nidus of infection at umbilicus or circumcision site. In neonates, a complete sepsis evaluation is mandatory. In addition to intravenous antibiotics for typical cutaneous organisms, neonates should also receive parenteral therapy with ampicillin and gentamicin.

Suggested Readings

Bolognia JL, Jorizzo JL, Rapini RP, eds. *Dermatology*. Vol. 1. 2nd Ed. St Louis, MO: Mosby; 2008:1084–1085.

Gorwitz RJ. A review of community-associated methicillin-resistant *Staphylococcus aureus* skin and soft tissue infections. *Pediatr Infect Dis J*. 2008;27:1–7.

Stevens DL, Bisno Al, Chambers HF, et al. Practice guidelines for the diagnosis and management of skin and soft-tissue infections. *Clin Infect Dis*. 2005;41(10):1373–1406.

◼◼ Diagnosis Synopsis

There are numerous cutaneous drug reaction patterns in the skin, many of which occur in the children. One recent review article found that the five most common types of cutaneous drug reactions in children are exanthematous, urticarial, fixed drug eruption, photosensitive, and serum sicknesslike reaction. Other drug reactions include acute generalized exanthematous pustulosis, acneiform and pseudoporphyria (not seen in neonates), and leukocytoclastic vasculitis. More serious reactions such as drug hypersensitivity, Stevens–Johnson syndrome (SJS), and toxic epidermal necrosis (TEN) occur as well.

Drug-induced eruptions should always be included in the differential of any diagnostic workup for skin abnormalities, dermatitis, or changes. Reactions occur as an adverse effect of a drug, often of unknown etiology and mechanism. Possible causes include metabolic reaction, immune response complications, manifestations of coexistent disease, or interactions of other medications. Sulfonamides, acetaminophen, ibuprofen, amoxicillin, cephalosporins, and other antibiotics are the most common cause of drug eruptions in this age group.

Exanthematous or morbilliform eruptions are the most common of all medication-induced eruptions. They consist of red, blanching macules and papules that begin on the head and trunk and spread symmetrically caudally and to the proximal extremities. In severe eruptions, lesions coalesce and may lead to generalized erythroderma. Palms, soles, and mucous membranes may also be involved. Pruritus is common, and fever may occur in more severe reactions. Onset is usually within 7 to 14 days of initiating a medication, although it is not uncommon for exanthematous penicillin reactions to develop after 2 weeks from the onset of exposure. Scarlatiniform (pinpoint papular) and sand-papery-feeling erythematous lesions may also be caused by drugs. In darker-skinned children, postinflammatory hyperpigmentation or hypopigmentation may take weeks to months to resolve.

Almost any oral agent can cause an exanthematous reaction, but it is most commonly seen with the use of antibiotics (penicillins and sulfas), allopurinol, phenytoin, barbiturates, chlorpromazine, carbamazepine, gold, d-penicillamine, captopril, naproxen, and piroxicam, among others.

◉ Look For

Red papules, erythema, urticaria, vesicles and bullae, pustules, plaques as well as edema, purpura, and petechiae following the use of a new medication (Figs. 4-286–4-292). Overall, the presentation is variable depending on the type of reaction.

●● Diagnostic Pearls

- Itching is commonly seen in older children but is not a reliable sign in infants.
- Transplacental transfer of drugs and drugs in maternal milk have both been reported and should be considered.

?? Differential Diagnosis and Pitfalls

- Viral exanthem
- Bacterial infection

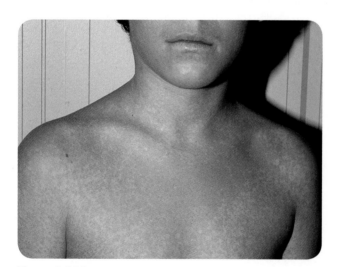

Figure 4-286 Exanthematous drug eruption due to phenytoin.

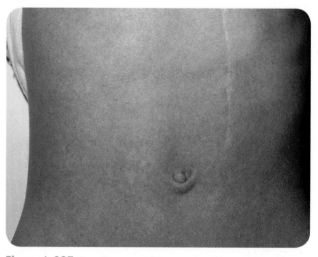

Figure 4-287 Exanthematous drug eruption due to phenytoin.

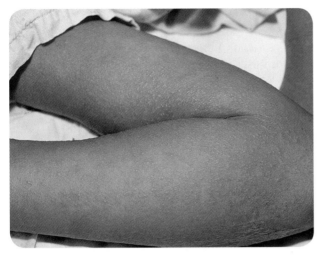

Figure 4-288 Exanthematous drug eruption due to phenytoin.

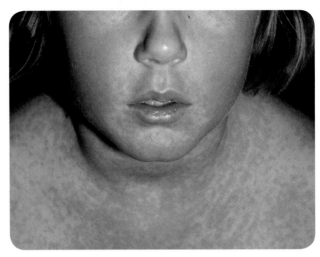

Figure 4-289 Exanthematous drug eruption due to penicillamine used for Wilson disease.

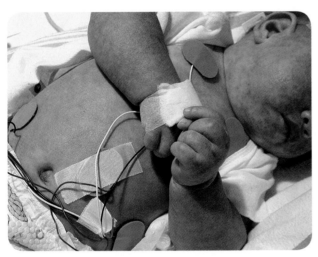

Figure 4-290 Generalized drug eruption due to phenobarbital.

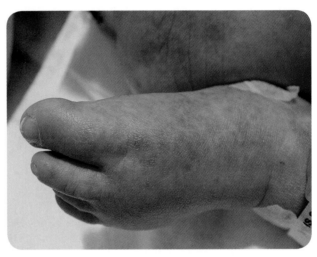

Figure 4-291 Generalized drug eruption due to phenobarbital.

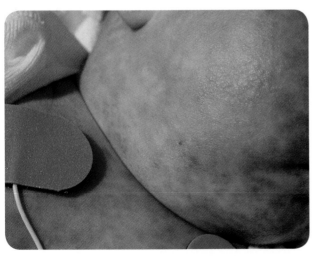

Figure 4-292 Generalized drug eruption due to phenobarbital.

- Henoch–Schönlein purpura
- Hemolytic uremic syndrome
- Acropustulosis
- Porphyria

✓ Best Tests

- A skin biopsy is helpful.
- A CBC may show eosinophilia.

▲▲ Management Pearls

The most important step is to identify and discontinue the offending agent.

Therapy

If possible, all medications should be discontinued. If all of the medications cannot be discontinued, then any non-essential medications should be stopped. For more severe reactions (SJS/TEN) the patient may need to be admitted to a burn unit.

Oral antihistamines can be used for pruritus if present. Topical corticosteroids may be helpful for localized reactions.

Suggested Readings

Segal AR, Doherty KM, Leggott J, et al. Cutaneous reactions to drugs in children. *Pediatrics*. 2007;120(4):e1082–e1096.

Sehgal VN, Srivastava G. Erythroderma/generalized exfoliative dermatitis in pediatric practice: An overview. *Int J Dermatol*. 2006;45(7):831–839.

Diagnosis Synopsis

The drug hypersensitivity syndrome (DHS) is a severe skin reaction with systemic manifestations. It is an idiosyncratic reaction consisting of fever, rash, and internal organ involvement, most typically hepatitis. The acronym DRESS, for drug reaction with eosinophilia and systemic symptoms, was proposed as a more specific term in 1996. However, because only 60% to 70% of patients demonstrate eosinophilia, many have suggested using DHS to avoid confusion. The specific underlying mechanisms of this condition are unknown, and they likely vary between patients and specific drugs. Defects in the detoxification of anticonvulsants and sulfonamides have been demonstrated in patients with DHS. HHV-6 and HHV-7 reactivations have also been demonstrated in many of these patients, although the pathogenic role of this viral reactivation, if any, is yet to be determined.

The most common drugs causing this syndrome are anticonvulsants such as phenytoin, carbamazepine, phenobarbital, and lamotrigine. Sulfonamide antibiotics, allopurinol, metronidazole, and abacavir (Ziagen) are also common causes. Any new drug taken in the preceding 2 months is considered suspect. The incidence of DHS has been estimated to be between 1 in 1,000 to 1 in 10,000 exposures to drugs such as sulfonamides and anticonvulsants. Clinically, symptoms develop 2 to 6 weeks after initiation of the responsible drug. If a patient is rechallenged with the drug, the reaction will occur within 24 h.

Look For

The condition frequently starts as a macular or morbilliform eruption beginning on the face and spreading to the upper trunk and extremities in a symmetrical fashion, which evolves through a dusky phase with confluent, papular lesions that are pruritic (Figs. 4-293–4-296). Periorbital and facial edema are characteristics and are found early along with cervical lymphadenopathy and pharyngitis. Additional cutaneous findings include vesicles and tense bullae induced by intense dermal edema as well as pustules, erythroderma, and purpuric lesions.

Eosinophilia and/or a mononucleosis-like atypical lymphocytosis are commonly observed. The liver is the most commonly and severely affected visceral site. Myocarditis, interstitial pneumonitis, interstitial nephritis, encephalitis, myositis, pancreatitis, and thyroiditis have all been observed. Cutaneous and visceral involvement may persist for several months after discontinuation of the offending drug. The cutaneous lesions of DHS will desquamate and often leave areas of hyperpigmentation and/or hypopigmentation that may persist for several months to 1 to 2 years. Hypothyroidism may develop several months after the acute phase of the illness.

Diagnostic Pearls

- The triad of fever, rash, and internal organ involvement is characteristic of the syndrome.
- Liver, hematologic, or renal systems are the most common internal systems involved.
- Facial edema, a frequent finding, is considered to be a hallmark of DHS.

?? Differential Diagnosis and Pitfalls

- The main problem is thinking that this syndrome is something else. It is often confused with mononucleosis because of the presence of atypical lymphocytes and may similarly be confused with leukemia or lymphoma. Patients can have very striking lymphadenopathy that leads one to the incorrect lymphoma diagnosis. Viral syndromes can mimic these reactions early in the course.

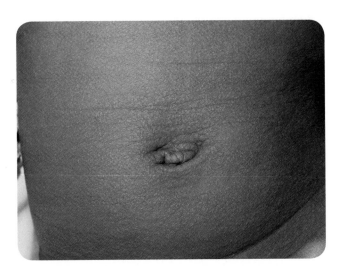

Figure 4-293 DHS (DRESS syndrome) due to phenytoin.

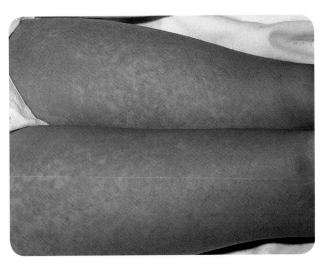

Figure 4-294 DHS (DRESS syndrome) due to phenytoin.

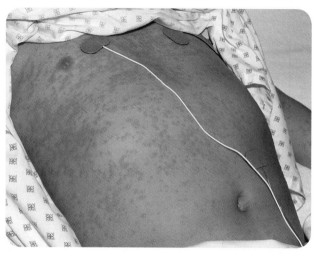

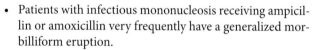

Figure 4-295 DHS (DRESS syndrome) with multiple discrete and confluent papules.

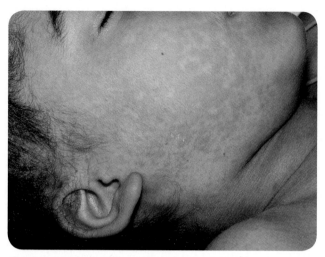

Figure 4-296 DHS (DRESS syndrome) due to phenytoin.

- Patients with infectious mononucleosis receiving ampicillin or amoxicillin very frequently have a generalized morbilliform eruption.
- The clinical appearance of DHS may at times overlap with toxic epidermal necrolysis (TEN) or Stevens–Johnson syndrome (SJS). These patients are best classified as having TEN or SJS.

✓ Best Tests

- Most importantly, look for internal organ involvement. Liver function tests, a CBC with differential (for eosinophilia), and urinalysis are the easiest and most useful tests.
- Other tests can be directed by symptoms such as coughing directing to chest X-ray.
- A skin biopsy in DHS typically shows a dense lymphocytic infiltrate in the superficial dermis with eosinophils and dermal edema.
- Evidence of keratinocyte necrosis is more indicative of erythema multiforme, SJS, or TEN.

▲▲ Management Pearls

- The inciting drug must be stopped.
- The search for systemic involvement is very important, especially liver involvement as manifested by increased serum transaminases. It is critical to recognize the reaction early.

Therapy

Most patients will recover spontaneously although slowly with discontinuation of the offending drug. Corticosteroids are the first line of therapy for DHS. High-potency topical steroids may be helpful for treatment of skin manifestations in mild cases. Systemic corticosteroids (1 to 2 mg/kg of prednisone) are indicated in patients with significant visceral disease. Inflammation in the lungs and heart has been shown to be the most steroid responsive, while kidney and liver involvement appear to be more resistant to treatment. Relapses can occur with tapering of steroids. Cases more consistent with TEN are best managed by admission to a burn unit, supportive care, and consideration of treatment with intravenous immunoglobulin.

Suggested Readings

Bolognia JL, Jorizzo JL, Rapini RP, eds. *Dermatology*. Vol. 1. 2nd Ed. St Louis, MO: Mosby; 2008:343–344.

James WD, Berger TG, Elston DM, eds. *Andrews' Diseases of the Skin*. 10th Ed. Philadelphia, PA: WB Saunders; 2006:117–118.

Gianotti–Crosti Syndrome

Diagnosis Synopsis

Gianotti–Crosti syndrome (papular acrodermatitis of childhood, papulovesicular acrolated syndrome) is a self-limiting dermatosis likely triggered by viral infection.

The eruption of Gianotti–Crosti syndrome typically lasts 3 to 4 weeks and is usually seen in preschool children but can be seen in children aged up to 13 years. It is most commonly diagnosed in children aged 6 months to 14 years. The lesions can last up to 8 weeks before resolving spontaneously.

Agents thought to be responsible for the typical eruption include hepatitis B virus, hepatitis A and C viruses, cytomegalovirus (CMV), Epstein–Barr virus (EBV), enteroviruses, rotavirus, respiratory syncytial virus, parvovirus B19, vaccinia virus, rubella virus, HIV-1, and parainfluenza virus. The syndrome has also been observed following immunizations against poliovirus, diphtheria, pertussis, Japanese encephalitis, influenza, and hepatitis B virus and measles (together). The clinical features of the syndrome are identical, independent of the triggering agent.

With widespread immunization, most cases of Gianotti–Crosti syndrome seen in the United States, Canada, Europe, and India are not associated with hepatitis B virus infection. Epstein–Barr virus is by far the most common cause in the United States.

Look For

Symmetrically distributed monomorphous, pink–brown, flat-topped papules or papulovesicles 1 to 10 mm in diameter on the face, extensor limbs, and buttocks (Figs. 4-297–4-300). Lesions initially appear on the buttocks and spread distally. The torso is typically spared or minimally affected, and scale is absent. Lesions may be pruritic. Mucous membranes are not involved.

Additional manifestations of the disease include low-grade fever, enlarged inguinal and axillary lymph nodes, and an enlarged spleen. When hepatitis B virus is implicated as a trigger, acute viral hepatitis occurs at the same time or 1 to 2 weeks after the onset of the skin eruption. Hepatomegaly may be prominent in these cases.

Diagnostic Pearls

Monomorphic, erythematous to brown papules involve the face, buttocks, and extensor extremities. Relative sparing of the torso and popliteal fossae.

Differential Diagnosis and Pitfalls

- Erythema multiforme presents with targetoid lesions, often best seen on the palms and soles. Patient may have coexisting herpes orolabialis.
- Henoch–Schönlein purpura presents with palpable purpura over the bilateral lower extremities.
- Lichen planus typically presents with pruritic, flat-topped, polygonal, violaceous papules on the volar wrists and

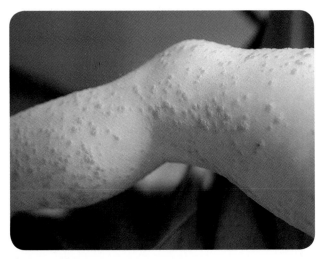

Figure 4-297 Gianotti–Crosti syndrome with multiple red and flesh-colored papules at the same stage in evolution.

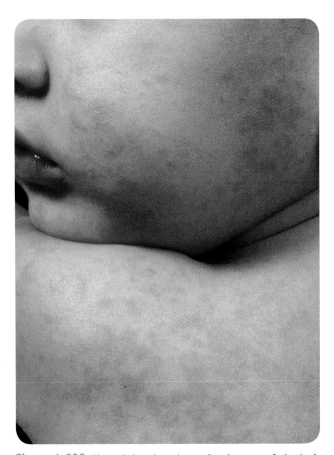

Figure 4-298 Gianotti–Crosti syndrome. Involvement of cheeks is common.

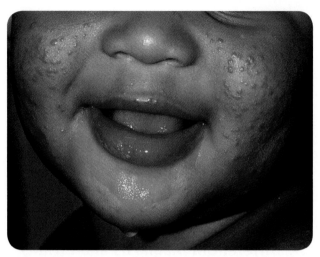

Figure 4-299 Gianotti–Crosti syndrome with monomorphic, dome-shaped papules favoring the cheeks.

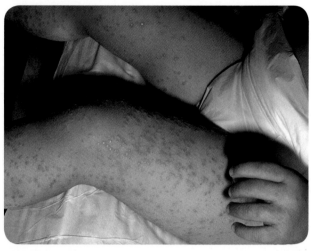

Figure 4-300 Gianotti–Crosti syndrome. Monomorphic, symmetric eruption commonly involves the extremities.

ankles. Mucosal and nail findings frequently aid in the clinical diagnosis.

- Inflamed lesions of molluscum contagiosum may mimic those seen in Gianotti–Crosti syndrome but tend to be concentrated within the groin, axillae, as well as antecubital and popliteal fossae. The presence of noninflamed molluscum lesions is a helpful clue.
- A detailed history is helpful in distinguishing this entity from a drug eruption.
- Id reaction (autoeczematization) secondary to a primary severe inflammatory dermatosis elsewhere (allergic contact dermatitis, dermatophytosis, and bacterial infection).

✓ Best Tests

Liver function tests and hepatitis serologies may be performed if the patient has not been immunized against hepatitis B virus previously.

▲▲ Management Pearls

- The eruption of Gianotti–Crosti syndrome spontaneously resolves, usually over a period of 3 to 4 weeks. Associated lymphadenopathy may persist for 2 to 3 months.
- Investigate for triggers such as viral hepatitis, CMV, and EBV, only if indicated.

Therapy

The treatment for Gianotti–Crosti syndrome is supportive. No treatment appears to shorten the course of the disease.

Suggested Readings

Brandt O, Abeck D, Gianotti R, et al. Gianotti–Crosti syndrome. *J Am Acad Dermatol.* 2006;54:136–145.

Diagnosis Synopsis

Hand-foot-and-mouth disease (HFM) is ordinarily an acute self-limited viral disease caused by one of the enteroviruses. The most common cause of HFM is Coxsackie virus A16, though HFM can be caused by enterovirus 71 or other enteroviruses. It primarily occurs in children aged 2 to 10 years, but adults may also be affected. The incubation period is short, from 3 to 6 days, and prodromes may be absent. The illness begins with a mild fever with temperature up to 38°C (101°F), sore throat, sore mouth, cough, headache, malaise, diarrhea, and occasionally arthralgia. One or two days after the beginning of fever, small oral vesicles develop.

The disease is highly contagious and often spreads from child to child and then from child to adult. Epidemic outbreaks usually occur from June to October. Though HFM is typically a relatively benign and self-limited disease, life-threatening complications such as encephalitis may rarely occur. Such complications were seen in outbreaks of HFM due to enterovirus 71 in Malaysia and Taiwan in 1997 and 1998, respectively, and during the spring of 2008 in China. Thousands of children were ill with HFM in the China epidemic, and more than 30 deaths were reported.

Look For

Small macules and papules on the oropharynx, which develop into 1 to 3 mm vesicles and rather rapidly ulcerate. Lesions develop a shallow yellow-gray base and a red areola. Oral lesions involve the buccal mucosa, tongue, soft palate, and gingival (Fig. 4-301). Lesions on extremities typically involve the palms and soles (Fig. 4-302). They begin as erythematous macules and vesiculate to produce 3- to 7-mm oval or elliptical vesicles surrounded by a red halo. The dorsal

surfaces of the fingers and toes are less frequently affected (Figs. 4-303 and 4-304).

Diagnostic Pearls

Individual oval or elliptical cutaneous vesicles run parallel to skin lines (dermatoglyphics).

?? Differential Diagnosis and Pitfalls

- The distribution of lesions as well as the morphology of individual lesions helps to differentiate it from cases of varicella.
- Dyshidrotic eczema is a more chronic dermatitis that presents as pruritic deep-seated vesicles involving the sides of the fingers.
- Erythema multiforme minor presents with targetoid lesions as opposed to the oval or elliptical vesicles seen in HFM. Patients frequently have coexisting herpes orolabialis.

For oral lesions consider

- Herpes stomatitis
- Aphthous ulcers
- Streptococcal infection
- *Candida*

For lesions on the hands consider

- Meningococcemia
- Rocky mountain spotted fever
- Subacute bacterial endocarditis
- Gonococcemia
- Disseminated herpes simplex/zoster
- Papular acrodermatitis of childhood

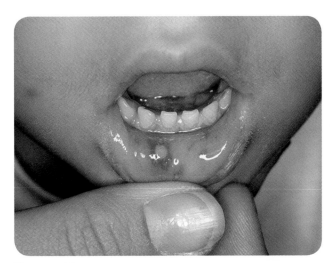

Figure 4-301 HFM with discrete ulcers on an erythematous base.

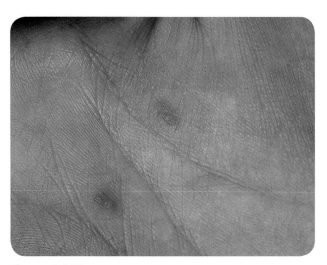

Figure 4-302 HFM with palmar vesicles with red rims oriented along dermatoglyphics.

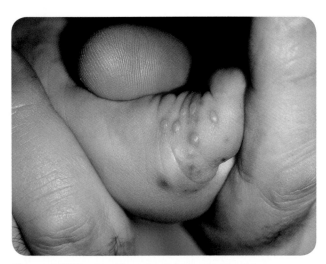

Figure 4-303 HFM with oval vesicles on the lateral foot.

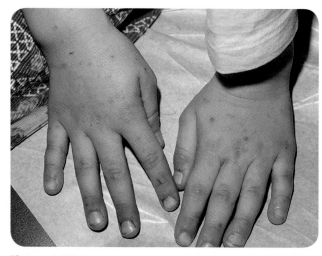

Figure 4-304 HFM. Discrete, flaccid vesicles with erythematous halos.

 Best Tests

Virus may be uncovered from vesicles. Given that HFM-associated CNS involvement has not yet been described in cases caused by Coxsackie A16, discrimination of viral types may be helpful in the setting of an HFM epidemic. However, this ordinarily self-limited condition is diagnosed clinically, and routine diagnostic testing with viral culture or serology is not needed.

▲▲ Management Pearls

This is a self-limited viral infection that needs to be treated only symptomatically.

Therapy

Supportive therapy and reassurance are generally all that are required. Encourage adequate hydration. Oral pain may interfere with alimentation. Therefore, judicious use of oral topical anesthetics may be needed.

Viscous lidocaine (Xylocaine 2% topical solution) may be applied directly with a swab to oral ulcers several times daily, as needed, for pain.

Antipyretics and oral analgesics (e.g., acetaminophen and ibuprofen) can be used to manage fever and arthralgias, if present.

Suggested Readings

Bolognia JL, Jorizzo JL, Rapini RP. *Dermatology*. Vol. 1. 2nd Ed. St Louis, MO: Mosby; 2008:1220.

James WD, Berger TG, Elston DM, eds. *Andrews' Diseases of the Skin*. 10th Ed. Philadelphia, PA: WB Saunders; 2006:398.

Wolff K, Goldsmith LA, Katz SI, et al., eds. *Fitzpatrick's Dermatology in General Medicine*. Vol. 2. 7th Ed. New York, NY: McGraw-Hill; 2008:1867–1869.

Henoch–Schönlein Purpura (HSP)

Diagnosis Synopsis

Henoch–Schönlein purpura (HSP) is an idiopathic, cutaneous small-vessel vasculitis characterized by IgA deposition in vessel walls. The disease occurs mostly in children, with a peak incidence at 5 to 6 years of age. The incidence of HSP is estimated to be approximately 10 in 100,000 children per year. A history of preceding upper respiratory tract infection is frequently elicited. Patients may experience a 2 to 3 week history of fever, headache, myalgias, arthralgias, and abdominal pain that precedes the skin eruption.

Extracutaneous manifestations include arthritis, gastrointestinal bleeding, pulmonary hemorrhage, and nephritis. Renal involvement is typically mild and self-limited with transient microscopic hematuria and minimal proteinuria. However, approximately 2% of patients progress to end-stage renal disease.

Consensus criteria for the diagnosis of HSP includes palpable purpura plus at least one of

- Diffuse abdominal pain
- Acute arthritis or arthralgias
- Renal involvement
- A skin biopsy showing IgA deposition

Look For

Erythematous macules and papules or urticarial lesions that quickly evolve into purpura within 24h (Figs. 4-305–4-308). Vesicles, bullae, and necrotic ulcers may also be seen. Lesions are symmetrically distributed over the buttocks, distal legs, and extensor extremities, but they may occasionally involve the trunk and face. Individual lesions resolve with hyperpigmentation over 5 to 7 days, but recurrent crops tend to appear over a period of 6 to 16 weeks.

Diagnostic Pearls

- The spread of purpura to the upper parts of the trunk portends a higher likelihood of renal involvement. In patients with severe abdominal pain, consider an acute surgical abdomen, intussusception, or paralytic ileus.
- Look for linear purpura in areas of externally applied pressure: elastic from top of sock on legs, wrinkles of hospital bed sheets on back in recumbent patient, etc.

?? Differential Diagnosis and Pitfalls

- A finding of palpable purpura suggests vasculitis (causes include infections, drugs, connective tissue disease, or malignancy). Children with HSP are usually systemically well, and these alternative etiologies should be strongly considered and evaluated for in the systemically unwell child.
- Erythema multiforme presents with target lesions with a predilection for acral surfaces. Patients often have coexisting herpes orolabialis.
- Patients with systemic lupus erythematosus (SLE) may also develop purpuric skin lesions, arthritis, and nephritis. Patients with HSP lack photosensitivity, though, as seen in SLE.
- Acute hemorrhagic edema of infancy can have a similar clinical appearance in the skin, but it presents in children aged between 4 months to 2 years, lacks systemic involvement, and resolves without sequelae within 1 to 3 weeks.
- Patients with other cutaneous small vessel vasculitides (Kawasaki disease, Wegener granulomatosis, Churg–Strauss syndrome, microscopic polyangiitis, or essential cryoglobulinemia) may also present with palpable purpura and systemic symptoms. Unlike these vasculitides, direct immunofluorescence of skin biopsies will reveal

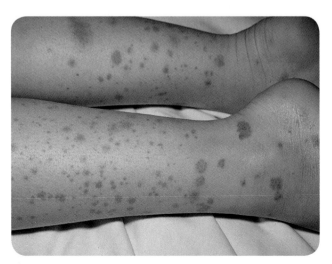

Figure 4-305 HSP with symmetric petechial and purpuric papules.

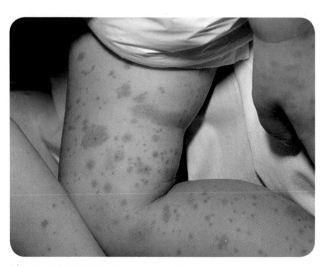

Figure 4-306 HSP with some lesions in a linear group due to external pressure.

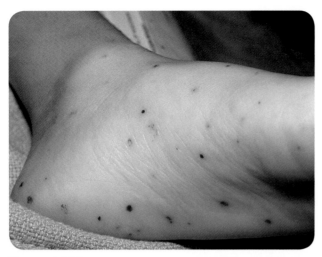

Figure 4-307 HSP with palpable purpura and petechiae with erythematous halos on a sole.

perivascular IgA deposition and basic immunologic investigations (ANA, dsDNA, ANCA, immunoglobulins, C3, and C4) will usually be normal in HSP.

- Drug therapy for prodromal lesions will raise the possibility of a drug eruption.

✓ Best Tests

- There is no specific laboratory test shown to help establish the diagnosis of HSP. Laboratory testing should be used to exclude other diagnoses and establish the extent of organ involvement. Leukocytosis, elevated ESR, hematuria, proteinuria, and positive stool Hemoccult test are consistent with HSP.
- Skin biopsy shows leukocytoclastic vasculitis, and direct immunofluorescence from lesional skin shows IgA deposits within blood vessel walls.

▲▲ Management Pearls

The long-term prognosis in patients with HSP is associated with the presence or absence of renal disease.

Therapy

HSP is generally benign and self-limited. Treatment is usually supportive. Corticosteroids may be effective in treating abdominal pain and arthritis, although reliable data on their effect on purpura, duration of the illness, or in mitigating potential long-term renal disease is lacking. Several reports point to a possible benefit of high-dose corticosteroids alone or in combination with other immunosuppressive agents in patients with HSP with progressive renal disease.

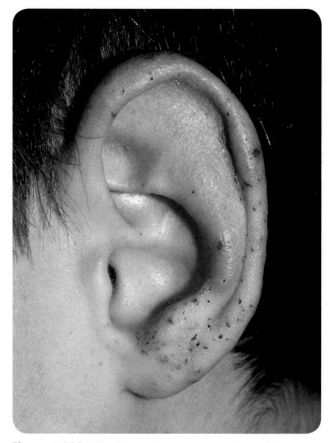

Figure 4-308 HSP with erosions, purpura, and petechiae on the helix of the ear.

Suggested Readings

Bolognia JL, Jorizzo JL, Rapini RP. *Dermatology* Vol. 1. 2nd Ed. St Louis, MO: Mosby; 2008:351–353.

Gibson KL, Amamoo MA, Primack WA. *Pediatrics*. 2008;121(4):870–871, author reply 871–872.

James WD, Berger TG, Elston DM, eds. *Andrews' Diseases of the Skin*. 10th Ed. Philadelphia, PA: WB Saunders; 2006:832–834.

Ozen S, Ruperto N, Dillon MJ, et al. EULAR/PReS endorsed consensus criteria for the classification of childhood vasculitides. *Ann Rheum Dis*. 2006;65(7):936–941.

Tizard EJ, Hamilton-Ayres MJ. Henoch Schonlein purpura. *Arch Dis Child Educ Pract Ed*. 2008;93:1–8.

Weiss PF, Feinstein JA, Luan X, et al. Effects of corticosteroid on Henoch-Schönlein purpura: A systematic review. *Pediatrics*. 2007;120(5):1079–1087.

■■ Diagnosis Synopsis

Kawasaki disease (KD), or mucocutaneous lymph node syndrome, is an idiopathic, small-vessel vasculitis characterized by fever and mucocutaneous inflammation. Although usually self-limited, potentially life-threatening coronary artery aneurysms may develop in 20% to 25% of children without treatment (versus <5% with appropriate therapy). Mortality most often occurs within the first weeks to a year after KD due to ischemic heart disease caused by myointimal proliferation within persistent aneurysms. The disease occurs primarily in children aged younger than 6 years.

The classic case definition of KD is

Fever lasting at least 5 days

Plus the presence of at least four of the following principal clinical criteria:

- Bilateral bulbar conjunctival injection without exudate
- Oral mucosa changes: cracked lips, "strawberry tongue," or diffuse erythema of the mucosa
- Changes in the extremities: erythema, induration, or periungual peeling
- Exanthem
- Cervical lymphadenopathy (>1.5 cm diameter)

◉ Look For

The classic case definition of KD should be used as a guideline to increase awareness of KD and prevent over diagnosis. However, one should remember that (i) the principal clinical criteria are all typically not present at a single point of time and (ii) children will often present with "incomplete" KD in which criteria are not fulfilled but coronary artery abnormalities do develop. Therefore, all suspected cases should be diagnosed based on (i) ruling out alternative diagnoses; (ii) assessment of principal clinical criteria over time; and (iii) supportive clinical features and laboratory data.

Principal Clinical Criteria

- Fever: Remittent and high spiking.
- Extremity changes: Erythema or firm induration of the palms and soles that may be painful is typical in the acute phase. Desquamation occurs 2 to 3 weeks after disease onset (Figs. 4-309 and 4-310).
- Exanthem: Within 5 days of fever onset, an erythematous, diffuse, nonspecific maculopapular eruption occurs, usually with accentuation in the perineal region. Occasionally, the rash is urticarial, scarlatiniform, erythema multiforme-like, or micropustular (Fig. 4-311).
- Bilateral conjunctival injection: Spares the limbus and is not associated with pain, exudate, conjunctival edema, or corneal ulceration.
- Oral mucosa changes: Lips may be erythematous, dry, peeling, cracked, and bleeding. The tongue may be erythematous with prominent fungiform papillae ("strawberry tongue"). The oropharyngeal mucosae may be diffusely erythematous (Fig. 4-312).
- Cervical lymphadenopathy: Nodes in the anterior cervical triangle may be unilaterally enlarged and are typically firm, nonfluctuant, and nontender.

Supportive Clinical Findings

- Cardiovascular: Cardiac findings may be prominent in the acute phase and may affect any structure of the heart.

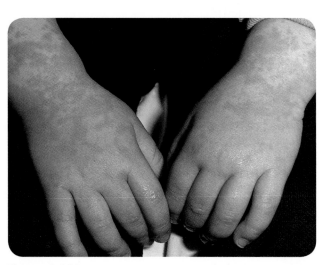

Figure 4-309 KD with finger edema and macular and papular erythema.

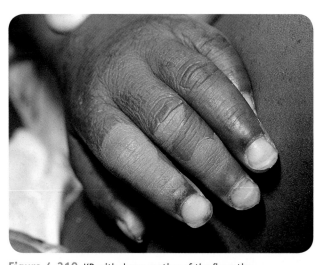

Figure 4-310 KD with desquamation of the fingertips.

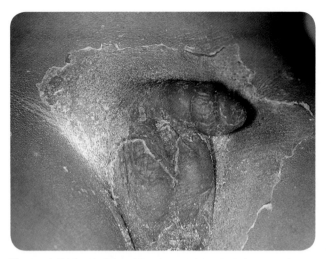

Figure 4-311 KD with penile edema and inguinal desquamation.

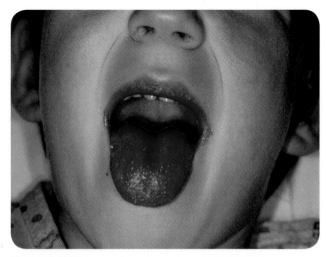

Figure 4-312 KD with prominent red tongue and lips.

- Musculoskeletal: Arthritis and arthralgias of small and large joints may occur in the first week of illness. Large joints are more often affected after the first week.
- Gastrointestinal: Various manifestations during the acute phase may include diarrhea, vomiting, abdominal pain, hepatic dysfunction, jaundice, hepatic enlargement, and hydrops of the gallbladder.
- Neurologic: Extreme irritability, aseptic meningitis, and transient sensorineural hearing loss.
- Genitourinary: Symptomatic or asymptomatic urethritis may be diagnosed by urinalysis.

Supportive Laboratory Findings

- Elevated erythrocyte sedimentation rate (ESR)
- Elevated C-reactive protein (CRP)
- Leukocytosis (>15,000 with granulocyte predominance)
- Thrombocytosis (>500,000 after the 1st week)
- Anemia
- Abnormal plasma lipids
- Mild to moderate elevation of serum transaminases
- Mild to moderate sterile pyuria
- Pleocytosis of cerebrospinal fluid
- Leukocytosis of synovial fluid

Diagnostic Pearls

- "Incomplete" KD should be strongly considered in any child with unexplained fever for 5 or more days associated with two or more of the principal clinical features and three or more supportive laboratory findings.
- KD is unlikely if platelet counts, ESR, and CRP are normal after 7 days of illness.

- Conjunctival exudates, pharyngeal exudates, discrete intraoral lesions, a bullous eruption, or significant generalized lymphadenopathy weigh strongly against KD.
- Perineal erythema with overlying scale frequently presents early in the disease course and provides a useful clue to the diagnosis.

?? Differential Diagnosis and Pitfalls

- Common pitfalls may include diagnosing an infection in an infant with fever and an enlarged cervical lymph node (bacterial lymphadenitis) or sterile pyuria (partially treated urinary tract infection). The subsequent exanthem and mucosal changes may be misdiagnosed as a drug reaction to the prescribed antibiotics. Viral meningitis may be misdiagnosed in a child with fever, rash, and cerebrospinal fluid pleocytosis.
- Patients with toxic shock syndrome most often have focal cutaneous skin infections, abscesses, infections associated with nasal packing, or a history of recent surgical procedures.
- Erythema multiforme presents with symmetrically distributed target lesions. Patients frequently have coexisting herpes orolabialis.
- Viral exanthems like measles may be difficult to distinguish from KD. However, patients with measles often display an exudative conjunctivitis and Koplik spots within the oral mucosa.
- The cutaneous and mucosal findings in scarlet fever may also easily be confused with KD. However, these patients respond to antistreptococcal antibiotic therapy.
- Staphylococcal scalded skin syndrome presents with erythema and desquamation accentuated within skin folds.

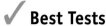

✓ Best Tests

As KD is idiopathic, no specific tests exist to confirm its diagnosis. Initial investigation should include tests to both support the diagnosis of KD and evaluate for alternative diagnoses. Testing should include a complete blood count with differential, ESR, CRP, urinalysis for blood and protein, liver function tests, an electrocardiogram, and echocardiogram.

▲▲▲ Management Pearls

- Echocardiography should be performed at diagnosis, at 2 weeks, and at 6 to 8 weeks after onset. Coronary artery morphology, left ventricular and left valvular function, and the presence of pericardial effusion should be evaluated with each examination. If there is persistent fever or any cardiac abnormalities, echocardiography should be repeated more frequently.
- Live virus vaccines (measles, mumps, rubella, and varicella) should be deferred for at least 11 months after IV Ig administration.
- Patients on long-term aspirin should be warned of the potential for Reye syndrome and should report to their physician any exposures or symptoms consistent with influenza or varicella. They should receive an annual influenza vaccine and consider alternative antiplatelet medications during the first 6 weeks after administration of the varicella vaccine.
- In the United States, KD is reportable in several states.

Therapy

The acute phase of KD is treated with high-dose IV Ig (2 g/kg infused over 10 to 12 h) and high anti-inflammatory doses of aspirin (80 to 100 mg/kg/day divided into four doses until afebrile for 48 to 72 h). Patients with persistent or recrudescent fever for 36 or more hours after completion of the first infusion of IV Ig should be considered for retreatment with high-dose IV Ig or corticosteroids (intravenous pulse methylprednisolone, 30 mg/kg once daily for 1 to 3 days). Low-dose aspirin (3 to 5 mg/kg/day) is continued until no evidence of coronary changes is found on echocardiography at 6 to 8 weeks after illness onset. Aspirin may be continued indefinitely for patients with coronary abnormalities. Long-term therapy should be provided under the guidance of a pediatric cardiologist.

Special Considerations in Infants

KD has a peak incidence in infants aged 9 to 11 months and is extremely rare in infants aged younger than 3 months. Infants aged younger than 6 months may be at increased risk for aneurysms.

Suggested Readings

Avshouri N, Takahashi M, Dorey F, et al. Risk factors for nonresponse to therapy in Kawasaki disease. *J Pediatr.* 2008 Sep; 153(3):365–368.

Bolognia JL, Jorizzo JL, Rapini RP. *Dermatology.* Vol. 1. 2nd Ed. St Louis, MO: Mosby; 2008:1232–1234.

Brogan PA, Bose A, Burgner D, et al. Kawasaki disease: An evidence based approach to diagnosis, treatment, and proposals for future research. *Arch Dis Child.* 2002;86(4):286–290.

Fong NC, Hui YW, Li CK, et al. Evaluation of the efficacy of treatment of Kawasaki disease before day 5 of illness. *Pediatr Cardiol.* 2004;25(1): 31–34.

James WD, Berger TG, Elston DM, eds. *Andrews' Diseases of the Skin.* 10th Ed. Philadelphia, PA: WB Saunders; 2006:843.

Newburger JW, Fulton DR. Kawasaki disease. *Curr Opin Pediatr.* 2004; 16(5):508–514.

Newburger JW, Takahashi M, Gerber MA, et al. Committee on Rheumatic Fever, Endocarditis, and Kawasaki Disease, Council on Cardiovascular Disease in the Young, American Heart Association. Diagnosis, treatment, and long-term management of Kawasaki disease: A statement for health professionals from the Committee on Rheumatic Fever, Endocarditis, and Kawasaki Disease, Council on Cardiovascular Disease in the Young, American Heart Association. *Pediatrics.* 2004;114(6):1708–1733.

Onouchi Y, Gunji T, Burns JC, et al. ITPKC functional polymorphism associated with Kawasaki disease susceptibility and formation of coronary artery aneurysms. *Nat Genet.* 2008;40:35–42.

Onouchi Y, Tamari M, Takahashi A, et al. A genomewide linkage analysis of Kawasaki disease: Evidence for linkage to chromosome 12. *J Hum Genet.* 2007;52(2):179–190.

Pickering LK, ed. *Red Book: 2003 Report of the Committee on Infectious Diseases.* 26th Ed. Elk Grove Village, IL: American Academy of Pediatrics; 2003:392–395.

Rosenfeld EA, Corydon KE, Shulman ST. Kawasaki disease in infants less than one year of age. *J Pediatr.* 1995;126(4):524–529.

◼◼ Diagnosis Synopsis

Systemic lupus erythematosus (SLE) is a disease of unclear etiology characterized by immune abnormalities and multisystem involvement. Approximately 15% to 20% of patients with SLE will present during the first two decades of life. Constitutional symptoms, fever, fatigue, weight loss, headache, mood disturbances, arthralgias, and skin findings may all be seen. Neurologic and renal involvement is prominent in childhood SLE. The onset of the disease is usually between the ages of 10 and 15; however, it can occur at any age. Girls outnumber boys 8:1 in adolescence, but the incidence nearly equalizes in younger ages.

The disease is more common in nonwhites. It is found worldwide. Genetic factors play a role, and a family history of SLE or lupus erythematosus or an inherited complement deficiency in any form is a risk factor for developing the disease.

There are drug-induced forms of the disease with a differing pattern of autoimmunity and clinical profile (discussed separately as drug-induced SLE).

◉ Look For

The classic cutaneous finding in SLE, the malar or "butterfly" blush, is more common in adolescents (Figs. 4-313–4-315). Erythema covering the nose and medial cheeks and sparing the perialar folds can occur after sun exposure and precede the systemic symptoms by weeks. The erythema often develops into fine, scaling, coalescing papules (Fig. 4-316). The erythema can become intense, and small infarcts and necrosis can develop in fulminant cases. An eruption can develop in a photodistribution with prominence on the dorsa of the hands and digits. This eruption can involve the arms and trunk. Nailfold erythema and even necrosis occur. Small mucous membrane ulcers, especially on the palate, can develop. Alopecia may also be seen.

●● Diagnostic Pearls

Constitutional symptoms are more common than skin findings in children and adolescents. Ulcers, photosensitivity, and alopecia are all less common in children than in adults.

?? Differential Diagnosis and Pitfalls

- Dermatomyositis and other rheumatic disease
- Viral illness
- Malignancy
- Polymorphous light eruption
- Seborrheic dermatitis

✓ Best Tests

- If SLE is suspected, a complete workup should be initiated to include ANA, anti-dsDNA, anti-SSA, anti-SSB, anti-RNP, and anti-Smith antibodies.
- Diagnosis is made on clinical and serologic grounds, using the ARA (American Rheumatologic Association) criteria for diagnosis. These criteria were revised in 1997.
- Skin biopsy can be diagnostic for lupus, as well as biopsy of uninvolved skin for direct immunofluorescence.
- Check BUN/Cr, liver urinalysis, function tests, and serum complement (CH50). Slight elevations in PTT and PT might suggest the presence of the lupus anticoagulant.

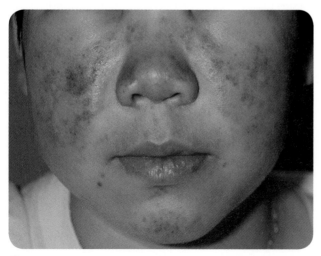

Figure 4-313 SLE with malar and mental eruption with purpura.

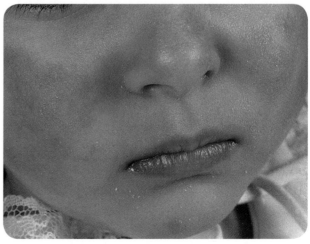

Figure 4-314 SLE with typical malar butterfly that stops at melolabial fold.

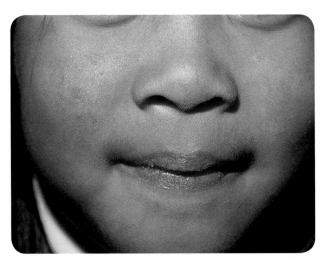

Figure 4-315 SLE with typical malar eruption.

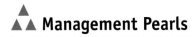 **Management Pearls**

A multidisciplinary approach is best. Patients should see a pediatric rheumatologist, ophthalmologist, and dermatologist. Prompt diagnosis is important so early treatment can be initiated.

Therapy

Oral corticosteroids are the mainstay of treatment. Steroid-sparing agents such as antimalarials, azathioprine, cyclophosphamide, cyclosporine, and mycophenolate mofetil are also used frequently. Anti-B-cell therapy with rituximab has also been successful. Interferon and anti-TNF therapies may also be considered.

Topically, all patients should use sunscreen daily, which provides both UVA and UVB blockage. High-potency topical corticosteroids can be used for localized areas of involvement.

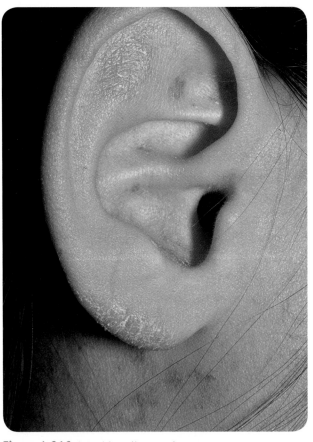

Figure 4-316 SLE with scaling ear plaques.

Suggested Readings

Hiraki LT, Benseler SM, Tyrrell PN, et al. Clinical and laboratory characteristics and long-term outcome of pediatric systemic lupus erythematosus: A longitudinal study. *J Pediatr*. 2008;152(4):550–556.

Macdermott EJ, Adams A, Lehman TJ. Systemic lupus erythematosus in children: Current and emerging therapies. *Lupus*. 2007;16(8):677–683.

Tucker LB. Making the diagnosis of systemic lupus erythematosus in children and adolescents. *Lupus*. 2007;16(8):546–549.

Meningococcemia, Acute

Diagnosis Synopsis

Meningococcal disease is a rapidly progressive infection caused by *Neisseria meningitides*, a Gram-negative diplococcus bacterium. Infection begins as a nonspecific viral-like illness that rapidly evolves (within hours) into one of two main presentations: meningitis or septicemia. Most cases are acquired through exposure to asymptomatic carriers via respiratory droplets. Children aged younger than 5 years and teenagers aged 15 to 19 years are predominantly affected.

Look For

Within 24 h, a typical patient has fever and nonspecific viral illness-like signs, then sepsis symptoms, and finally petechial rash and central nervous system (CNS) signs.

The early rash is erythematous and blanchable and may be macular or macular and papular. Scattered petechiae may be found in areas subject to friction, body folds, flexor surfaces, ankles, or mucosal surfaces. Within hours, the petechiae coalesce into well-demarcated, large ecchymoses, usually concentrated on the limbs and trunk (Figs. 4-317–4-320). Digits and limbs may become gangrenous with well-demarcated gun-metal-gray discoloration. At this stage, patients will have significant CNS abnormalities and signs of severe sepsis.

Diagnostic Pearls

- Fever and a petechial rash is meningococcal disease until proven otherwise.
- Most patients with blanching eruptions have a benign self-limited illness; therefore, a careful search for the

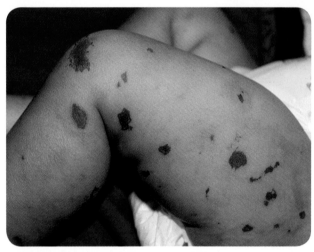

Figure 4-317 Acute meningococcemia with multiple gun-metal-gray lesions.

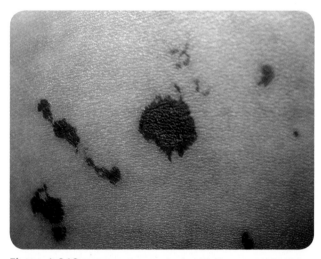

Figure 4-318 Acute meningococcemia with linear area of purpura. (Close-up of Fig. 4-317.)

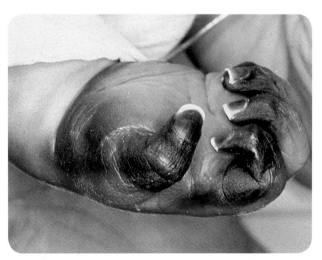

Figure 4-319 Acute meningococcemia with digital gangrene from disseminated intravascular coagulation.

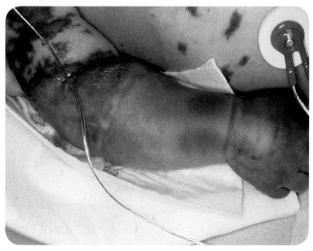

Figure 4-320 Acute meningococcemia with areas of purpura and deep vascular thrombosis.

presence of signs of meningitis, sepsis, or severe illness is key to identifying meningococcal disease.

- Meningococcal disease is less likely if illness lasts longer than 24 h without progressing.

?? Differential Diagnosis and Pitfalls

- Clotting factor deficiency—ecchymoses are ill-defined and subcutaneous and are not associated with necrosis.
- Traumatic ecchymoses—ill-defined, subcutaneous, history of trauma.
- Post-tussive petechiae—localized to the face and upper chest rather than diffusely over the torso and extremities.
- Rocky mountain spotted fever—petechiae first appear distally on the extremities, including the palms and soles; appears after a prodrome of 3 to 5 days; associated with tick exposure in an endemic region.
- Bacterial sepsis—shock and purpuric rash; cultures will confirm the diagnosis.
- Hypersensitivity vasculitis—palpable, usually do not coalesce into ecchymoses; leukocytoclastic vasculitis on biopsy.
- Henoch-Schönlein purpura—palpable, usually concentrated on legs; leukocytoclastic vasculitis on biopsy.
- Kawasaki disease—evolves over days rather than hours, significant mucous membrane changes, purpura is not typical, negative cultures.

✓ Best Tests

- Meningococcal disease should be confirmed by isolation of *N. meningitidis* from normally sterile sites (i.e., blood and CSF Gram stain and cultures).
- Meningococcal PCR should also be obtained from whole blood (EDTA specimen) and CSF to increase the sensitivity and specificity and allow rapid diagnosis.
- Histology of skin lesions will show leukocytoclastic vasculitis with hemorrhage and vascular thromboses. Diplococci may be seen in Gram-stained sections.

▲▲ Management Pearls

- All children with a petechial eruption and signs of sepsis should be admitted and treated for meningococcal disease without delay.
- Household contacts should receive prophylactic rifampin, ceftriaxone, or ciprofloxacin.
- Blood cultures should be taken at the time of intravenous cannula insertion before giving antibiotics, if possible. However, treatment should not be delayed in order to obtain cultures.
- **Precautions:** Standard, droplet (isolate patient, wear a mask, and limit patient transport).
- In the United States, meningococcemia is reportable in the District of Columbia.

- Per the CDC, meningococcal disease is a nationally notifiable disease via the National Notifiable Diseases Surveillance System (NNDSS).

Therapy

Intravenous benzylpenicillin 300 mg, cefotaxime 50 mg/kg, or ceftriaxone 80 mg/kg should be administered immediately to all suspected cases of meningococcal disease unless there is a history of anaphylaxis to penicillin. If the etiology of sepsis or meningitis is unknown at admission (usual scenario), ceftriaxone or cefotaxime should be given for the first 24 to 48 h. Chloramphenicol should be administered to those with a history of anaphylaxis to penicillin or cephalosporins.

Special Considerations in Infants

Classic signs of meningismus (photophobia and nuchal rigidity) are often absent in children aged <2 years, and it is often very difficult to clinically differentiate septicemia from meningitis in infants; however, certain clinical clues are helpful in early recognition and distinction between sepsis and meningitis in infants. Systemic signs of sepsis include (i) early signs: tachycardia (>160 beats per minute), poor capillary refill (>4 s), pallor and mottling, rigors, oliguria (<1 mL/kg/h), and tachypnea (>40 breaths per minute); and (ii) late signs: drowsiness, agitation, and hypotension (<70 mm Hg systolic blood pressure). Signs of meningitis include (i) early signs: a full or bulging fontanelle, abnormal tone (floppy or very stiff), irritability (even handling directed toward soothing the infant causes distress), lethargy, vacant staring, and poor responsiveness; and (ii) late signs: Abnormal breathing patterns, bradycardia, hypertension, twitching, and convulsions.

Suggested Readings

Carrol ED, Thompson AP, Shears P, et al. Performance characteristics of the polymerase chain reaction assay to confirm clinical meningococcal disease. *Arch Dis Child.* 2000;83(3):271–273.

Cartwright KA, Jones DM. ACP Broadsheet 121: June 1989. Investigation of meningococcal disease. *J Clin Pathol.* 1989;42(6):634–639.

van Deuren M, van Dijke BJ, Koopman RJ, et al. Rapid diagnosis of acute meningococcal infections by needle aspiration or biopsy of skin lesions. *BMJ.* 1993;306(6887):1229–1232.

Pollard AJ, Britto J, Nadel S, et al. Emergency management of meningococcal disease. *Arch Dis Child.* 1999;80(3):290–296.

Ramesh V, Mukherjee A, Chandra M, et al. Clinical, histopathologic and immunologic features of cutaneous lesions in acute meningococcaemia. *Ind J Med Res.* 1990;91:27–32.

Thompson MJ, Ninis N, Perera R, et al. Clinical recognition of meningococcal disease in children and adolescents. *Lancet.* 2006;367(9508):397–403.

Staphylococcal Scalded Skin Syndrome

■■ Diagnosis Synopsis

Staphylococcal scalded skin syndrome (SSSS) is an acute, potentially life-threatening condition caused by epidermolytic toxins released by phage group II strains of *Staphylococcus aureus*. Any systemic or cutaneous infection with epidermolytic toxin-producing *S. aureus* may induce SSSS. Children aged <6 years are believed to have increased susceptibility to SSSS due to their decreased renal ability to excrete the toxin. The severity ranges from limited cutaneous involvement to diffuse skin disease and sepsis.

◉ Look For

SSSS typically begins with a sudden onset of fever, irritability, cutaneous tenderness, and diffuse erythema that is accentuated at the flexures and perioral area. This is followed within days by the development of large, fragile bullae or desquamation that is also accentuated at the flexures and perioral area (Figs. 4-321–4-324). The underlying skin is moist and erythematous. Patients classically develop radial fissuring around the eyes, mouth, and nose. In more severe cases, the entire cutaneous surface may be involved with bullae and erosions. Mild cases may display only mild erythema and superficial desquamation in flexural areas. Mucosal surfaces are never affected.

●● Diagnostic Pearls

- The source of the infection is rarely found. Consider the nasopharynx, urinary tract, surgical site, umbilicus, and/or conjunctiva. Very mild forms of the disease exist, with desquamation and circumoral pallor as the major findings.

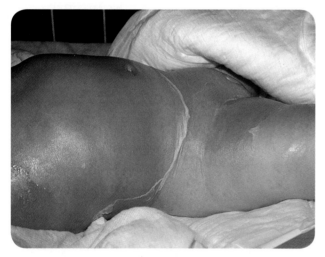

Figure 4-321 SSSS with typical peeling at the edge of the lesion.

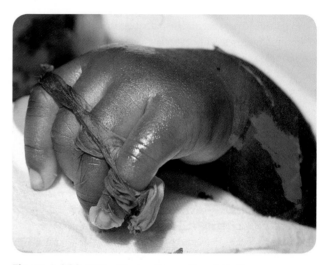

Figure 4-322 SSSS with glovelike peeling of the fingers.

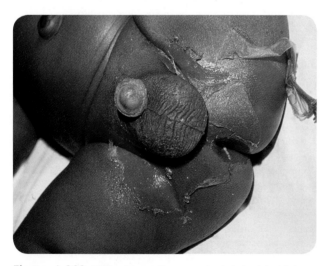

Figure 4-323 SSSS with peeling accentuated in intertriginous regions.

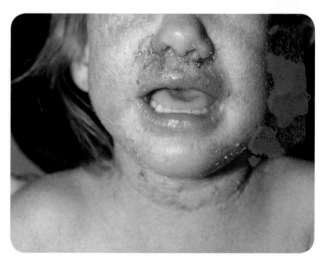

Figure 4-324 SSSS with redness and some scaling early in the course.

- The bullae of SSSS are very fragile and rupture easily with gentle pressure, unlike many other bullous diseases in which bullae are tense and do not rupture with gentle pressure.
- Bullae and Nikolsky sign (extension of bullae with gentle pressure) may be present over erythematous and nonerythematous skin.
- A typical early patient is an irritable child with skin tenderness and erythema around mouth and localized to the neck, axillae, and perineal creases.

?? Differential Diagnosis and Pitfalls

- Toxic shock syndrome—associated with shock and multiorgan failure.
- Toxic epidermal necrolysis—Nikolsky sign in only erythematous areas and mucous membrane involvement.
- Graft-versus-host disease—history of transplant or transfusion in an immunodeficient child.
- Epidermolysis bullosa—onset at birth, does not improve with antibiotics.
- Nutritional deficiency—subacute to chronic onset with failure to thrive and systemic symptoms.
- Keratolysis exfoliativa—acrally limited.
- Drug eruption-associated desquamation—history of drug rash, desquamation occurs as erythema resolves, Nikolsky negative, and limited to areas of prior erythema.

✓ Best Tests

- Cultures should be obtained from the nasopharynx, nostrils, conjunctivae, blood, and any suspected sites of infection. Fluid from bullae is sterile.
- Sloughed skin can be snipped and examined by frozen sections. SSSS will reveal cleavage at the level of the granular layer, whereas toxic epidermal necrolysis will reveal full thickness necrosis down to the dermal–epidermal junction.
- Skin biopsy is usually unnecessary but will reveal a noninflammatory subcorneal split at the level of the stratum granulosum.

▲▲ Management Pearls

- The underlying focus of staphylococcal infection is not always obvious, and treatment is often initiated based on the characteristic clinical picture. Cover eroded areas with Aquaphor ointment or petroleum jelly.

- The skin is very tender, like with sunburns. Minimize handling and apply ointments only as tolerated.
- The blister is superficial and does not cause scarring. Full recovery occurs in 1 to 2 weeks.
- **Precautions:** Standard and contact (isolate patient, wear gloves and a gown, limit patient transport, and avoid sharing patient-care equipment).
- In the United States, outbreaks of staphylococcal skin infections are reportable in OH and UT.
- In the United States, infections due to methicillin-resistant *S. aureus* (MRSA), VRSA, vancomycin-intermediate *S. aureus* (VISA), vancomycin-resistant *Enterococcus* sp., or vancomycin resistant *S. epidermidis* are reportable in many states.
- Per the CDC, infections due to VISA and VRSA are nationally notifiable via the National Notifiable Diseases Surveillance System (NNDSS).

Therapy

Children with moderate to severe disease require hospitalization and intravenous penicillinase-resistant antistaphylococcal antibiotics (i.e., nafcillin or methicillin). Mild cases can be treated with oral antibiotics (i.e., dicloxacillin, cephalexin, or clindamycin) as outpatients but need to be followed closely. If MRSA is isolated, then treatment should be based on sensitivity testing and local resistance patterns. Other general measures include fluid and electrolyte management, minimizing handling of the infant, pain control, and copious use of emollients (petrolatum).

Special Considerations in Infants

In the newborn, a majority of cases present between 3 and 7 days of age.

Suggested Readings

Amagai M, Matsuyoshi N, Wang ZA, et al. Toxin in bullous impetigo and staphylococcal scalded skin syndrome targets desmoglein 1. *Nature Med.* 2000;6(11):1275–1277.

Amagai M, Yamaguchi T, Hanakawa Y, et al. Staphylococcal exfoliative toxin B specifically cleaves desmoglein 1. *J Invest Dermatol.* 2002;118(5):845–850.

Ladhani S, Joannou C. Difficulties in diagnosis and management of the staphylococcal scalded skin syndrome. *Pediatr Infect Dis J.* 2000;19(9):819–821.

Patel GK, Finlay AY. Staphylococcal scalded skin syndrome: Diagnosis and management. *Am J Clin Dermatol.* 2003;4(3):165–175.

Stevens–Johnson Syndrome

Diagnosis Synopsis

Stevens–Johnson syndrome (also called erythema multiforme major) is an acute, severe hypersensitivity reaction usually triggered by medications and occasionally, infection. Presentation during infancy is rare. Implicated medications include sulfonamides, phenytoin, and other anticonvulsants, allopurinol, penicillins, and nonsteroidal anti-inflammatory drugs. More severe cases may be expected with Stevens–Johnson syndrome related to sulfa drugs, gold, and phenylbutazone. The best-documented association of Stevens–Johnson syndrome is with mycoplasma pneumonia. Herpes simplex virus infection may be associated. Other viral associations include influenza, orf, Coxsackie, ECHO, and Epstein–Barr virus. Yersinia, tuberculosis, histoplasmosis, coccidioidomycosis, and X-ray therapy of certain tumors are well-documented associations.

Stevens–Johnson syndrome is distinguished from erythema multiforme minor by the extent of the cutaneous and mucous membrane involvement. Patients with Stevens–Johnson syndrome typically have greater involvement of the mucous membranes.

Fever, malaise, rhinitis, pharyngitis, and cough may precede the rash. Myalgias, vomiting, diarrhea, and arthralgias may also occur. Cases with pneumonia or characteristics of toxic epidermal necrolysis may result in death. Recurrences of Stevens–Johnson syndrome are uncommon.

With secondary infection or severe involvement of the eyes, photophobia, uveitis, panophthalmitis, ulceration, pseudomembrane formation, and scarring may occur. Corneal perforation, lacrimal scarring, xerophthalmia, immobile eyelids, symblepharon, entropion, trichiasis, and blindness may result.

Esophageal strictures, anal strictures, vaginal stenosis, and urethral meatal stenosis may be seen. Gastrointestinal bleeding, hepatitis, urinary retention, nephritis, anuria (from dehydration or genitourinary injury), myocarditis, pneumothorax, obtundation, and seizures are rare complications. Other involvement includes GI lesions with diarrhea, cystitis, splenic inflammation, arthritis, pneumonitis, otitis media, paronychia, and nail shedding.

Look For

In contrast to erythema multiforme minor, the skin lesions of Stevens–Johnson syndrome rapidly evolve into large, erythematous areas with bullae formation, purpura, and epidermal necrosis. The initial lesions are flat, atypical target and purpuric macules. Often, the eruption is widespread with the predominance of lesions on the trunk, with less involvement of the acral surface. The skin surrounding the bullae may be red and tender, and blisters may be hemorrhagic. Widespread shedding of blisters may result in large areas of eroded skin creating a clinical picture that overlaps with that of toxic epidermal necrolysis (often designated when >30% of the body surface area is involved).

In Stevens–Johnson syndrome, the mouth is affected in virtually all cases. The lips can appear blackened and crusted and are often held slightly open (Figs. 4-325 and 4-326). Buccal and labial bullae, erosions, and hemorrhagic crusting may be painful, making eating, talking, and swallowing difficult. Severe oral pain, hypersalivation, and trismus may be observed. Cervical lymphadenopathy correlates with the degree of oral involvement.

Conjunctivitis is the most common eye finding (Fig. 4-327). Blisters and erosions characterize genital involvement (Fig. 4-328). Swelling of the hands, feet, and lips may be seen. Urethral or vaginal bleeding may occur. A positive Nikolsky sign (shearing of the epithelium with lateral pressure applied to previously unblistered skin) may be present.

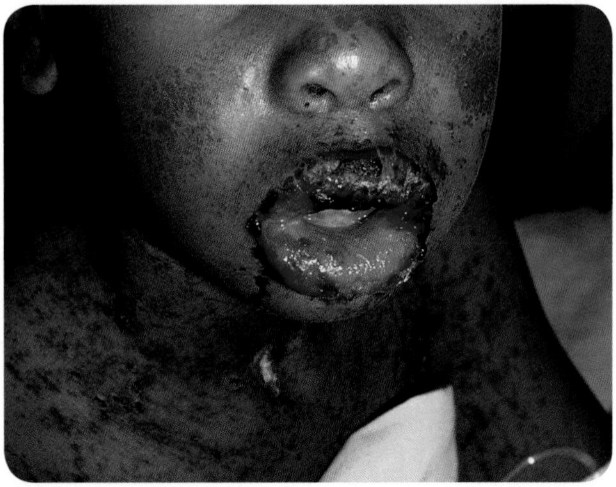

Figure 4-325 Stevens–Johnson syndrome with lip edema and ulceration.

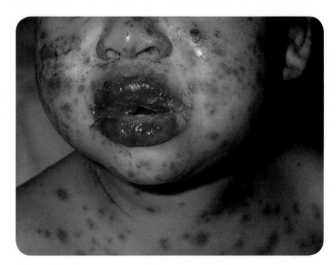

Figure 4-326 Stevens–Johnson syndrome with erosions and no obvious target lesions.

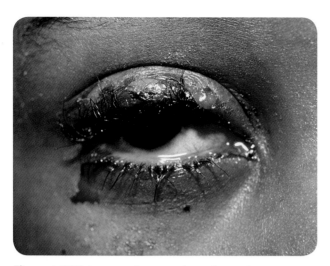

Figure 4-327 Stevens–Johnson syndrome due to phenytoin.

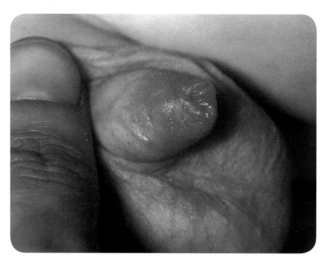

Figure 4-328 Stevens–Johnson syndrome due to lamotrigine.

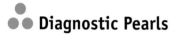 ## Diagnostic Pearls

- Consider Stevens–Johnson syndrome in cases of mucosal pain, crusting, or hemorrhagic bullae.
- The distinction of the severe form of Stevens–Johnson syndrome from toxic epidermal necrolysis may be nosological and may not be clinically important.

?? Differential Diagnosis and Pitfalls

- Staphylococcal scalded skin syndrome presents in neonates and young children, with fever and widespread superficial desquamation accentuated in skin folds.
- Patients with erythema multiforme minor typically have milder mucosal involvement and lack systemic symptoms. The rash of erythema multiforme is characterized by typical acral, symmetrical true target-like lesions. Erythema multiforme minor is most commonly associated with herpes simplex infections and less so with drugs.
- Bullous pemphigoid is rare in children and presents with tense bullae arising within urticarial plaques. If necessary, immunofluorescence studies help confirm this diagnosis.
- Pemphigus vulgaris is extremely rare in children and presents with flaccid blisters and erosions. If necessary, immunofluorescence studies help confirm this diagnosis.
- Paraneoplastic pemphigus is extremely rare in children and presents with extensive, severe mucosal lesions. Like other autoimmune blistering diseases, characteristic immunofluorescence findings help confirm the diagnosis.

✓ Best Tests

- Skin biopsy and clinical picture.
- Elevated ESR, leukocytosis, and eosinophilia are common. Proteinuria or hematuria may be seen.

- An abnormal chest X-ray may indicate mycoplasma pneumonia, other infections responsible for the syndrome, or occasionally inflammation secondary to the Stevens–Johnson syndrome.
- Look for cold agglutinins to investigate for mycoplasma.

▲▲ Management Pearls

- The patient usually requires hospitalization, often in intensive care or a burn unit, depending on the severity and extent of bullae and erosions. The primary goals are to provide fluid/nutritional support, monitor for infection, and pain control.
- Unless used at the onset (this is controversial), systemic steroids offer no clinical benefit and may increase the rate of complications.

Therapy

Withdraw the triggering medication if it is known or suspected. Diagnose and treat potential underlying infection. If herpes simplex is suspected as the trigger, treat with acyclovir. A suppressive regimen may be required if the eruption is recurrent.

The use of steroids or IV Ig is controversial with mixed study results.

Suggested Readings

Bolognia JL, Jorizzo JL, Rapini RP, eds. *Dermatology*. Vol. 1. 2nd Ed. St Louis, MO: Mosby; 2008:291–299.

Cohen BA, ed. *Pediatric Dermatology*. 3rd Ed. St Louis, MO: Mosby; 2005:115–117.

James WD, Berger TG, Elston DM, eds. *Andrews' Diseases of the Skin*. 10th Ed. Philadelphia, PA: WB Saunders; 2006:140–142.

■ Diagnosis Synopsis

Toxic epidermal necrolysis (TEN) is a mucocutaneous disease characterized by the acute onset of diffuse, full-thickness epidermal necrosis leading to extensive epidermal detachment and systemic toxicity. Drugs are the major etiology in children and adults, most commonly sulfonamides, anticonvulsants, NSAIDs, and penicillins. *Mycoplasma pneumoniae*, other infections, vaccinations, and connective tissue diseases also occasionally cause TEN in children. TEN is fatal in up to 25% of patients with significant comorbidities (cancer), increased cutaneous involvement, and internal organ involvement portraying a worse prognosis.

◉ Look For

Symmetric eruption of erythematous to dusky, irregularly shaped macules and bullae that, within hours, progress to widespread, painful, sheetlike sloughing of the epidermis (Figs. 4-329–4-332). The face, upper trunk, and proximal extremities are most severely affected. The mucous membranes are involved in 90% of patients with painful erosions and hemorrhagic crusts of the oral and genital mucosa. Patients typically report a 1- to 14-day prodrome of nonspecific viral-like symptoms.

Other organ systems that may be involved include the eyes (hyperemia, photophobia, lacrimation, erosions, and purulent conjunctivitis), lungs (dyspnea, hypoxemia, hemoptysis, and expectoration of mucosa), gastrointestinal tract (profuse diarrhea, melena, and colonic perforation), and kidneys (proteinuria, hematuria, and azotemia).

●● Diagnostic Pearls

- Nikolsky sign (sloughing of epidermis) is positive only at sites of erythema.

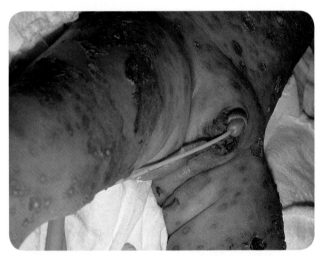

Figure 4-329 TEN, due to amoxicillin, with large erosions.

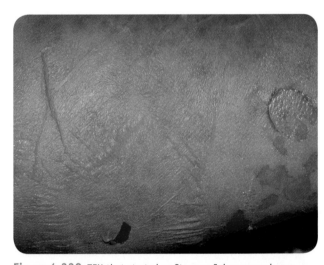

Figure 4-330 TEN that started as Stevens–Johnson syndrome.

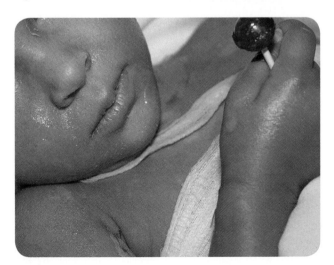

Figure 4-331 TEN with extensive healing nerosions.

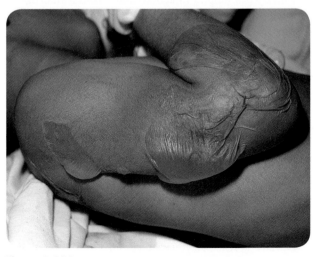

Figure 4-332 TEN, due to diazepam, with large bullae.

- TEN is usually induced by drugs started within 1 to 4 weeks of presentation.
- The **SCORTEN** provides an estimate of prognosis and is reliable at any time after admission:

Prognostic Factor

Aged >40 years: 1 point
Heart rate >120 beats per minute: 1 point
Cancer/hematologic malignancy: 1 point
>10% body surface area involved: 1 point
Serum urea level >10 mM: 1 point
Serum bicarbonate level <20 mM: 1 point
Serum glucose level >14 mM: 1 point

Mortality Rate

0 to 1 points: 3.2% mortality rate
2 points: 12.1% mortality rate
3 points: 35.8% mortality rate
4 points: 58.3% mortality rate
>5 points: 90% mortality rate

?? Differential Diagnosis and Pitfalls

- Kawasaki disease
- Acute, generalized exanthematous pustulosis
- Autoimmune blistering disease
- Graft-versus-host disease (GVHD)
- Staphylococcal scalded skin syndrome
- Epidermolysis bullosa
- Thermal burns
- Chemical burns
- Methotrexate overdose
- Postdrug eruption desquamation

✓ Best Tests

Skin biopsy of affected areas will show full-thickness necrosis.

▲▲ Management Pearls

Necrotic epidermal tissue should not be extensively debrided. It provides a natural barrier to the environment and may promote wound healing.

Therapy

Therapy consists of prompt recognition and removal of the offending drug and supportive care. Patients should be transferred to a burn unit or pediatric intensive care unit where standard burn protocols should be followed.

Patients require early fluid replacement, nutritional support, and increased environmental temperature (28°C to 30°C [82.4°F to 86°F]). Skin, blood, and urine should be cultured regularly for bacteria and fungi. Children with extensive oropharyngeal involvement should be prophylactically intubated. Ophthalmology should also follow patients regularly from the day of admission.

Special Considerations in Infants

Unlike children and adults, in whom drugs are the major etiology, all reported cases in infants aged younger than 6 months have been due to either bacterial sepsis combined with multiantibiotic regimens or acute GVHD. Acute GVHD is usually secondary to engraftment of maternally transmitted or transfusion-derived T lymphocytes in infants with severe combined immunodeficiency (SCID). When secondary to acute GVHD, infants may have associated alopecia, diarrhea, splenomegaly, eosinophilia, failure to thrive, and a history of multiple infections.

One should also recognize that TEN is extremely rare in infants and other diagnoses should be strongly considered. Staphylococcal scalded skin syndrome is the most common disease confused for TEN. Staphylococcal scalded skin syndrome is often associated with rhinitis, it tends to favor intertriginous areas, and it is much more common in infants than TEN. Other diagnoses to consider in neonates with large erosions include intrauterine epidermal necrosis, aplasia cutis congenita, epidermolytic hyperkeratosis, and congenital erosive and vesicular dermatosis.

Suggested Readings

Alain G, Carrier C, Beaumier L, et al. In utero acute graft-versus-host disease in a neonate with severe combined immunodeficiency. *J Am Acad Dermatol.* 1993;29(5 Pt 2):862–865.

Bastuji-Garin S, Fouchard N, Bertocchi M, et al. SCORTEN: A severity-of-illness score for toxic epidermal necrolysis. *J Invest Dermatol.* 2000;115(2):149–153.

Guégan S, Bastuji-Garin S, Poszepczynska-Guigné E, et al. Performance of the SCORTEN during the first five days of hospitalization to predict the prognosis of epidermal necrolysis. *J Invest Dermatol.* 2006;126(2):272–276.

Lohmeier K, Megahed M, Schulte KW, et al. Toxic epidermal necrolysis in a premature infant of 27 weeks' gestational age. *Br J Dermatol.* 2005;152:150–151.

Roujeau JC, Stern RS. Severe adverse cutaneous reactions to drugs. *N Engl J Med.* 1994;331(19):1272–1285.

Scully MC, Frieden IJ. Toxic epidermal necrolysis in early infancy. *J Am Acad Dermatol.* 1992;27(2 Pt 2):340–344.

Valeyrie-Allanore L, Roujeau JC. Epidermal necrolysis (Stevens–Johnson syndrome and toxic epidermal necrolysis). In: Wolff K, Goldsmith LA, Katz SI, et al., eds. *Fitzpatrick's Dermatology in General Medicine.* Vol. 1. 7th Ed. New York, NY: McGraw-Hill; 2008:349–355.

Toxic Shock Syndrome

Diagnosis Synopsis

Toxic shock syndrome (TSS) is an acute toxin-mediated illness characterized by fever, hypotension, multisystem involvement, and rash. It is caused by superantigens (e.g., TSS toxin 1 [TSST-1] or staphylococcal enterotoxins) released by toxin-producing strains of *Staphylococcus aureus*. Superantigens activate T lymphocytes by linking T-cell receptors to class II major histocompatibility complex antigens on the surface of antigen-presenting cells, resulting in massive cytokine release. The extent of subsequent multiorgan system dysfunction is directly related to the severity of hypotension.

TSS may result from surgical wounds, burns, or any other type of mucous membrane, skin, or soft tissue infection with *S. aureus*. The Center for Disease Control (CDC) has developed criteria for the diagnosis of TSS (see next section).

Look For

Patients present with fever and rapid development of diarrhea and severe prostration within hours. Children have an associated diffuse scarlatiniform erythroderma primarily located on the face, trunk, and proximal extremities that is accentuated at the skin folds (Figs. 4-333–4-336). There are no discrete lesions, cutaneous tenderness, or induration. Evaluation of the mucous membranes reveals nonexudative conjunctival erythema, pharyngeal inflammation, and "strawberry tongue." Children will also have hypotension and evidence of multiple organ involvement (see CDC definition of staphylococcal TSS). One to two weeks after the onset of illness, thick desquamation occurs mainly on the digits, palms, and soles.

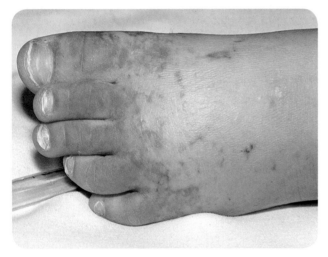

Figure 4-333 TSS with disseminated intravascular coagulation.

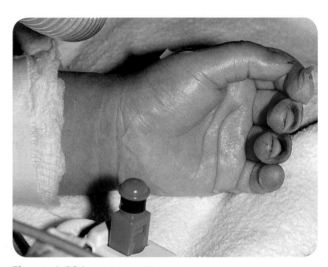

Figure 4-334 TSS with diffuse erythema. (Same patient as in Fig. 4-333.)

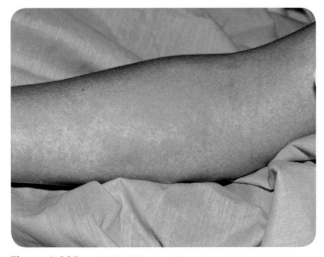

Figure 4-335 TSS with diffuse erythema.

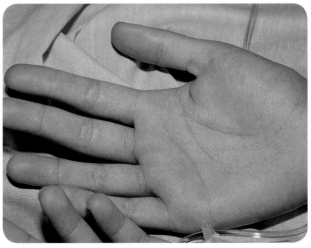

Figure 4-336 TSS. (Same patient as in Fig. 4-335.)

CDC Definition of Staphylococcal TSS

Definite diagnosis: All six criteria; probable diagnosis: Five of six criteria

1. Temperature >38.9°C (102°F)
2. Diffuse macular erythroderma
3. Desquamation 1 to 2 weeks after onset of illness
4. Hypotension (systolic blood pressure less than or equal to fifth percentile for age)
5. Involvement of three or more of the following organ systems:
   - Gastrointestinal (vomiting or diarrhea at onset)
   - Muscular (severe myalgia or creatinine phosphokinase greater than two times the upper limit of normal)
   - Mucous membrane (vaginal, oropharyngeal, or conjunctival hyperemia)
   - Renal system (BUN or creatinine two times or more than the upper limit of normal, or five or more white blood cells per high-power field in the absence of a urinary tract infection)
   - Hepatic (total bilirubin, aspartate aminotransferase, or ALT greater than two times the upper limits of normal)
   - Hematologic (platelets equal to <100,000/μL)
   - Central nervous system (altered consciousness without focal neurologic signs when fever and hypotension are absent)
6. Negative results for the following:
   - Blood cultures (except *S. aureus*)
   - Another explanation (e.g., rise in titer for Rocky Mountain spotted fever, leptospirosis, or measles)

Diagnostic Pearls

- The causative *S. aureus* infection may be occult (sinusitis).
- Toxin-mediated exanthems may overlap, and TSS can develop in patients with staphylococcal scalded skin syndrome or scarlet fever (likely due to the production of multiple toxins).

?? Differential Diagnosis and Pitfalls

- Streptococcal TSS
- Kawasaki disease
- Staphylococcal scalded skin syndrome
- Scarlet fever
- Drug reaction
- Viral exanthem
- Stevens–Johnson syndrome
- Toxic epidermal necrolysis
- Rubeola (measles)
- Leptospirosis
- Rocky Mountain spotted fever
- Acute meningococcemia

✓ Best Tests

Every child with fever and erythroderma should have a complete septic workup, including a complete blood cell count, urinalysis, erythrocyte sedimentation rate, C-reactive protein, complete metabolic profile, and cultures of the blood, urine, cerebrospinal fluid, and any potentially infected sites.

▲▲ Management Pearls

- Decreased vascular volume is the primary derangement in TSS, and one should remember that peripheral edema is usually due to toxin-mediated capillary leakage and is not a sign of fluid overload.
- Decreased vascular volume will manifest as dry mucous membranes, tachycardia, tachypnea, metabolic acidosis, and mental status changes.
- Depending on the stage of shock, peripheral pulses may be bounding or weak; distal extremities may be warm with capillary congestion or cool and pale; and urinary volume may be adequate or decreased.
- Fluids should be restricted only if central venous pressure or pulmonary wedge pressure is elevated.

Therapy

Treatment is divided into (i) treatment of the primary disease; (ii) management of secondary organ dysfunction; and (iii) adjunctive therapy.

Primary disease is first managed by rapid and aggressive fluid resuscitation followed by volume maintenance. The causative focus of infection should then be drained, débrided, and treated with intravenous anti-staphylococcal, β-lactamase-resistant antibiotics (i.e., nafcillin or cefazolin). When suspicion for methicillin-resistant *S. aureus* (MRSA) is high, vancomycin should be given.

Management of secondary organ dysfunction includes intubation for respiratory distress syndrome, ionotropic agents (dopamine or dobutamine) for myocardial failure, and dialysis or fluid restriction for renal failure.

Adjunctive therapies are unproven but may include intravenous immune globulin to neutralize bacterial toxins, stress dose corticosteroids for possible relative or absolute adrenal insufficiency, and clindamycin to inhibit toxin production.

Special Considerations in Infants

If the CDC criteria are strictly followed, TSS is extremely rare in infants. Partial expression may be due to passive immunity conferred by maternal antibodies during the first 3 to 6 months of life; the increased tolerance of infantile T cells to superantigens; and early treatment leading to a blunted course. Names for these partial expressions of toxin-mediated disease include neonatal TSS-like exanthematous disease (NTED) and staphylococcal toxemia.

Suggested Readings

Childs C, Edwards Jones V, Dawson M, et al. Toxic shock syndrome toxin-1 (TSST-1) antibody levels in burned children. *Burns*. 1999;25(6):473–476.

Davis JP, Osterholm MT, Helms CM, et al. Tri-state toxic-shock syndrome study. II. Clinical and laboratory findings. *J Infect Dis*. 1982;145(4):441–448.

McAllister RM, Mercer NS, Morgan BD, et al. Early diagnosis of staphylococcal toxaemia in burned children. *Burns*. 1993;19(1):22–25.

Takahashi N. Neonatal toxic shock syndrome-like exanthematous disease (NTED). *Pediatr Int*. 2003;45(2):233–237.

Takahashi N, Imanishi K, Nishida H, et al. Evidence for immunologic immaturity of cord blood T cells. Cord blood T cells are susceptible to tolerance induction to in vitro stimulation with a superantigen. *J Immunol*. 1995;155(11):5213–5219.

White MC, Thornton K, Young AE. Early diagnosis and treatment of toxic shock syndrome in paediatric burns. *Burns*. 2005;31(2):193–197.

■■ Diagnosis Synopsis

Viral exanthems are eruptive skin rashes caused by viral illnesses usually associated with constitutional symptoms. Some viruses may be associated with specific clinical syndromes (e.g., roseola, rubella, erythema infectiosum [page 32], exanthema subitum, and varicella [page 169]). Most viral exanthems, however, are nonspecific in both symptoms and signs. These nonspecific viral exanthems tend to be self-limited, resolve over 1 to 2 weeks, and are not associated with any long-term morbidity.

◉ Look For

Viral exanthems may be any combination of erythematous macules, erythematous papules, vesicles, petechiae, pustules, or urticaria (Figs. 4-337–4-340). A full history and physical examination should be performed looking for signs and symptoms of specific viral exanthems. (See sections on individual viral illnesses.) Often, a specific viral syndrome cannot be determined and the patient is diagnosed with a nonspecific viral exanthem. The most common presentation of nonspecific viral exanthems is a combination of blanching macules and papules that favors the trunk (morbilliform).

●● Diagnostic Pearls

- The patient may be ill or well except for the nonspecific exanthem. The rash is often the most significant finding.
- Mucous membranes should always be evaluated, as many viral and viral-like syndromes have specific mucous membrane lesions (i.e., roseola; rubeola; hand, foot, and mouth disease; scarlet fever; mononucleosis; and Kawasaki syndrome).

?? Differential Diagnosis and Pitfalls

- Morbilliform drug rash
- Rubella
- Rubeola
- Mononucleosis
- Urticaria
- Stevens–Johnson syndrome
- Kawasaki syndrome
- Scarlet fever
- *Mycoplasma* infection
- *Rickettsial* illness
- Meningococcemia
- Staphylococcal scalded skin syndrome
- Toxic shock syndrome
- Toxic exposure, such as acrodynia
- Graft-versus-host disease

✓ Best Tests

- Most laboratory tests are nonspecific: Elevated erythrocyte sedimentation rate, normochromic normocytic anemia, thrombocytosis, and sometimes leukocytosis.
- IgM and IgG acute and convalescent sera may be obtained to confirm specific viral infections.

▲▲ Management Pearls

As no combination of clinical assessment and diagnostic testing can guarantee the diagnosis of a benign viral exanthem, parents should be instructed to return to the emergency department or medical office for any deterioration in the child's medical condition.

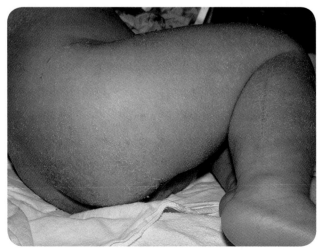

Figure 4-337 Viral exanthem with diffuse erythema and desquamation.

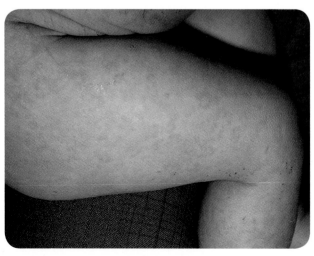

Figure 4-338 Viral exanthem with discrete and confluent papules.

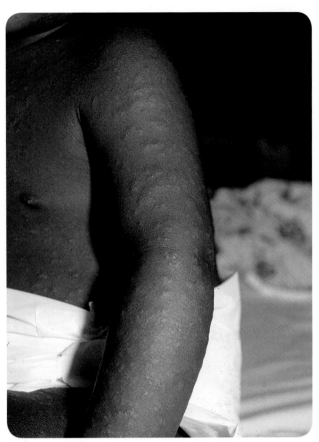

Figure 4-339 Viral exanthem with multiple nonscaling papules.

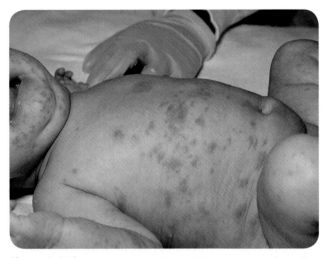

Figure 4-340 Viral exanthem with multiple large and small papules.

Suggested Readings

Drago F, Rampini E, Rebora A. Atypical exanthems: Morphology and laboratory investigations may lead to an aetiological diagnosis in about 70% of cases. *Br J Dermatol*. 2002;147(2):255–260.

Paller AS, Mancini AJ. Bites and infestations. In: Paller AS, Mancini AJ, eds. *Hurwitz Clinical Pediatric Dermatology. A Textbook of Skin Disorders of Childhood and Adolescence*. 3rd Ed. Philadelphia, PA: Elsevier Saunders; 2006:479–502.

Schachner LA, Hansen RC, eds. *Pediatric Dermatology*. 3rd Ed. Edinburgh, NY: Mosby; 2003:1059–1071.

Therapy

Treat supportively. Consider topical steroids and antihistamines for pruritus, and acetaminophen (15 mg/kg every 4 to 6 h) for fever.

Abscess

Diagnosis Synopsis

An abscess is a localized inflammatory process in which the white blood cells accumulate at the site of infection in the dermis and/or subcutaneous tissue. Lesions evolve over days to 1 or 2 weeks. They are usually painful and are sometimes associated with fever. Abscesses are typically caused by *Staphylococcus* sp.

Methicillin-resistant *Staphylococcus aureus* (MRSA) first emerged as an important nosocomial pathogen in the 1960s. In more recent years, community-acquired outbreaks of MRSA have been described increasingly among healthy individuals lacking the traditional risk factors for such infections (IV drug use, incarceration, participation in contact sports, etc.). These strains have a propensity for causing abscesses, furunculosis, and folliculitis and have a unique antibiotic susceptibility profile from health care-associated strains of MRSA.

Look For

A red, tender, hard or fluctuant mass (Figs. 4-341–4-344). Oozing pus is not generally seen; the lesion sometimes appears as a multiheaded pustule. The abscess may have multiple interconnected portions, especially in the back of the neck. The lesion evolves over days to 1 to 2 weeks. It is usually painful and sometimes associated with fever.

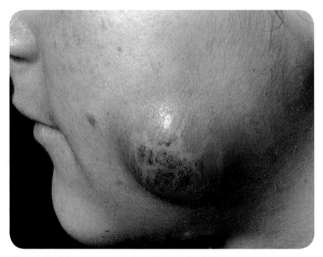

Figure 4-341 Abscess. Firm nodule with erythema and crust.

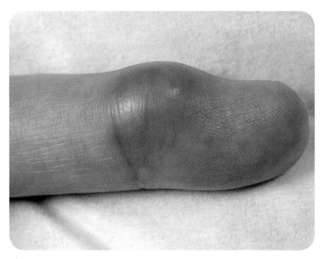

Figure 4-342 Abscess on distal finger. Herpetic whitlow is within the differential diagnosis.

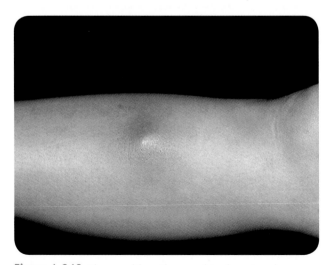

Figure 4-343 Abscess with erythema and tenderness on leg.

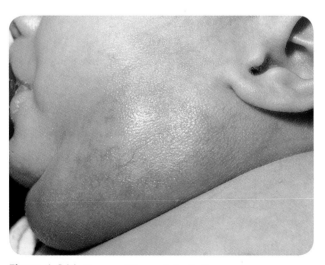

Figure 4-344 Abscess of the neck due to *S. aureus*.

Diagnostic Pearls

- In the immunosuppressed patient (from disease or medications), inflammation may be decreased or absent. Gentle pressure often reveals an opaque white core.
- If the lesion is within the scalp, look for other signs of scalp dermatophyte infection, such as broken hairs (black dot fungus) or fine scales. In a child, a scalp abscess is more likely fungal than bacterial. Fungal scalp infections have more pruritus than bacterial infections.
- Childhood perianal abscesses are often associated with chronic granulomatous diseases or inflammatory bowel disease.
- Abscesses can occur at the site of insulin injections as a result of poor sterile technique.

?? Differential Diagnosis and Pitfalls

- Kerions on the scalp are fungal-induced hypersensitivity reactions, commonly associated with adenopathy and difficult to tell from bacterial-induced abscesses.
- In a normal host, a noninflammatory abscess is "classic" for mycobacterial infections.
- Large dermal nodules of pseudolymphoma (rare in childhood) or subcutaneous granuloma annulare may resemble an abscess.
- Sterile abscesses or soft tissue hypertrophy "insulin tumors" can develop at the site of insulin injections. These nodules are noninflammatory.
- A brisk inflammatory response to molluscum virus can resemble abscesses. Look for other evidence of molluscum contagiosum lesions and the nontoxic appearance of the patient.

✓ Best Tests

- If the nature of a subcutaneous mass is uncertain, an ultrasound can be used to delineate the nature (cystic, solid, vascular).
- Incision and Gram and fungal stains of the exudate may yield immediate diagnosis. Cultures will take a few days (bacterial) or weeks (fungal).
- Sensitivities should be performed on any *S. aureus* isolates to determine antibiotic resistance.

▲▲ Management Pearls

- Incision and drainage is the mainstay of therapy for treatment of cutaneous abscesses.

- Given the prevalence of MRSA, maintain a high index of suspicion for this diagnosis and make the initial choice of empiric antibiotic therapy accordingly. It is helpful to be aware of the patterns of antimicrobial resistance within your community (check with your local hospital microbiology lab).
- Eradication of MRSA nasal carriage may be accomplished with application of 2% mupirocin cream to the nares. The combination of rifampin and trimethoprim–sulfamethoxazole (TMP–SMX) has also been shown to eradicate MRSA colonization.
- **Precautions:** Standard and contact (isolate patient, wear gloves and a gown, limit patient transport, and avoid sharing patient-care equipment).
- In the United States, infections due to MRSA, VRSA, vancomycin-intermediate *S. aureus* (VISA), vancomycin-resistant *Enterococcus* sp., or vancomycin-resistant *S. epidermidis* are reportable in several states.
- Per the CDC, infections due to VISA and VRSA are nationally notifiable via the National Notifiable Diseases Surveillance System (NNDSS).

Therapy

Incision and drainage is the mainstay of therapy. Locally anesthetize with 1% lidocaine and use a no. 11 blade to incise the fluctuant mass. Probing may be necessary if there is a suggestion of a foreign body. Consider using a ribbon of iodoform gauze to pack the cavity if it is large.

Antibiotics such as a semisynthetic penicillin p.o. every 4 to 6 h by body weight and erythromycin four times daily for 10 days is a standard course of therapy.

Standard cephalosporins and penicillins are of no benefit in treating MRSA. In recent studies, community-acquired MRSA demonstrated a high degree of susceptibility to TMP–SMX and rifampin (100%), clindamycin (95%), and tetracycline (92%). However, tetracycline should not be used in children aged younger than 8 years. Inducible resistance to clindamycin should be excluded by performing a D-zone disk-diffusion test. Critically ill patients with MRSA or suspected MRSA should receive vancomycin or linezolid.

Implementation of dilute bleach baths (1/2 to 1 cup of bleach in a full-size tub of water) two to three times per week is helpful in reducing the number of recurrent infections.

Special Considerations in Infants

In infants, consider other causes of abscesses secondary to neutrophil dysfunctions and immunological dysfunctions, as seen in hyperimmunoglobulin E syndrome and chronic granulomatous disease. Bacteremia is rare but can occur in newborns or in association with malnutrition. Sites of predilection are around the umbilicus and circumcision sites. In the neonatal period, subcutaneous masses can be cystic (dermoid cysts), solid (cutaneous metastases), or vascular (hemangiomas or malformations). Distinguishing a fungal from a bacterial-induced lesion is the first step of management. Enlarged nodes do not suggest one over the other. In the neonatal period, consideration of intravenous antibiotics and acquisition of other cultures (blood and CSF) are mandatory, as the neonate is essentially immunocompromised.

Suggested Readings

Cohen PR. Community-acquired methicillin-resistant *Staphylococcus aureus* skin infections: Implications for patients and practitioners. *Am J Clin Dermatol.* 2007;8(5):259–270.

Elston DM. Community-acquired methicillin-resistant *Staphylococcus aureus*. *J Am Acad Dermatol.* 2007;56:1–16.

Fortunov RM, Hulten KG, Hammerman WA, et al. Community-acquired *Staphylococcus aureus* infections in term and near-term previously healthy neonates. *Pediatrics.* 2006;118(3):874–881.

Fortunov RM, Hulten KG, Hammerman WA, et al. Evaluation and treatment of community-acquired *Staphylococcus aureus* infections in term and late-preterm previously healthy neonates. *Pediatrics.* 2007;120(5):937–945.

Cyst, Epidermoid (Sebaceous Cyst)

Diagnosis Synopsis

Epidermoid cysts (epidermal cyst, epidermal inclusion cysts, keratin cysts) are frequently incorrectly called sebaceous cysts. One of the most common benign skin tumors in adults, epidermoid cysts are rare in childhood and infancy. These semisolid cysts are lined by a keratinizing epithelium and filled mostly with macerated keratin, which has a cheeselike consistency and pungent odor. They frequently appear to arise spontaneously. Alternatively, they may result from disruption of follicular structures or by implantation of the epidermis via a penetrating injury.

Look For

A dome-shaped, skin-colored protuberance, freely movable over underlying tissue on palpation, and sometimes with a small comedo-like central punctum through which cyst contents may be expressed with pressure (Figs. 4-345–4-348). Generally one-half to several centimeters in diameter, the cyst can be well defined or irregular due to prior rupture, scarring, and regrowth. Epidermoid cysts can be located almost anywhere but are most common on the face, neck, or trunk. If manipulated or inflamed, the cyst can appear infected, with erythema and tenderness.

Diagnostic Pearls

- Careful examination frequently demonstrates a porelike opening (punctum). The lesion is usually firm and has consistency a little firmer than the adult eyeball.

- Sudden pain or swelling may be related to the rupture of the cyst contents into the surrounding tissue, leading to a vigorous foreign body inflammatory response and not true infection.

Differential Diagnosis and Pitfalls

- Epidermoid cysts are rare before puberty, and alternative diagnoses should be strongly considered in infancy and childhood.
- The presence of multiple epidermoid cysts and a family history of the same should lead to the consideration of Gardner syndrome, a heritable disorder associated with GI malignancy.
- Cyst rupture with associated inflammation is often misdiagnosed as an "infection" of the cyst. Cultures are usually negative and treatment with antibiotics is not required.
- Superficial lymph nodes are palpated within the subcutaneous fat and are found within the course of lymphatics.
- Lipomas are soft, mobile subcutaneous nodules with normal overlying epidermis.
- Pilar cysts (trichilemmal cysts) may be clinically indistinguishable from epidermoid cysts, but are more common in childhood and are typically found on the scalp.
- Pilomatricoma usually presents as a solitary skin-colored to faint-blue nodule, frequently found on the head or upper trunk in children. Firmness is a reflection of calcification within this benign tumor.
- Steatocystomas occur as asymptomatic single or multiple cysts on the chest, axillae, and/or groin that may drain an oily substance if punctured. Multiple steatocystomas are seen in some patients with pachyonychia congenital.

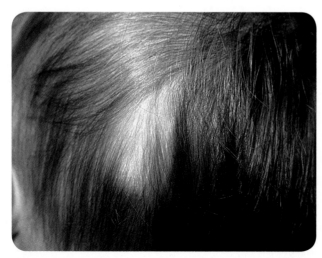

Figure 4-345 Pilar cyst is common on the scalp and is usually painless.

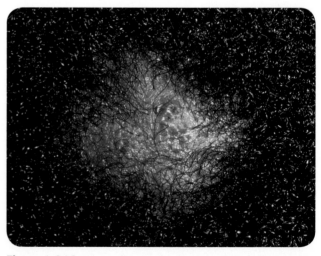

Figure 4-346 Pilar cyst in scalp may have an indistinct border.

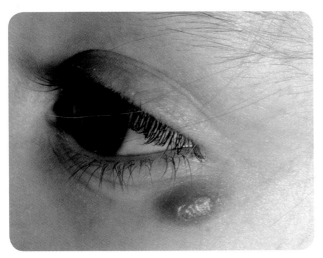

Figure 4-347 Cyst that has ruptured and may need excision after the inflammation has subsided.

- Dermoid cysts result from anomalies in embryonic closure zones. Surgical removal or biopsy of a cyst over the midline should not be attempted without proper imaging to rule out intraspinal or intracranial connection.
- Bronchogenic cysts are most frequently found in the suprasternal notch, and they represent sequestered respiratory epithelium during embryological development.
- Thyroglossal duct cysts present as midline cystic nodules on the neck in children.
- Branchial cleft cysts present in the second or third decade as a nodule in the preauricular area, mandibular region, or along the anterior border of the sternocleidomastoid muscle.

✓ Best Tests

- If the punctum is present over a typical lesion, no test is necessary.
- Skin biopsy may be performed if diagnosis is unclear.
- Cystic lesions present over the midline may require imaging to rule out central nervous system connection prior to surgical intervention.

▲▲ Management Pearls

If the child is young, defer therapy of an asymptomatic, stable, nonfacial cyst until older. Incision and drainage can provide immediate reduction in the cyst, but without removing the epidermal lining, the cyst is likely to refill with layers of soft keratin and significant scarring.

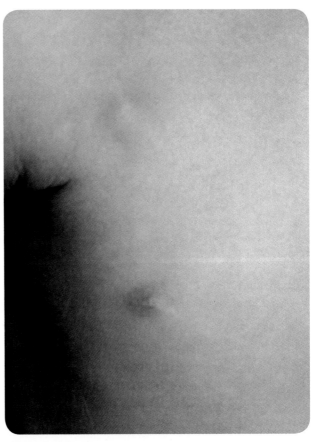

Figure 4-348 Epidermoid cyst with central punctum.

Therapy

Surgical dissection around the wall of a noninflammatory cyst is the best way to permanently remove lesions.

Some have used a punch biopsy to create a small skin opening and then curetted the cyst wall. This technique is sometimes effective and can reduce the incision size.

If the cyst is inflamed, resist the urge to incise and express (usually results only in temporary relief). Intralesional triamcinolone (3 to 5 mg/mL) and oral tetracycline (only in children older than 8 years) can be effective in decreasing inflammation of a symptomatic/ruptured lesion.

Suggested Readings

Bolognia JL, Jorizzo JL, Rapini RP, eds. *Dermatology*. Vol. 1. 2nd Ed. St Louis, MO: Mosby; 2008:1199–1204.

Cohen BA, ed. *Pediatric Dermatology*. 3rd Ed. St Louis, MO: Mosby; 2005:129.

James WD, Berger TG, Elston DM, eds. *Andrews' Diseases of the Skin*. 10th Ed. Philadelphia, PA: WB Saunders; 2006:677.

Granuloma, Pyogenic

Diagnosis Synopsis

Pyogenic granulomas are rapidly growing, usually single, benign vascular growths. The etiology is unknown. They can bleed profusely even after a minor trauma. While they can occur in patients aged younger than 6 months, they generally occur in older children. One recent study reported an average age of 5.9 years.

Look For

Red, small (typically about 1 mm), raspberrylike, friable papules (Figs. 4-349–4-352). The base may have a well-circumscribed collarette. Pyogenic granulomas occur most often on exposed surfaces, such as the hands, forearms, and face, although the condition can appear in the mouth as well.

Fingers are a frequent location. Pyogenic granulomas may be a complication of isotretinoin therapy and can occur within port-wine stains.

Diagnostic Pearls

- Occasionally, there is a history of preceding trauma.
- Pyogenic granuloma should be on your differential in any patient who presents with a rapidly growing lesion that bleeds easily.

Differential Diagnosis and Pitfalls

- Infantile hemangioma
- Amelanotic melanoma
- Bacillary angiomatosis

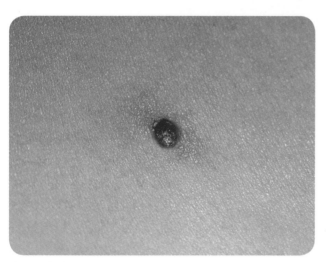

Figure 4-349 Pyogenic granuloma is often a red papule that easily bleeds.

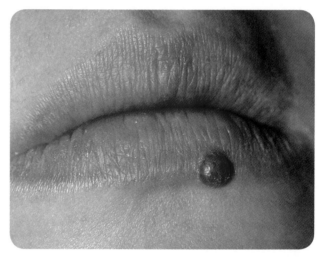

Figure 4-350 Pyogenic granuloma on the vermillion border.

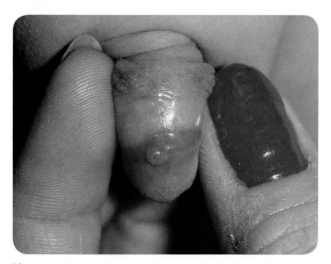

Figure 4-351 Pyogenic granuloma can occur on the genitals.

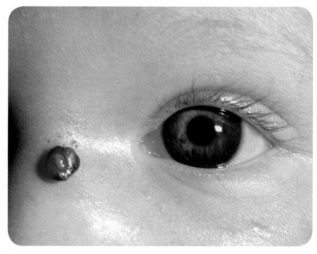

Figure 4-352 Pyogenic granuloma. Friable papule in a common location.

Best Tests

A biopsy is necessary and is both curative and diagnostic.

▲▲ Management Pearls

Always send the lesion for pathologic diagnosis, as amelanotic melanoma can also present as a rapidly growing papule that bleeds easily.

Therapy

Shave excision followed by electrodesiccation of the base is the most commonly reported treatment. Other treatments that have been reported to be successful include cryotherapy, imiquimod, and both pulsed dye and CO_2 lasers.

Suggested Readings

Fallah H, Fischer G, Zagarella S. Pyogenic granuloma in children: Treatment with topical imiquimod. *Australas J Dermatol.* 2007;48(4):217–220.

Pagliai KA, Cohen BA. Pyogenic granuloma in children. *Pediatr Dermatol.* 2004;21:10–13.

■■ Diagnosis Synopsis

Hemangiomas are the most common tumor of childhood. They occur in up to 10% of infants. Female sex, prematurity, white skin, history of chorionic villus sampling, and prenatal factors such as older maternal age, placenta previa, and pre-eclampsia are the risk factors for the development of hemangiomas. Superficial hemangiomas are noticed by 3 weeks of life. They have an initial proliferative phase lasting for about 3 to 6 months followed by a stage of regression (occurs at a rate of 10% per year) over a period of many years. They usually subside by 10 years of age, and they may leave behind some residual changes such as telangiectasia, scarring, atrophy, and fibrosis. Hemangiomas are usually solitary (focal), involving the head and neck region, but they may also be segmental or disseminated.

◉ Look For

Hemangiomas are classified as superficial, deep, or mixed types.

- Superficial—bright red, dome-shaped, lobulated vascular papules, plaques, or nodules (Fig. 4-353)
- Deep—usually noted at 3 months of age as subcutaneous firm to rubbery, compressible, bluish vascular plaques or nodules with overlying telangiectasia or surrounding venous network
- Mixed—has features of both

In children aged more than 2 years, most hemangiomas will be in the stage of involution (Figs. 4-354–4-356). Regressing superficial hemangiomas are soft and have color changes from bright red to dull red and central graying.

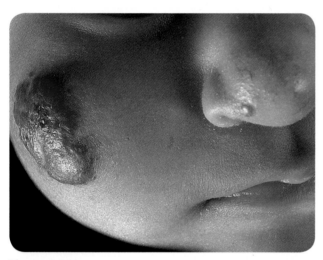

Figure 4-353 Infantile hemangioma. Superficial and deep, on the cheek and nasal tip.

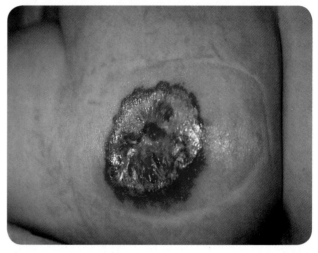

Figure 4-354 Infantile hemangioma on the buttocks, a common area for ulceration.

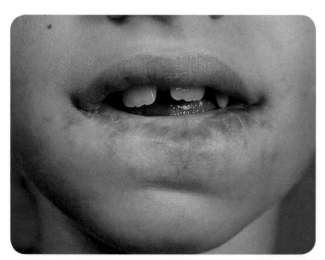

Figure 4-355 Infantile hemangioma. Involuted stage with permanent deformity of the lower lip.

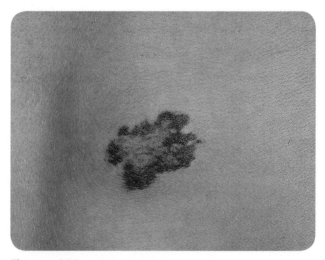

Figure 4-356 Infantile hemangioma. Superficial, with early involution noted centrally by grayish hue.

Diagnostic Pearls

- Regressing deep hemangiomas will be marked by softening of the vascular plaque or nodule.
- Children with multiple hemangiomas (greater than five) and segmental types are more likely to have extracutaneous lesions in other organs, notably, the liver, lungs, CNS, eye, etc.
- Segmental hemangiomas may also be associated with structural malformations (PHACES syndrome: **P**osterior fossa malformation, **H**emangiomas, **A**rterial anomalies, **C**oarctation of the aorta and other cardiac defects, and **E**ye abnormalities, **S**ternal defects, and **S**upraumbilical raphe). Lumbosacral hemangiomas may be a marker of an underlying spinal dysraphism. Lesions in the "beard" region may be associated with airway hemangiomas.

Differential Diagnosis and Pitfalls

The differential diagnosis for infantile hemangioma is broad depending on the type and its stage of growth. Precursor lesions provide the most diagnostic challenge. When in doubt, questionable lesions should be followed over time as the common similar-appearing lesions (contusions, vascular malformations, pigmentary changes, and cysts) do not rapidly proliferate like infantile hemangiomas.

Vascular Malformations

Capillary malformation (port-wine stain)—borders are usually well defined, does not proliferate postnatally.
Venous malformation
Lymphatic malformation
Glomuvenous malformation
Arteriovenous malformation

Vascular Tumors

Rapidly involuting congenital hemangioma (RICH)—fully formed at birth, does not proliferate postnatally
Noninvoluting congenital hemangioma (NICH)—fully formed at birth, does not proliferate postnatally
Tufted angioma
Kaposiform hemangioendothelioma

Nonvascular Tumors

Neuroblastoma
Infantile myofibromatosis
Rhabdomyosarcoma
Plexiform neurofibroma
Lipoma

Other

Cyst
Glioma
Contusion
Nevus anemicus
Pigmentary mosaicism (nevus depigmentosus)
Leukemia cutis/lymphoma cutis

Best Tests

- Skin biopsy is indicated only to exclude other vascular or soft tissue tumors. GLUT-1 immunoreactivity is positive in infantile hemangiomas.
- Doppler ultrasound and magnetic resonance imaging may be used to confirm the diagnosis and determine the extent of an infantile hemangioma.

Management Pearls

- Most of the stable focal hemangiomas in older children do not need any specific treatment.
- Treatment of large facial hemangiomas and lesions in certain anatomical locations—such as lip, nasal tip, eyes, and ears—is needed during infancy. Treat lesions that interfere with feeding, vision, cosmesis, or obstruct the airways.
- Evaluate children with large, segmental, or multiple hemangiomas. Look for complications such as high output failure, hypothyroidism, and visceral hemorrhage.
- Ulceration is common in the intertriginous areas, such as genitalia, perineum, and perianal region, and should be treated immediately.

Therapy

Active nonintervention is sufficient for uncomplicated infantile hemangiomas.

Steroids are the mainstay of therapy in complicated infantile hemangiomas. Oral steroids (prednisone or prednisolone 2 to 4 mg/kg/day) are the first-line systemic therapy. The treatment (including the tapering dose) duration usually varies from 3 to 9 months. Topical or intralesional steroids may be considered for small, isolated, and localized lesions. There may be a role for propanolol during aggressive proliferation.

Life-threatening steroid-resistant infantile hemangiomas may be treated with vincristine, cyclophosphamide, interferon α-2a, or interferon α-2b.

Ulcerated hemangiomas require local wound care (i.e., nonstick dressings, topical antibiotics, regular dressing changes) and pain control (i.e., acetaminophen, ibuprofen, topical lidocaine). Persistent, large, or deep ulcerations may require the addition of systemic or local steroids, pulsed dye laser, becaplermin gel, or excision.

Special Considerations in Infants

Focal, or localized, infantile hemangiomas are discrete papules, nodules, or plaques that appear to arise from a central focus. Segmental infantile hemangiomas are small or large plaques that appear to affect an embryological or developmental segment of the body. Segmental infantile hemangiomas often have many surface telangiectases and irregular, ill-defined borders. Infants with multiple or segmental infantile hemangiomas are more likely to have extracutaneous hemangiomas. The liver is the most commonly affected site; however, any organ may be involved. Refer any segmental, facial, or perineal infantile hemangioma to a local vascular lesion expert before proliferation begins.

If following without active treatment, follow monthly from birth through at least 6 months of age to monitor for potential aggressive proliferation.

Palpate the liver in all infants with infantile hemangiomas. If palpable, obtain hepatic ultrasound for potential systemic involvement.

Be aware of complications such as high output failure, hypothyroidism, and visceral hemorrhage in infants with multiple and segmental lesions.

Aggressively treat lesions that interfere with function (feeding, vision, or obstruct airways), are cosmetically deforming (lips, nasal tip, eyes, and ears), or ulcerate.

If treating with systemic steroids, minor transient side effects are common. These include the development of a cushingoid facies, insomnia, personality changes, temporary, delayed skeletal growth, gastric upset, hypertension, and decreased immunity. While on systemic steroids, blood pressure should be monitored monthly; live virus vaccines (rotavirus vaccine) should be avoided; and antacids (ranitidine) should be provided for infants with gastric upset.

Suggested Readings

Bennett ML, Fleischer AB Jr, Chamlin SL, et al. Oral corticosteroid use is effective for cutaneous hemangiomas: an evidence-based evaluation. *Arch Dermatol*. 2001;137(9):1208–1213.

Bruckner AL, Frieden IJ. Hemangiomas of infancy. *J Am Acad Dermatol*. 2003;48(4):477–493.

Haggstrom AN, Drolet BA, Baselga E, et al. Prospective study of infantile hemangiomas: Clinical characteristics predicting complications and treatment. *Pediatrics*. 2006;118(3):882–887.

Haggstrom AN, Drolet BA, Baselga E, et al. Hemangioma Investigator Group. Prospective study of infantile hemangiomas: demographic, prenatal, and perinatal characteristics. *J Pediatr*. 2007;150(3):291–294.

Léauté-Labrèze C, Dumas de la Roque E, Hubiche T, et al. Propranolol for severe hemangiomas of infancy. *N Engl J Med*. 2008;358(24):2649–2651.

■■ Diagnosis Synopsis

Keloids are raised scars that spread beyond the margins of the original wound. They arise in areas of previous trauma (e.g., burns and lacerations) or inflammation (e.g., acne, folliculitis, and varicella). The risk for keloidal scarring is highest in those aged 10 years and above. Over several months, keloids may become erythematous, pruritic, and grow to become very large. They can be unsightly, and parents frequently seek removal. Keloids are most frequent in dark-skinned individuals, but they may appear in any individual.

◉ Look For

Smooth and shiny; firm to the touch; red, hyperpigmented, or skin-colored nodules with regular or irregularly shaped ridges (Figs. 4-357–4-360). Keloids, by definition, develop projections that extend beyond the area of original trauma. Their growth is usually seen on the neck, ear lobes, extremities, and upper trunk.

●● Diagnostic Pearls

Keloids often develop months after wound repair, unlike hypertrophic scars, which develop within weeks after cutaneous injury.

?? Differential Diagnosis and Pitfalls

- Keloids and hypertrophic scars may initially appear similar, but keloids progress and extend beyond the boundary of the original injury, whereas hypertrophic scars always stay within the boundaries of the original scar.

- Sarcoidosis can localize in scars and form nodules that appear similar to keloids, but patients will have other cutaneous lesions (i.e., red-orange papules on the face in areas not subject to trauma) and systemic signs (e.g., pulmonary, ocular, rheumatic, etc.) consistent with sarcoidosis.
- Foreign body reactions may become elevated but remain localized to the areas of foreign body deposition.
- Dermatofibromas are localized (usually smaller than 1 cm in diameter) benign dermal tumors that do not grow after their initial appearance.

✓ Best Tests

The diagnosis is based on history and lesion morphology. If there is doubt, a biopsy will confirm the clinical diagnosis.

▲▲ Management Pearls

- Surgical excision of keloids is inevitably fraught with the possibility of keloid recurrence and expansion. Surgical excision is advised only if there is a postoperative plan that includes regular follow-up for adjunctive therapy.

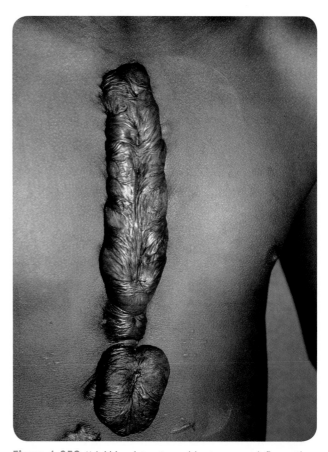

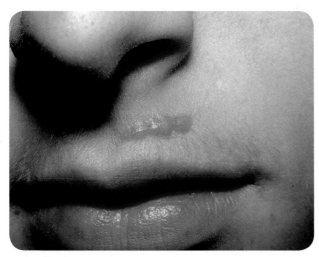

Figure 4-357 Keloid with shiny red, linear plaque.

Figure 4-358 Keloid in a later stage without apparent inflammation.

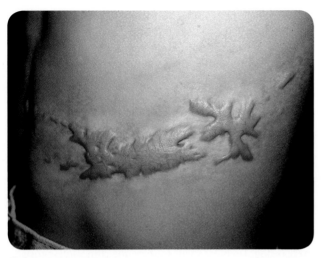

Figure 4-359 Keloid with erythema and a clawlike configuration.

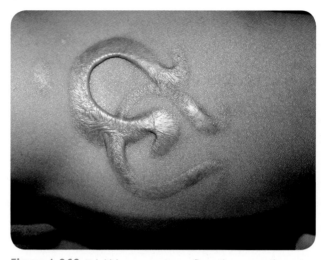

Figure 4-360 Keloid in an arcuate configuration suggesting external etiology.

- Pedunculated earlobe keloids tend to have better response to excision than keloids of other locations. Pre-excision serial intralesional steroid injections monthly for 3 to 5 months can reduce the chance of recurrent earlobe keloids after excision.

Therapy

There is no consistently effective modality for the treatment of keloids. Intralesional triamcinolone (0.1 to 1 mL at 20 to 40 mg/kg) is the most widely accepted first-line therapy to treat and prevent keloidal growth. Although clear evidence for a beneficial effect of silicone is lacking, many providers also utilize silicone gel sheeting to reduce and prevent keloidal or hypertrophic scarring. Prevention is also attempted with pressure therapy (i.e., compression garments or "clip-on" earrings for earlobe keloids).

Less-accepted Alternative Therapies Include

Intralesional interferon, α and γ: 0.01 to 0.1 mg three times per week

Cryosurgery plus intralesional steroids

Re-excision with adjunctive therapy (radiation, imiquimod, or corticosteroids)

Carbon dioxide (CO_2) laser

Pulsed dye laser to actively expanding lesions

Suggested Readings

Bolognia JL, Jorizzo JL, Rapini RP. *Dermatology*. Vol. 2. 2nd Ed. St Louis, MO: Mosby; 2008:2291–2292.

James WD, Berger TG, Elston DM, eds. *Andrews' Diseases of the Skin*. 10th Ed. Philadelphia, PA: WB Saunders; 2006:602–604.

O'Brien L, Pandit A. Silicon gel sheeting for preventing and treating hypertrophic and keloid scars. *Cochrane Database Syst Rev*. 2006;(1):CD003826.

Wood F, Rea S, Tuckerman JL, et al. Interventions for treating keloid disease. *Cochrane Database Syst Rev*. 2008;(3):CD006805.

Lipoma

Diagnosis Synopsis

Lipomas are benign tumors of fat cells that usually occur in those aged between 30 and 60 years. The possible predisposing factors are obesity, diabetes, and genetic predisposition (familial lipomatosis). They are commonly found on the neck, shoulders, back, and abdomen. The lesions can be single or multiple.

The clinical variants of lipoma are nevus lipomatosus superficialis, angiolipomas, and many others.

In lipomatosis, numerous lipomas can occur in subcutaneous tissue. Familial lipomatosis occurs in adulthood. Lipomatoses in children include *Proteus* syndrome, Bannayan–Riley–Ruvalcaba syndrome, and encephalocraniocutaneous lipomatosis.

Look For

Solitary or multiple soft, round to ovoid, lobulated tumors with the typical slippery edge (Figs. 4-361 and 4-362). The tumors are painless and freely movable. Overlying skin can be pinched up.

Nevus lipomatosus superficialis—clusters of soft skin-colored to yellowish papuloplaques or nodules on the thighs, gluteal region, and lumbosacral region (Fig. 4-363).

Look for spinal dysraphism in the case of congenital, centrally located lumbosacral lipomas (Fig. 4-364).

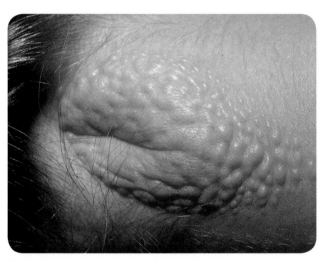

Figure 4-361 Lipoma with a corrugated surface.

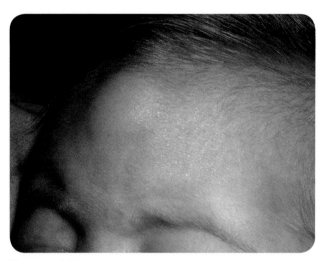

Figure 4-362 Lipoma in a common location.

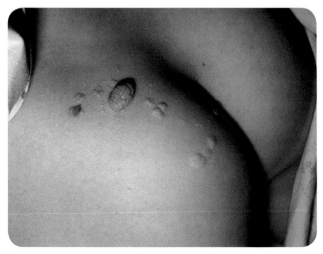

Figure 4-363 Nevus superficialis lipomatosus is a connective tissue nevus with fat differentiation.

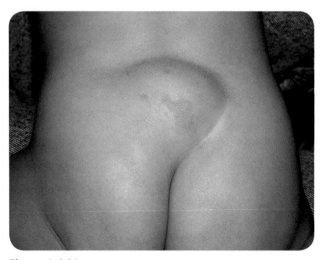

Figure 4-364 Lipoma in midline of lower back requires imaging to investigate spinal dysraphism.

Diagnostic Pearls

Lipomas are not tender; angiolipomas are tender and may have a faint overlying erythema.

 Differential Diagnosis and Pitfalls

- Neurofibroma—soft flesh-colored papule or papulonodule that can be moved in lateral (side to side) but not along the direction of the nerve. The pathognomonic "buttonhole" sign is positive.
- Epidermal cyst—cystic swelling with dilated pores or punctum. Overlying skin cannot be pinched upward.

✓ **Best Tests**

- Biopsy the lesion.
- Ultrasound may be used to distinguish from vascular and cystic lesions.

 Management Pearls

Lipomas can be left alone. Malignant transformation of cutaneous lipomas is extremely rare.

Therapy

A lipoma can often be fully excised through a small skin opening. A 6-mm punch biopsy can be used over the lipoma and then, through a combination of manual expression and curettage, the entire lipoma can be removed through the small opening.

Liposuction has been used for treatment of larger lesions.

Suggested Readings

Dalal KM, Antonescu CR, Singer S. Diagnosis and management of lipomatous tumors. *J Surg Oncol*. 2008;97(4):298–313.

Mentzel T. Cutaneous lipomatous neoplasms. *Semin Diagn Pathol*. 2001;18(4):250–257.

Pilomatricoma

Diagnosis Synopsis

Pilomatricoma, also known as calcifying epithelioma of Malherbe or pilomatrixoma, is a small benign tumor of hair cortex cell origin. A molecular defect in β-catenin is present in the lesions. Pilomatricoma tends to arise during early childhood as solitary, asymptomatic tumors. Although usually sporadic in incidence, familial cases of pilomatricomas have been reported. Additionally, multiple pilomatricomas have been observed in patients with myotonic dystrophy and Gardner syndrome.

Look For

Usually single (sometimes multiple), small tumors or cystlike lesions, with either normal overlying skin or a bluish-red surface color (Figs. 4-365–4-368). Lesions typically range between <1 and 3 cm in size. These hard, cystlike growths are usually found on the face, scalp, or upper extremities.

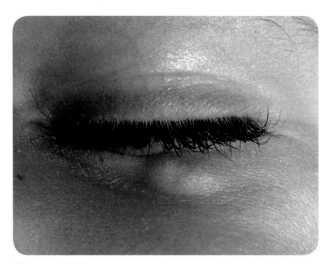

Figure 4-367 Pilomatricoma presenting as a bifid nodule.

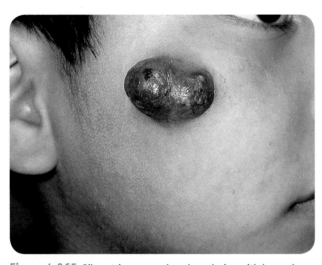

Figure 4-365 Pilomatricoma may be a large lesion with hemorrhage.

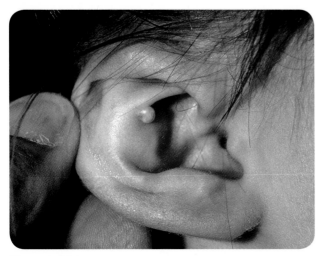

Figure 4-366 Pilomatricoma presenting as a raised papule.

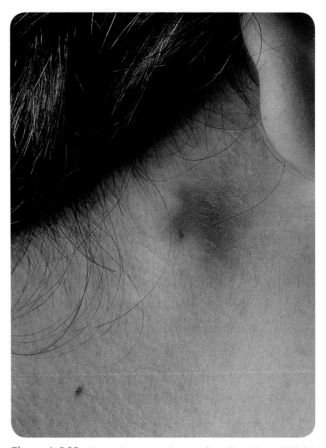

Figure 4-368 Pilomatricoma may have surface distortion and bluish hue, as in this nodule.

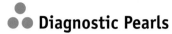
Diagnostic Pearls

- When superficial, they may have a chalky-white appearance. Often, the lesions assume an angulated shape (tent sign).
- Multiple lesions can be associated with myotonic dystrophy.
- If deep in the skin, the lesion may appear blue.
- On palpation, lesions have an irregular "meteorite"-like topography.

?? Differential Diagnosis and Pitfalls

- Epidermoid cyst can frequently be identified by observing an overlying punctum.
- A pilomatricoma is typically firmer and less regular in shape than a dermoid cyst.
- Glomus tumor is painful and tends to involve the nail unit.
- Osteoma cutis presents as a firm dermal nodule and may be clinically indistinguishable from pilomatricoma.
- Calcinosis cutis also presents as a firm dermal nodule and may be clinically indistinguishable from pilomatricoma.

Best Tests

Skin biopsy will reveal an encapsulated dermal tumor with characteristic "shadow cells."

▲▲ Management Pearls

Incompletely excised lesions may recur.

Therapy

Simple excision is the best way to remove the growth.

Suggested Readings

Bolognia JL, Jorizzo JL, Rapini RP, eds. *Dermatology.* Vol. 2. 2nd Ed. St Louis, MO: Mosby; 2008:1698–1699.

Cohen BA, ed. *Pediatric dermatology.* 3rd Ed. St Louis, MO: Mosby; 2005:129–130.

James WD, Berger TG, Elston DM, eds. *Andrews' Diseases of the Skin.* 10th Ed. Philadelphia, PA: WB Saunders; 2006:670–671.

Spider Angioma

Diagnosis Synopsis

A spider angioma, also known as nevus araneus or spider nevus, is the most common telangiectasia in childhood. It is composed of a central arteriole with numerous radiating telangiectases. Lesions are never present at birth but may arise spontaneously at any time after 2 years of age. The etiology in children is unknown, although trauma and sun exposure are hypothesized to play a role in their development. It is estimated that 50% of spider angiomas will spontaneously regress by adulthood.

Look For

Bright red lesions consisting of a small central papule surrounded by small radiating vessels (Figs. 4-369–4-372).

Spider angiomas occur most commonly on the sun-exposed areas of the face, neck, trunk, and arms.

Diagnostic Pearls

Lesions blanch completely on diascopy and rapidly refill from the central arteriole when pressure is released.

?? Differential Diagnosis and Pitfalls

- Insect bites
- Hereditary hemorrhagic telangiectasia
- Pyogenic granuloma
- Cherry angioma
- Angiokeratoma corporis circumscriptum
- Ataxia telangiectatica

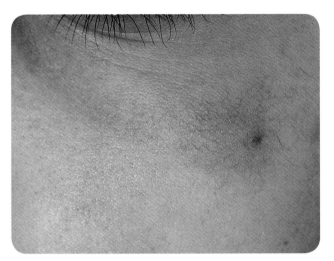

Figure 4-369 Spider angioma with a raised red punctum and dilated vessels in a common location.

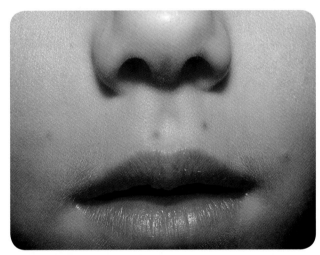

Figure 4-370 Spider angioma on the upper lip.

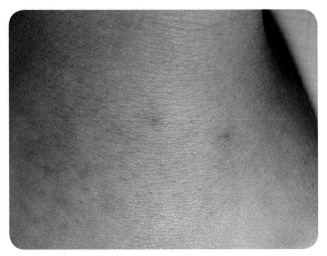

Figure 4-371 Spider angiomas.

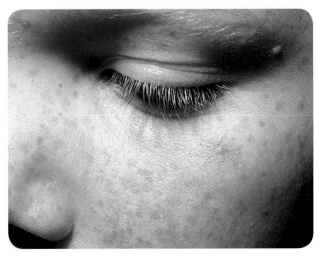

Figure 4-372 Spider angioma with dilated vessels.

- Rendu–Osler–Weber syndrome
- Capillaritis

 Best Tests

This is a clinical diagnosis.

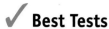 **Management Pearls**

Strict sun protection may prevent the development of new lesions.

Therapy

Electrodesiccation
The central arteriole can be ablated using fine needle electrodesiccation. This involves sealing of the blood vessels by monopolar, high-frequency electric current. A pinpoint scar is often produced by this method.

Laser Treatment
Pulsed dye laser therapy will completely remove spider angiomas in one to two treatments. Proper application results in complete removal of the angioma without scarring. Local anesthesia is unnecessary and decreases the effectiveness of the laser.

Special Considerations in Infants

Spider angiomas do not occur in infancy, and other diagnoses should be strongly considered.

Suggested Readings

Frieden I, Enjolras O, Esterly N. Vascular birthmarks and other abnormalities of blood vessels and lymphatics. In: Schachner LA, Hansen RC, eds. *Pediatric Dermatology*. 3rd Ed. Edinburgh, Scotland: Mosby; 2003: 833–862.

Mancini AJ, Paller AS. *Hurwitz Clinical Pediatric Dermatology*. 3rd Ed. Philadelphia, PA: Elsevier Saunders; 2006:307–344.

■■ Diagnosis Synopsis

Giant congenital nevi occur in approximately 1 in 20,000 newborns. These giant congenital nevi most often occur on the trunk, followed by the extremities, the head, and the neck. The definition of giant congenital nevus varies but may include those that measure 20 cm or larger in greatest diameter in an adult, those that cover more than 1% of the surface of the head or neck, or those that cannot be excised in a single operation.

The lifetime risk of melanoma has been reported to range anywhere from 5% to 10%, usually with very large lesions with higher risks of malignancy. Another reported complication is neurocutaneous melanosis, which is defined by the presence of benign or malignant melanocytic proliferations in the central nervous system, most commonly involving the leptomeninges.

◉ Look For

Extensive areas of hyperpigmentation on the trunk with possible areas on the head and neck or extremities (Figs. 4-373 and 4-374). Black patches and plaques are common. Satellite lesions, away from the main lesion, may be seen as well (Figs. 4-375 and 4-376). The areas may have darker and less pigmentation such that within the entire lesion, colors range from tan or pink to black; erosions in large nevi are not uncommon. As with small and medium congenital nevi, they grow proportionally with the child.

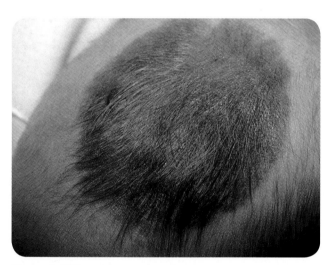

Figure 4-373 Giant congenital nevus in the scalp.

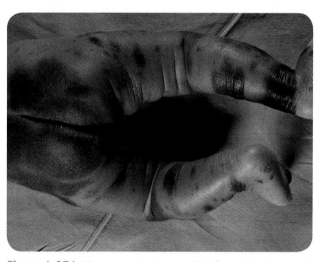

Figure 4-374 Giant congenital nevus with large scattered congenital nevi.

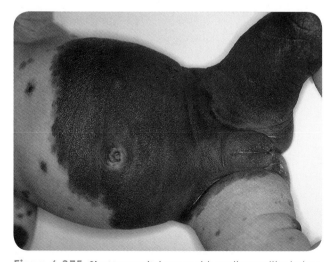

Figure 4-375 Giant congenital nevus with smaller satellite lesions. Color of such lesions varies from brown to black.

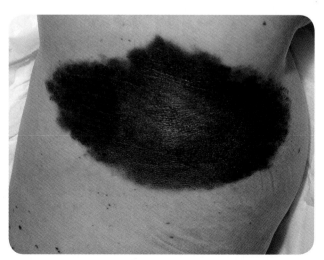

Figure 4-376 Giant congenital nevus with very small satellite lesions. The back is a common location.

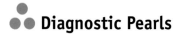

Diagnostic Pearls

- Large dark brown or black patches or plaques on the newborn are typical.
- Multiple satellite lesions or nevi overlying the midline or calvaria raise the concern for potential neurocutaneous melanosis.

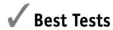

Differential Diagnosis and Pitfalls

- Café au lait macules can be similar to early lightly pigmented congenital melanocytic nevi; however, they do not progressively darken with time
- Mongolian spot
- Nevus of Ota
- Nevus spilus

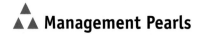

Best Tests

Clinical diagnosis with biopsy of irregular regions.

Management Pearls

Giant congenital nevi are best managed with a multidisciplinary approach. Consultations should be obtained from pediatrics, dermatology, and plastic surgery. Psychiatry should be involved for the parents and caregivers, as well as the patients themselves as they get older. If neurocutaneous melanosis is suspected, neurology and neurosurgery should be consulted as well.

Therapy

Fifty percent of melanomas in these lesions occur before the age of three, 60% in childhood, and 70% by puberty, so early and frequent screening is recommended. Multiple different treatments have been proposed to include surgical excision, curettage, dermabrasion, chemical peeling, and lasers. Surgical excision, sometimes in conjunction with tissue expansion, is the therapy most often recommended. Decisions are best made on a case-by-case basis after discussion involving the entire treatment team. For patients in whom neurocutaneous melanosis is suspected, an MRI of the brain and spinal cord should be obtained.

Suggested Readings

Arneja JS, Gosain AK. Giant congenital melanocytic nevi. *Plastic Reconst Surg.* 2007;120(2):26e–40e.

DeRaeve LE, Roseeuw DI. Curettage of giant congenital melanocytic nevi in neonates: a decade later. *Arch Dermatol.* 2002;138(7):943–947.

Krengel S, Hauschild A, Schäfer T. Melanoma risk in congenital melanocytic naevi: A systematic review. *Br J Dermatol.* 2006;155(1):1–8.

Tannous ZS, Mihm MC Jr, Sober AJ, et al. Congenital melanocytic nevi: Clinical and histopathologic features, risk of melanoma, and clinical management. *J Am Acad Dermatol.* 2005;52(2):197–203.

Lentigo Simplex

  ## Diagnosis Synopsis

Lentigo simplex is a common pigmented macule seen in childhood or, less frequently, at birth. The macule has little or no relationship with sun exposure and is the result of an increased number of melanocytes that manifest clinically as small hyperpigmented macules. Lentigo simplex can occur anywhere on the body. Multiple lentigos can occur with or without an underlying syndrome. Single lesions may also be seen on the lips, genitals, or gums.

Look For

Look for brown to almost black, regular, small macules, typically 3 mm or smaller in diameter (Fig. 4-377).

Diagnostic Pearls

Lentigo simplex is more regular than freckles (ephelides) that tend to darken with summer sun exposure.

?? Differential Diagnosis and Pitfalls

- Nevus spilus appears as a circumscribed patch of light brown hyperpigmentation with smaller, darker pigmented macules or papules within the patch.
- In children with multiple lentigines, consider LEOPARD syndrome, which consists of
  – Lentigines
  – EKG abnormalities
  – Ocular hypertelorism
  – Pulmonary stenosis
  – Abnormal genitalia
  – Retarded growth
  – Deafness
- Also consider Peutz–Jeghers syndrome, especially with multiple facial and perioral lentigines; GI hamartomatous polyps are part of the syndrome.
- African–Americans frequently have centrofacial lentiginosis that are inherited as an autosomal dominant trait.
- Solar lentigo typically occurs on sun-exposed surfaces with increasing age and is less regular in appearance.
- A café-au-lait macule is macular, even-colored, and present from early childhood.
- An oral mucosal lesion may be difficult to distinguish from an amalgam tattoo.

✓ Best Tests

Clinical exam is generally sufficient.

▲▲ Management Pearls

The ABCDEs of melanoma should be reviewed with the parents (and the patient if he/she is old enough). The patient may be followed annually in the office or at home by the patient or his/her parents with instructions to return if any suspicious changes are noted.

A—asymmetry
B—border irregularity
C—color variation
D—diameter >6 mm
E—evolution (change in appearance)

Therapy

For a simple lentigo, no treatment is required. A biopsy (preferably a punch biopsy) should be performed if there is any concern about melanoma.

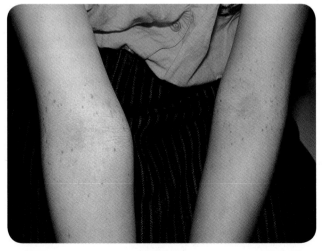

Figure 4-377 Lentigo simplex lesions are often darker than freckles and, when multiple, may be associated with systemic diseases.

Suggested Readings

Bolognia JL, Jorizzo JL, Rapini RP, eds. *Dermatology.* Vol. 1. 2nd Ed. St Louis, MO: Mosby; 2008:1717–1720.

■■ Diagnosis Synopsis

Melanoma is a life-threatening skin cancer seen with increasing frequency worldwide. Patients aged 20 years and younger represent 1% of all patients diagnosed with melanoma.

Predisposing conditions for melanoma in children include giant congenital melanocytic nevi, dysplastic nevus syndromes, xeroderma pigmentosum, or immunodeficiency states (either inherited or iatrogenic). A family history of melanoma, history of severe sunburns, multiple atypical nevi, inability to tan, or red hair color are predisposing conditions to adult melanoma; the relevance to development of childhood melanoma is unknown. Approximately 30% of pediatric melanomas arise from giant congenital nevi, while another 50% arise de novo.

In a review comparing pediatric melanoma with adult melanoma, it was found that pediatric patients often have a thicker depth of invasion at the time of diagnosis as well as a higher incidence of positive lymph node metastasis. Interestingly, however, there was no statistical difference in the 5- and 10-year survival between the two groups.

◉ Look For

Typical features such as asymmetry, irregular borders, color variation, and diameter >6 mm are helpful but are not always present in the pediatric population (Figs. 4-378–4-381). Pediatric melanomas are often amelanotic (nonpigmented). Change in size is not often reliable as children are growing, but any lesion that grows out of proportion with the patient raises concern. Lesions that ulcerate, bleed, or change in color are also worrisome.

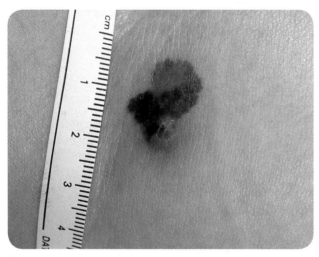

Figure 4-378 Melanoma with irregular pigmentation.

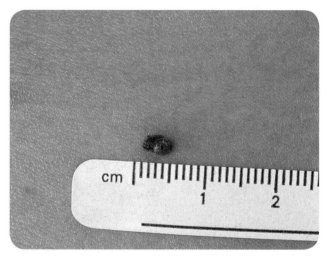

Figure 4-379 Spitz nevus. Gray color and black rim suggest melanoma.

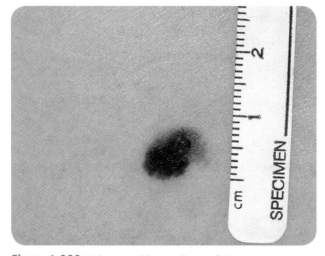

Figure 4-380 Melanoma with a small area of pigment spread.

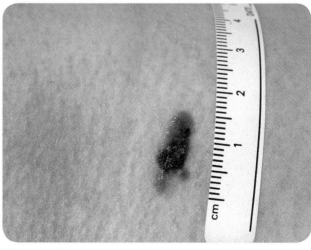

Figure 4-381 Melanoma with multiple colors and small nodule.

Diagnostic Pearls

Amelanotic melanomas can be very atypical in appearance and will not have the usual color changes seen in other melanomas. Any suspected melanoma will need a biopsy to establish diagnosis.

Differential Diagnosis and Pitfalls

- Spitz nevi—sometimes called juvenile melanoma—are often a source of confusion for doctor and patient.
- Compound nevi
- Dysplastic nevi
- Congenital nevi
- Blue nevi
- Lentigines
- Pyogenic granulomas
- Angiokeratoma

Best Tests

A punch or excisional biopsy should be performed on any suspicious lesion.

Management Pearls

- Dermoscopic examination allows rapid examination of the pigment pattern in a large number of lesions. Whole body photographs establish an objective baseline for follow-up. Early diagnosis with prompt surgical excision is crucial as there is no truly effective therapy for metastatic melanoma.

- Individuals with one melanoma have a higher frequency of another melanoma occurring and should have careful and regular follow-up.
- Family members of the patients with a melanoma and multiple atypical nevi should also be examined.

Therapy

Excision of suspicious lesions after biopsy.

- 0.5 cm margin for in situ melanoma
- 1 cm margins for lesions <2 mm in thickness
- 2 cm margins for lesions >2 mm in thickness

Recent reviews have demonstrated a role for both sentinel lymph node biopsy and adjuvant interferon. The role of PET scans or PET/CT is less clear in the pediatric population.

Suggested Readings

Abdulla FR, Feldman SR, Williford PM, et al. Tanning and skin cancer. *Pediatr Dermatol.* 2005;22(6):501–512.

Bütter A, Hui T, Chapdelaine J, et al. Melanoma in children and the use of sentinel lymph node biopsy. *J Pediatr Surg.* 2005;40(5):797–800.

Downard CD, Rapkin LB, Gow KW. Melanoma in children and adolescents. *Surg Oncol.* 2007;16(3):215–220.

French JC, Rowe MR, Lee TJ, et al. Pediatric melanoma of the head and neck: A single institutions experience. *Laryngoscope.* 2006;116(12): 2216–2220.

Livestro DP, Kaine EM, Michaelson JS, et al. Melanoma in the young: differences and similarities with adult melanoma: A case matched control analysis. *Cancer.* 2007;110:614–624.

Schaffer JV. Pigmented lesions in children: When to worry. *Curr Opin Pediatr.* 2007;19(4):430–440.

Diagnosis Synopsis

Atypical, or dysplastic, nevi are benign acquired melanocytic nevi characterized by aggregation of melanocytes that have an abnormal architecture and cellular atypia. These pigmented melanocytic lesions fall on the continuum between benign nevi and melanoma.

Atypical nevi usually begin to appear during puberty and may be seen anywhere, but they most often occur on sun-exposed areas. Clinically, atypical nevi share some of the features of melanoma, including asymmetry, color variegation, border irregularity, and larger size.

Look For

Asymmetric shape along two axes
Border that is irregular or "fuzzy"
Color variegation containing pink, tan, brown, and dark brown
Diameter >5 mm
Dysplastic nevi may occur anywhere, but they occur more often on sun-exposed areas
Evolution.

In atypical nevus syndrome, hundreds of nevi of varying size and color are seen (Figs. 4-382–4-385).

Diagnostic Pearls

- The occurrence of a new pigmented lesion in a child is common. Discerning an atypical nevus from a normal nevus can be difficult. Maintain a very low threshold of suspicion for any new pigmented lesions that have a much darker color than other nevi, multiple colors, asymmetry, symptoms, or irregular border.
- If indicated, plan for excisional biopsy early to rule out atypical nevus or melanoma. If a parent or child states a nevus is symptomatic or has changed, have a very low threshold to remove.
- Question the parents about a family history of melanoma and examine first-degree relatives.
- There is a high incidence of clinically appearing atypical nevi on the scalp and forehead in children and adolescents. Most pediatric dermatologists feel that these lesions have worse clinical appearance than biologic behavior. Careful clinical examination and monitoring are prudent. Multiple scalp excisions, however, are likely unnecessary.

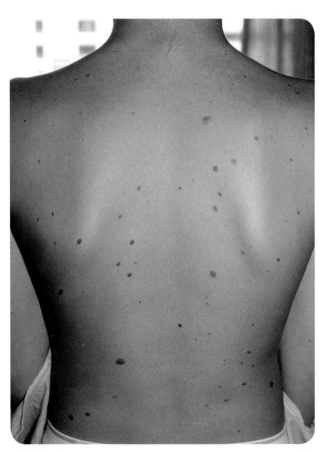

Figure 4-382 Atypical nevi with multiple lesions.

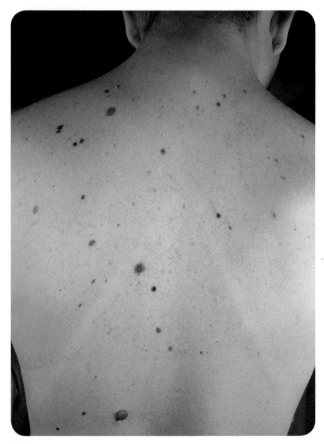

Figure 4-383 Atypical nevi with multiple sizes and shapes.

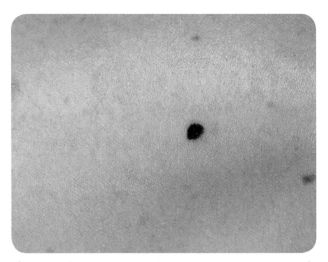

Figure 4-384 Spitz nevus with black pigmentation.

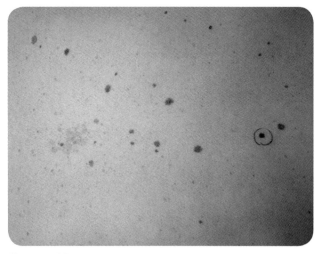

Figure 4-385 Atypical nevus in a child with multiple nevi. The circled nevus is darker in pigmentation than all the surrounding nevi; has a notched, irregular border; and has variegated pigmentation.

?? Differential Diagnosis and Pitfalls

- Melanoma—rapidly enlarging papule or nodule, often bluish-black or brownish-black in color. Bleeding, itching, ulceration, and crusting may be present. Many have the typical ABCDEs of melanoma.
- Compound nevus—flesh-colored to brown, smooth or papillomatous papule with dark, coarse hairs within them.
- Blue nevus—uniformly pigmented (dark blue or bluish-black), round or oval, smooth-surfaced, dome-shaped, solitary papule.
- Spitz nevi—pinkish, tan, or red-brown; smooth-surfaced; dome-shaped; solitary papule, often with surface telangiectasia.

✓ Best Tests

Excisional skin biopsy is indicated to exclude other lesions such as melanoma. Partial biopsy only provides histology of the section removed.

▲▲ Management Pearls

- Atypical nevi and melanoma frequently run in families. Therefore, question the parents about a family history of melanoma and examine first-degree relatives.
- Children with multiple nevi and atypical nevi should be examined by a dermatologist every 6 to 12 months,

depending on the patient's past medical and family history as well as the morphology of the lesion(s). If atypical nevi are seen in a child with a family history of melanoma, careful follow-up is appropriate. (Whole body and specific nevus photographs may be useful.)
- Dermoscopy offers better characterization of the atypical nevi and the pigment distribution. Atypical nevi that show eccentric peripheral hyperpigmentation should be assessed carefully.

Therapy

Surgical removal is indicated when the nevus becomes symptomatic or changes in shape or color.

Sun-protective measures, including assiduous use of sunscreens (SPF 30 at a minimum).

Suggested Readings

Fernandez M, Raimer SS, Sánchez RL. Dysplastic nevi of the scalp and forehead in children. *Pediatr Dermatol.* 2001;18:5–8.

Haley JC, Hood AF, Chuang TY, et al. The frequency of histologically dysplastic nevi in 199 pediatric patients. *Pediatr Dermatol.* 2000;17(4): 266–269.

Hofmann-Wellenhof R, et al Dermoscopic classification of atypical melanocytic nevi (Clark nevi). *Arch Dermatol.* 2001;137(12):1575–1580.

Schaffer JV. Pigmented lesions in children: When to worry. *Curr Opin Pediatr.* 2007;19(4):430–440.

■■ Diagnosis Synopsis

Aplasia cutis congenita is a congenital disorder seen in newborns. It typically manifests as an absence of the skin of the scalp but can occur in any location. While most children have no other associated abnormalities, cleft lip and palate, tracheoesophageal fistula, double cervix and uterus, patent ductus arteriosus, coarctation of the aorta, cutis marmorata telangiectatica congenita, AV fistulas, CNS dysraphisms, and intestinal lymphangiectasia have been reported with the anomaly. The newborn can present with open erosion or a healed, depressed scar.

◉ Look For

A localized alopecia with scarred and atrophic epidermis (Figs. 4-386–4-389). There may be a "hair collar sign"

(presence of hypertrichosis or coarse hair at the rim of the lesion). Although typically seen as a depressed scar, some may have a hypertrophic scar.

●● Diagnostic Pearls

- Aplasia cutis congenita may present as single or sometimes overlapping papules resembling a barbell. It lacks the pinkish cobblestoned surface of sebaceus nevi.
- If the lesion is associated with lipoma or vascular stain, the likelihood of the underlying CNS malformation is significantly greater.

?? Differential Diagnosis and Pitfalls

- Most cases of aplasia cutis congenita do not have other associated findings. However, the lesion has been associated

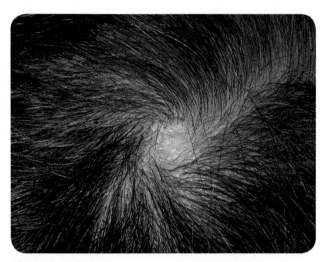

Figure 4-386 Aplasia cutis congenita heals with atrophic scarring with no hair follicles.

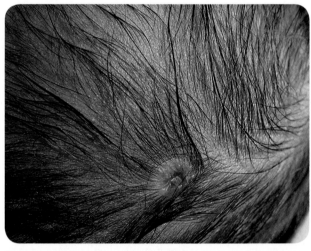

Figure 4-387 Aplasia cutis congenita in a neonate with a small, punched-out ulceration in a typical location near the vertex.

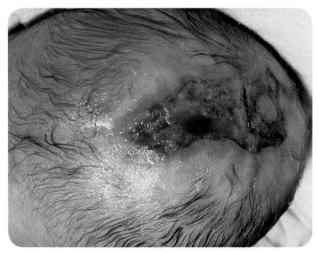

Figure 4-388 Aplasia cutis congenita with large, irregularly shaped ulceration.

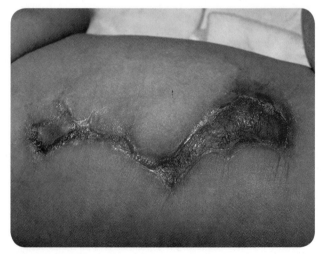

Figure 4-389 Stellate aplasia cutis congenita with partial healing and wound retraction.

with trisomy 13, which should be considered if other signs and symptoms of trisomy 13 are present. Aplasia cutis congenita is also seen in focal dermal hypoplasia (Goltz syndrome) and epidermolysis bullosa.
- Erosions from herpes simplex infection
- Ulceration from application of scalp electrodes or forceps
- Neonatal lupus
- Nevus sebaceus
- Pyoderma

✔ Best Tests

- Observation.
- On rare occasions, an X-ray may be indicated if large or stellate scalp lesions are present.
- CNS imaging if hair collar sign is present.

▲▲ Management Pearls

- Scalp defects are self-limiting and heal spontaneously with scarring. In severe cases, surgery is necessary to close the defect.

- Hypertrophic lesions respond to intralesional steroid injections (10 mg/mL, 0.1 to 0.3 mL).

Therapy

Standard good wound care until completely healed.

Special Considerations in Infants

In neonates, aplasia cutis congenita can present as moist open erosions or healed and atrophic scars. Bullous lesions can drain, then refill. Hair collar sign may be associated with underlying CNS dysraphism.

Suggested Readings

Frieden IJ. Aplasia cutis congenita: A clinical review and proposal for classification. *J Am Acad Dermatol*. 1986;14(4):646–660.

Spraker MK, Garcia-Gonzalez E, Tamayo Sanchez L. Sclerosing and atrophying conditions. In: Schachner LA, Hansen RC, eds. *Pediatric Dermatology*. 3rd Ed. Edinburgh, Scotland: Mosby; 2003:793–795.

▪️ Diagnosis Synopsis

Alopecia areata is a T-lymphocyte mediated autoimmune disease of the hair follicle resulting in nonscarring hair loss. Most cases are limited to one to two small patches of alopecia, but in severe cases all the hair on the scalp may be lost (alopecia totalis) or all body hair may be lost (alopecia universalis). Hair in most patients will spontaneously regrow, though recurrences are also typical. Alopecia areata is seen equally in both sexes and in patients of all ethnic groups and ages, though it is seen most commonly in the first three decades. There is an increased incidence of alopecia areata in patients with Down syndrome; in those with autoimmune diseases, such as vitiligo; and the autoimmune polyglandular syndrome. Patients with alopecia areata are also more likely to have atopy (atopic dermatitis, seasonal allergies, and asthma). The condition is treatable but cannot be cured.

◉ Look For

Round, patchy areas of nonscarring hair loss (Figs. 4-390–4-392). Although it usually affects the scalp, the condition can also target the eyebrows, eyelashes, beard, and other body sites. Typically, gray or white hairs are not affected. Additionally, pitting and ridging of the fingernails can occur with this disease (Fig. 4-393). Hairs that grow back are often hypopigmented; the hypopigmentation is usually temporary but may be permanent. This hypopigmentation is not seen in other forms of alopecia.

● Diagnostic Pearls

- Scalp burning, with or without redness, can accompany the lesions.

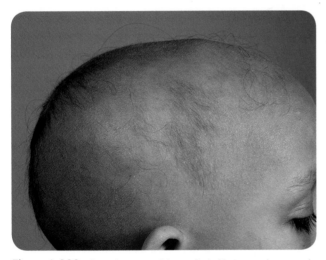

Figure 4-390 Alopecia areata with rare foci of hair growth approaching alopecia totalis.

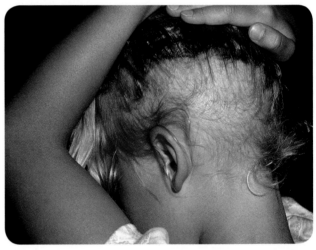

Figure 4-391 Alopecia areata with hair loss extending as a band from the posterior occiput, the ophiasis pattern.

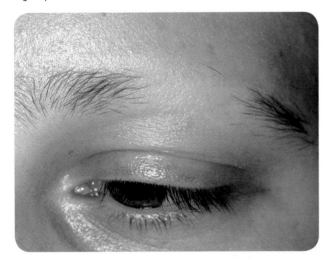

Figure 4-392 Alopecia areata in a focal location in the eyebrow.

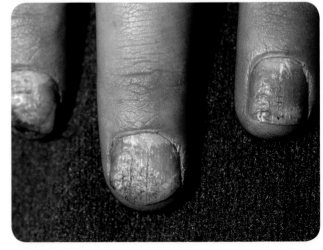

Figure 4-393 Alopecia areata with involvement of the nail plate and coarse stippling.

- Exclamation point hairs with a tapering base and a ragged proximal portion are diagnostic of the disease. They are frequently at the border of the lesions and can be seen with the aid of a magnifying glass. The ragged end is easily seen under the microscope.
- A hair-pull test (gentle pulling on the hairs with fingers) is often positive at the periphery of active areas.

?? Differential Diagnosis and Pitfalls

- Trichotillomania—from the twisting and pulling of hair, may mimic alopecia areata. Hairs are broken off at varying lengths.
- Telogen effluvium—usually secondary to recent major illness, surgery, or malnutrition. The loss is diffuse, not localized.
- Tinea capitis—usually associated with lymphadenopathy and pruritus.
- Syphilis.
- Loose anagen syndrome.

✓ Best Tests

- This diagnosis can usually be made clinically, though scalp biopsy can be helpful if the diagnosis is in question. Biopsy appearance will vary depending on the age of the area that is sampled.

If the clinical situation warrants, tests for associated conditions may be fruitful:

- Ferritin (to rule out iron deficiency)
- Thyroid stimulating hormone

▲▲ Management Pearls

- It is important to help the patient understand the nature of the disease and that there is often a chance of regrowth. The condition is benign but can be psychosocially devastating to the patient or family; therefore, treatment is best made on a case-by-case basis.
- Support groups, wigs, hats, caps, and scarves are important options for some patients.
- Patients with severe atopy often have a poorer prognosis for regrowth.

Therapy

Think and counsel carefully before attempting treatment, which can be unsuccessful. A recent Cochrane review, which included 17 trials with a total of 540 patients, found no interventions that showed significant treatment benefit in terms of hair regrowth when compared to placebo. Patients with limited areas of loss in regions of no cosmetic importance are often best left untreated as spontaneous regrowth often occurs within a year.

First-line therapy includes topical steroids (clobetasol propionate solution twice daily). A trial of at least 1 month should be attempted before other therapies are considered.

If topical steroids are ineffective, intralesional corticosteroids may be considered. The most commonly used is triamcinolone acetonide aqueous suspension injected in a subdermal fashion at a concentration of 3 to 5 mg/mL at 1-month intervals. No more than 3 mL should be injected per visit. Concentrations greater then 5 mg/mL are associated with cutaneous atrophy and should be avoided.

Topical immunotherapy offers another approach if topical or intralesional steroids are ineffective or not well tolerated. One study found some success using squaric acid dibutyl ester in acetone. This treatment is not FDA approved for any age group.

For extensive disease, consider PUVA or topical steroids plus minoxidil (each applied twice daily). The efficacy of each is debated. Systemic corticosteroids may offer short-term help, but they have no long-term benefit and should be avoided. A small recently published study compared the use of methotrexate with or without systemic steroids; this approach may be considered when widespread involvement is noted and no other treatments have been helpful.

Suggested Readings

Ajith C, Gupta S, Kanwar AJ. Efficacy and safety of the topical sensitizer squaric acid dibutyl ester in alopecia areata and factors influencing the outcome. *J Drugs Dermatol.* 2006;5(3):262–266.

Delamere FM, Sladden MM, Dobbins HM, et al. Interventions for alopecia areata. *Cochrane Database Sys Rev.* 2008;2:CD004413.

Joly P. The use of methotrexate alone or in combination with low doses of oral corticosteroids in the treatment of alopecia totalis or universalis. *J Am Acad Dermatol.* 2006;55(4):632–636.

Wolff K, Goldsmith LA, Katz SI, et al., eds. *Fitzpatrick's Dermatology in General Medicine.* Vol 1. 7th Ed. New York, NY: McGraw-Hill; 2008:762–765.

Nevus Sebaceus

■■ Diagnosis Synopsis

Nevus sebaceus (nevus sebaceus of Jadassohn) is a congenital growth that usually presents at birth or early childhood. It is typically found on the scalp as a hairless lesion that persists indefinitely. Numerous benign intralesional neoplasms may arise, most commonly after adolescence. True basal cell carcinomas may also arise but are only thought to eventually affect <1% of lesions. Removal is generally recommended before adolescence.

◉ Look For

A solitary pink to yellow-orange, hairless plaque at birth, which may darken or thicken into a rubbery, cobblestone quality at puberty (Figs. 4-394–4-397).

●● Diagnostic Pearls

- The lesion is often raised and cobblestoned in the neonate.
- As maternal hormones decrease, the lesion flattens but maintains its orange color.
- As children enter pubertal years, sebaceous gland proliferation (in response to changing hormones) makes the lesion thicken.

?? Differential Diagnosis and Pitfalls

- Perinatal trauma to the scalp from forceps, scalp blood sampling, or monitor electrode placement may result in scarring with associated alopecia.

- Aplasia cutis congenita presents at birth as a focal erosion or ulceration in the scalp. Lesions eventually heal with atrophy and scarring with associated alopecia. A ring of long, coarse, dark hair (hair collar sign) suggests associated underlying neural tube closure defect.

✓ Best Tests

This is usually a clinical diagnosis. Skin biopsy is diagnostic.

▲▲ Management Pearls

- In the adult years, benign adnexal neoplasms, basaloid neoplasms, true basal cell carcinomas, or, rarely, squamous cell carcinoma can develop within a nevus sebaceus. Prophylactic excision of the entire lesion is reasonable.
- For larger (larger than 1.5 cm) or facial lesions, early removal (first 3 years of life) results in overall better cosmetic outcome.

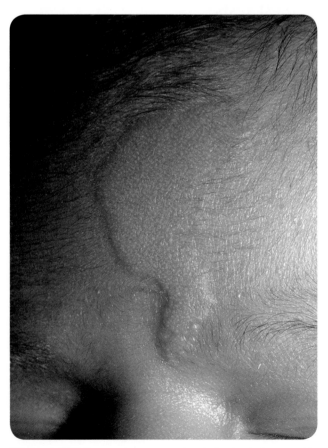

Figure 4-395 Nevus sebaceus as a sharply bordered plaque on the forehead.

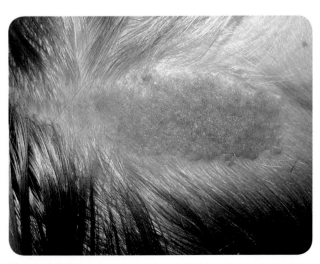

Figure 4-394 Nevus sebaceus in a typical location on the scalp.

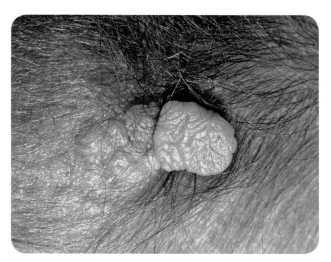

Figure 4-396 Nevus sebaceus with irregular hairless surface.

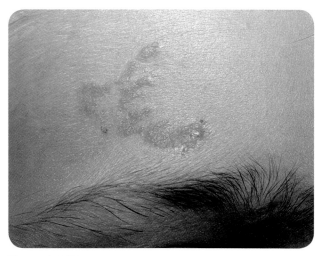

Figure 4-397 Nevus sebaceus with orange-brown color.

Therapy

Surgical removal is reasonable; it can be delayed for adolescence with small lesions (smaller than 8 mm). Consider
early excision for larger lesions to minimize scar and
deformity.

Suggested Readings

Cohen BA, ed. *Pediatric Dermatology*. 3rd Ed. St Louis, MO: Mosby;
2005:55.

James WD, Berger TG, Elston DM, eds. *Andrews' Diseases of the Skin*.
10th Ed. Philadelphia, PA: WB Saunders; 2006:661–662.

Pediculosis Capitis (Head Lice)

◼◼ Diagnosis Synopsis

Pediculosis capitis, also known as head lice, is caused by *Pediculus humanus capitis* (head lice). Pediculosis typically affects children between ages 3 to 11 of all socioeconomic groups. Transmission is by close contact (direct head-to-head contact) and fomites (e.g., on clothes, brushes, linens, combs, hats, etc.). Lice live approximately 30 days on the host and 1 to 3 days off the host. Eggs (nits) hatch within 7 to 10 days.

Resistance to permethrin, pyrethrins, malathion, and lindane has been documented.

◉ Look For

Lice and nits in the scalp and hair (**Figs. 4-398 and 4-399**).

The adult lice are small wingless ectoparasites. They are 1 to 3 mm long with elongated bodies and three pairs of claw-like legs (**Figs. 4-400 and 4-401**).

Nits appear as 0.5 to 1 mm gray-white specks that are firmly attached to individual hair shafts. Microscopy will reveal an oblong structure attached to the hair at an acute angle with a lobular breathing apparatus at its superior end.

Cervical and occipital lymphadenopathy may occur as a result of secondary infection.

●● Diagnostic Pearls

Pyodermas in the scalp along with occipital and cervical lymphadenopathy suggest possible pediculosis infestation.

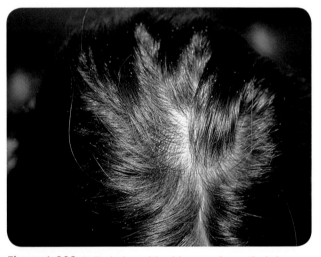

Figure 4-398 Pediculosis capitis with many nits on the hair.

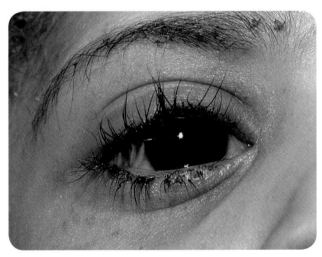

Figure 4-399 Pediculosis capitis occurring on the eyelashes.

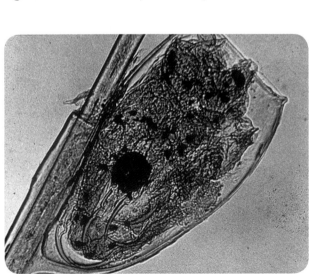

Figure 4-400 Pediculosis capitis with nit (egg case and larvae) of *P. humanus* on scalp hair.

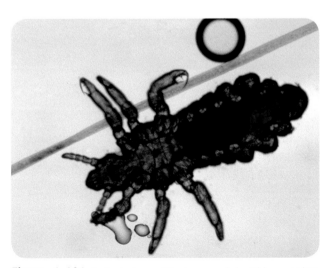

Figure 4-401 Pediculosis capitis is caused by this organism: *P. humanus*.

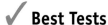 Differential Diagnosis and Pitfalls

- The scales of seborrheic dermatitis may be mistaken for pediculosis capitis, though these scales are greasy, yellow, irregular in shape and are easily removable.
- Tinea capitis has similar pruritus and lymphadenopathy but is associated with alopecia. Nits are not found on close examination of the hair.

✓ Best Tests

Demonstration of lice or nits on hair visually or under microscope.

▲▲ Management Pearls

- All household contacts should be examined and treated concurrently.
- On the day of treatment, clothing worn that day and bed linens can be machine washed or dry cleaned to decrease the risk of fomite transmission.
- Most "resistant" infestations are due to improper use of pediculicides or misdiagnosis of active infestations. After treatment, only individuals found to have living lice (move extremities when stimulated) should be considered to have an active infestation. Read all product labels for over-the-counter topical pediculicides and use exactly as directed by the manufacturer.

Therapy

Multiple topical and oral therapies are available for pediculosis. Prescription products should be reserved for patients with proven infestations that do not respond to proper application of over-the-counter pediculicides. Manual nit removal may be used as an adjuvant to topical therapy. Most herbal and home remedies are unproven in effectiveness and safety.

Over-the-Counter Pediculicides
- Permethrin 1% (Nix): Apply to dry hair and rinse after 10 min. Repeat in 1 to 2 weeks.
- Pyrethrins with piperonyl butoxide (RID and Pronto): Apply to dry hair and rinse after 10 min. Repeat in 1 to 2 weeks.

Prescription Products
- Malathion 0.5% lotion (Ovide): Apply to dry hair and rinse after 8 to 12 h. A repeat application is recommended after 1 to 2 weeks. Not indicated in children aged younger than 6 years.
- Permethrin 5% (Elimite): Apply to dry hair and rinse after 8 to 12 h. Repeat in 1 to 2 weeks. Not indicated in infants aged younger than 2 months.
- Oral ivermectin: Administer 200 µg/kg in one oral dose. Repeat in 7 to 10 days. Not indicated in children aged younger than 5 years or weighing <15 kg.
- Lindane, DDT, and carbaryl: Use of these products is rarely recommended due to potential systemic toxicity and limited effectiveness.

Suggested Readings

Chosidow O. Scabies and pediculosis. *Lancet.* 2000;355(9206):819–826.

Goates BM, Atkin JS, Wilding KG, et al. *Pediatrics.* 2006;118(5):1962–1970.

Meinking TL, Burkhart CN, Burkhart CG, et al. Infestations. In: Bolognia JL, Jorizzo JL, Rapini RP, eds. *Dermatology.* Vol. 1. 2nd Ed. St Louis, MO: Mosby; 2008:1291–1302.

Tebruegge M, Runnacles J. Is wet combing effective in children with pediculosis capitis infestation? *Arch Dis Child.* 2007;92(9):818–820.

Yoon KS, Gao JR, Lee SH, et al. *Arch Dermatol.* 2003;139(8):994–1000.

Tinea Capitis

■ Diagnosis Synopsis

Tinea capitis (scalp ringworm) is a fungal infection of the scalp caused by different species of dermatophytes. Most cases occur between the ages of 3 to 7 years, though it has been reported in infants and older children as well. In the United States and Great Britain, the most common causative agent is *Trichophyton tonsurans*. The most common agent worldwide, however, is *Microsporum canis*. It presents as numerous scaly macules and patches of broken hairs and alopecia on the scalp. More severe forms are associated with inflammatory papules, pustules, and plaques as well as systemic symptoms (i.e., fever and malaise).

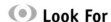 Look For

Areas of alopecia and scale on the scalp (Figs. 4-402–4-404). Inflammatory lesions are often seen (Fig. 4-405). Cervical and occipital lymph nodes may be palpable as well.

●● Diagnostic Pearls

- Tinea capitis should be within the differential in any child who presents with alopecia.
- Secondary bacterial infections can occur and should be considered in any patient with purulent discharge.

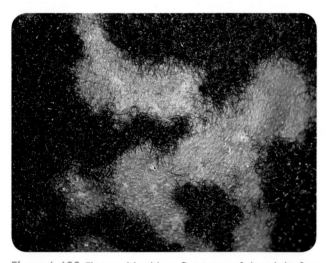

Figure 4-402 Tinea capitis with confluent areas of alopecia is often caused by *T. tonsurans*.

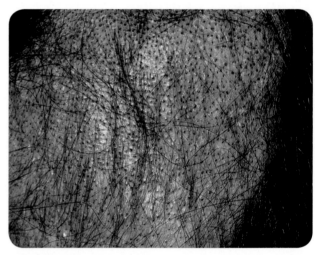

Figure 4-403 Tinea capitis with multiple broken hairs resembling black dots on the scalp is usually due to *T. tonsurans*.

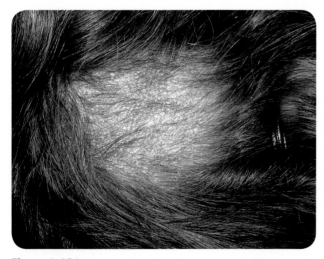

Figure 4-404 Tinea capitis with scaling and alopecia (that is usually reversible).

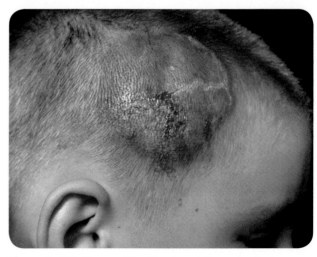

Figure 4-405 Tinea capitis with a large inflammatory kerion.

?? Differential Diagnosis and Pitfalls

- Bacterial folliculitis
- Seborrheic dermatitis
- Psoriasis
- Alopecia areata
- Trichotillomania

✔ Best Tests

- Light microscopy may be performed using a plucked hair, though this cannot determine the causative organism.
- Fungal culture allows for the determination of the causative organism.

▲▲▲ Management Pearls

- Tinea capitis must be treated with systemic antifungal agents because the organisms invade the hair follicle and cannot be reached by topical therapies.
- Pruritus is the first symptom to improve with therapy.
- New onset of pruritic papules on the forehead, ears, and extremities after 1 to 3 weeks of systemic therapy is typically an id reaction to effective treatment and does not represent an allergic reaction to the medication. Symptomatic care of the id reaction (oral antihistamines and topical steroids) with continued oral antifungal therapy will eradicate the id reaction and fungal infection.

Therapy

Griseofulvin is the treatment of choice. It should be dosed at 20 to 25 mg/kg/day for a minimum 8-week course. Other options include terbinafine, itraconazole, and fluconazole. Topical antifungal shampoos may be used in conjunction with systemic therapy to decrease scale and contagiousness. Secondary bacterial infection should be treated with oral antibiotics.

Suggested Readings

Gilaberte Y, Rezusta A, Gil J, et al. Tinea capitis in infants in their first year of life. *Br J Dermatol*. 2004;151(4):886–890.

Möhrenschlager M, Seidl HP, Ring J, et al. Pediatric tinea capitis: Recognition and management. *Am J Clin Dermatol*. 2005;6(4):203–213.

Sethi A, Antaya R. Systemic antifungal therapy for cutaneous infections in children. *Pediatr Infect Dis J*. 2006;25(7):643–644.

◼◼ Diagnosis Synopsis

Onychomycosis refers to fungal infection of the nails caused by fungi. Onychomycosis accounts for approximately 30% of all nail diseases in children. The prevalence of onychomycosis in children varies from 0.2% to 2.6% (mean 0.3%).

The predisposing factors are a family history of dermatophytosis, Down syndrome, diabetes, and immunosuppression due to HIV infection or medications.

Onychomycosis is classified by the mode and site of invasion, leading to five separate types of onychomycosis.

Distal lateral subungual onychomycosis (DLSO), the most common form, begins with fungal invasion of the hyponychium and spreads proximally along the nail bed and the lateral nail grooves. In Western countries, DLSO is mainly due to *Trichophyton rubrum*.

Endonyx onychomycosis (EO) is a form of distal lateral onychomycosis that involves the nail plate as well as the nail bed. EO is caused by organisms that normally cause endothrix scalp infections, including *T. soudanense* and *T. violaceum*.

Superficial onychomycosis (SO) is due to fungal invasion of the dorsal plate. Superficial white onychomycosis (SWO) is typically caused by *T. mentagrophytes* var. *interdigitale* while *T. rubrum* var. *melanoides* or *Scytalidium dimidiatum* causes a rare variety of black SO.

Proximal subungual onychomycosis (PSO) is caused by invasion of the proximal nail fold spreading distally along the nail plate. In the absence of paronychia, PSO is typically due to *T. rubrum*, rarely other dermatophytes or *Candida*. PSO with an extension to the nail plate leading to SWO is seen in patients with AIDS and is caused by *T. rubrum*. PSO with paronychia may be seen in the setting of *Candida albicans* or nondermatophyte mold infection from *Fusarium* sp. and *Scopulariopsis brevicaulis*.

Total dystrophic onychomycosis (TDO) is the most severe form and is rarely seen in children. It may be primarily seen in the setting of an immunodeficiency such as chronic mucocutaneous candidiasis, or it may be secondary to the culmination of any of the other types of onychomycosis.

Mixed clinical pictures involving more than one type may occur.

While *Candida* sp. are frequently cultured from nails, these species are not thought to be the primary pathogen, as topical or systemic antifungals do not cure the associated nail abnormalities. True nail invasion by *Candida* is seen almost exclusively in chronic mucocutaneous candidiasis.

◉ Look For

DLSO—toenails are more frequently affected than fingernails; if fingernails are involved, it is almost always in association with toenail disease. Nails show yellowish-white discoloration, nail thickening, subungual hyperkeratosis, and onycholysis **(Figs. 4-406–4-408)**. Paronychia may be involved.

EO—fingernails are more commonly involved than toenails. The nails may show milky white patches, nail pitting, lamellar splitting, ridging, or nail thickening. There is frequently coexisting skin or scalp disease.

SO—toenails are mainly affected with either opaque white or black powdery discoloration, which should be scraped off the nail surface **(Fig. 4-409)**.

PSO—fingernail involvement is rare. PSO appears as an area of leukonychia under the lunula that may spread distally along the nail plate. Later, there may be destruction of the proximal nail plate along with subungual hyperkeratosis and discoloration. Sometimes in the setting of AIDS or in young children, fungal invasion may spread to the dorsal nail layers, giving the appearance of SWO. PSO due to

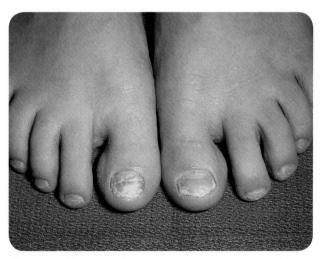

Figure 4-406 Onychomycosis with onycholysis on great nails and destruction of nail plate.

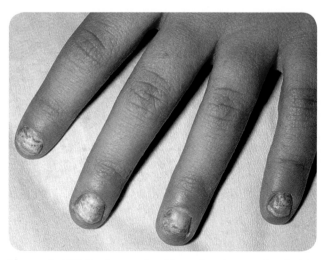

Figure 4-407 Onychomycosis with varying degrees of nail plate destruction.

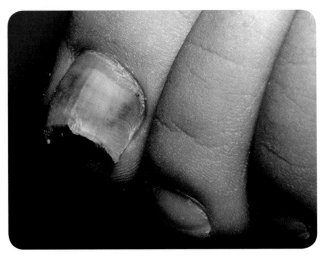

Figure 4-408 Onychomycosis with discolored, thickened nail plate.

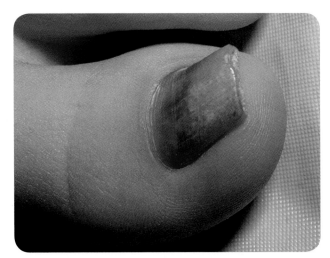

Figure 4-409 Onychomycosis with a discolored, thickened nail plate on the great nail.

nondermatophyte molds or *Candida* frequently presents with an associated paronychia. In *Aspergillus* infection, the proximal nail plate may show green or black discoloration.

TDO—if TDO is primary, it may involve all nails. Nails crumble and there is total destruction of the nail plate, leaving a thickened nail bed with retained fragments of the nail plate. Periungual skin may appear inflamed.

In the setting of dermatophyte infection, there is frequently concomitant tinea pedis, marked by scaly erythematous patches in the web spaces of the toes and on the soles or sides of the feet. Maceration of the web spaces may lead to painful fissures and secondary bacterial infection. Infection with *T. mentagrophytes* var. *interdigitale* may show bullae. There may also be concomitant tinea corporis or tinea capitis.

Diagnostic Pearls

- Onychomycosis is usually asymmetrical, involving one to three nails of only one hand or foot. In case of symmetrical involvement of all the nails, an alternative diagnosis or immunodeficiency should be considered.
- Always check the skin—particularly the feet and scalp—for coexistent infection and screen family members.
- Apparent SWO due to *T. rubrum* should raise concern for possible HIV/AIDS.

Differential Diagnosis and Pitfalls

- Psoriasis—multiple large, coarse, and deep pits randomly scattered on the nail plate; onycholysis (detachment of the nail plate from the nail bed) surrounded by an erythematous border; yellowish or salmon pink patches on the nail bed; subungual hyperkeratosis; and splinter hemorrhages.

- Lichen planus—thinning or ridging of the nail plate, dystrophic changes, and pterygium.
- Alopecia areata—fine, shallow pits regularly arranged either in horizontal or vertical rows, fine stippling, onychomadesis (proximal shedding of the nail plate), longitudinal riding, opacification, and serration of the free edges.
- Twenty nail dystrophy or trachyonychia—clinical sign is characterized by rough nail surface with marked longitudinal striations resulting in splitting.
- Pachyonychia congenita—marked subungual hyperkeratosis with accumulation of hard keratinous material, resulting in uplifting of the nail plate.

✓ Best Tests

- Laboratory confirmation with direct microscopy (KOH) and/or fungal culture.
- Material should be collected from the nail clippings, subungual debris, nail bed, or undersurface of the nail plate.
- Direct microscopy is the most inexpensive method and has a sensitivity of approximately 80%, but it cannot identify the specific genus or species of fungus.
- Fungal culture allows for identification of a viable, specific pathogen but has a sensitivity of only 50% to 70% and may show false-positive results due to contamination.
- Histopathology with a PAS stain is the most sensitive method, though it cannot identify viable or specific pathogens. Histopathology is generally reserved for cases in which direct microscopy and culture have failed to confirm infection.

▲▲ Management Pearls

- Although approximately 30% of nail dystrophies are due to onychomycosis, a patient should never be treated with systemic antifungal agents without confirmed infection based on direct microscopy, fungal culture, or histopathology because of the cost and potential morbidity associated with systemic antifungal agents.

- Measurement of the distance from proximal nail fold to proximal edge of onycholysis will monitor the response to treatment.

Therapy

Oral antifungal treatments offer the best mycologic cure rates in documented dermatophyte infections. The safety and efficacy of terbinafine and itraconazole have not been established in pediatric patients. Both medications are approved by the FDA in adults.

Antifungal medications itraconazole and terbinafine have better cure and relapse rates than griseofulvin. Moreover, the duration of treatment is shorter (2 to 5 months). Clinical trials show that itraconazole and terbinafine appear to be safe and effective.

Itraconazole is fungistatic against dermatophytes, molds, and yeasts, and it can be given as daily continuous therapy for 12 weeks.

- Dosage: 5 mg/kg/day (capsules)

Terbinafine is fungicidal against dermatophytes, *Aspergillus*, and *Scopulariopsis*, usually given as continuous therapy.

- Dosage:
  - <20 kg—125 mg every other day
  - 20 to 40 kg—125 mg/day
  - >40 kg—250 mg/day
- Duration of therapy:
  - 6 to 12 weeks for fingernails, 12 weeks for toenails

Other Medications

Fluconazole is fungistatic against dermatophytes, *Candida*, and some nondermatophyte molds, given as weekly intermittent therapy.

- Dose: 3 to 6 mg/kg/dose
- Duration: 12 weeks for fingernails, 26 weeks for toenails

Topical Therapy

Used in mild to moderate cases, topical therapy with ciclopirox 8% nail lacquer alone requires daily application for 9 to 12 months as well as amorolfine 5% (once a week application).

Mechanical debridement with total or partial surgical nail avulsion or chemical nail avulsion with topical 40% urea ointment under occlusion is a useful adjunct to either topical or oral antifungal agents.

Suggested Readings

Faergemann J, Baran R. Epidemiology, clinical presentation and diagnosis of onychomycosis. *Br J Dermatol.* 2003;149(Suppl. 65):1–4.

Gupta AK, Sibbald RG, Lynde CW, et al. Onsychomycosis in children: Prevalence and treatment strategies. *J Am Acad Dermatol.* 1997;36(3 Pt 1): 395–402.

Gupta AK, Skinner AR. Onychomycosis in children: A brief overview with treatment strategies. *Pediatr Dermatol.* 2004;21(1):74–79.

Lange M, Roszkiewicz J, Szczerkowska-Dobosz A, et al. Onychomycosis is no longer a rare finding in children. *Mycoses.* 2006;49(1):55–59.

Lateur N, Mortaki A, André J. Two hundred ninety-six cases of onychomycosis in children and teenagers: A 10-year laboratory survey. *Pediatr Dermatol.* 2003;20(5):385–388.

Paronychia, Candidal

◼◼ Diagnosis Synopsis

Paronychia presents as an acute or chronic painful, often purulent, tender swelling with marked inflammation involving the folds surrounding the fingernail. Several organisms may be recovered from involved sites, including *Candida albicans*. Regardless of the bacteria or yeast cultured, a predisposing factor is separation of the proximal nail fold from the nail plate with loss of the cuticle. The cause of this separation is moisture-induced maceration. In infants, this is most frequently caused by thumbsucking. *C. albicans* is the most frequently recovered organism in chronic paronychia; however, its actual role in the development of chronic paronychia is debated.

◉ Look For

Erythema, edema, and sometimes pus at the lateral and proximal nail folds with loss of the cuticle (Figs. 4-410–4-413). Discoloration and distortion of the nail are common.

●● Diagnostic Pearls

- Chronic paronychia can cause transverse ridging of the nail plates. There is no subungual debris as in nail psoriasis or onychomycosis. Loss of the cuticle is a helpful clue.
- Due to the slow rate of nail growth, acute paronychia (usually bacterial) does not cause nail plate changes.

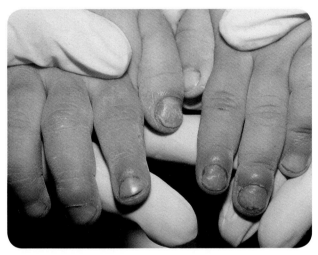

Figure 4-410 Candidal paronychia with inflamed proximal and lateral nail folds as well as some nail plate destruction.

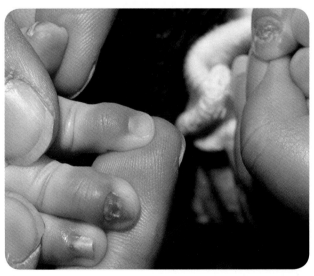

Figure 4-411 Candidal paronychia with redness of distal digits, nail plate destruction, and onycholysis.

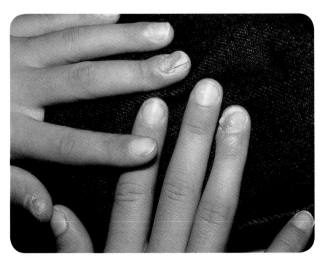

Figure 4-412 Candidal paronychia with posterior nail fold inflammation and onycholysis.

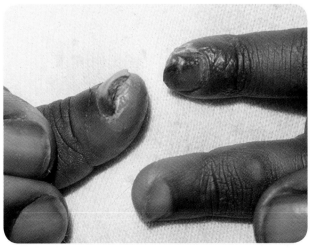

Figure 4-413 Candidal paronychia with nail plate distortion, destruction, and hyperpigmentation from chronic disease.

?? Differential Diagnosis and Pitfalls

- Bacterial paronychia tends to be more acute and tender, with redness and frank pus. *Staphylococcus aureus*, *Streptococcus pyogenes*, and *Pseudomonas* sp. are the most frequently recovered organisms.
- In newborns, when several nails are involved, the differential diagnosis includes epidermolysis bullosa, psoriasis, and acrodermatitis.
- Chronic mucocutaneous candidiasis should also be considered with chronic candidal paronychia.

✓ Best Tests

Culture for yeast is often unnecessary, as this diagnosis may be made clinically. KOH preparation.

▲▲▲ Management Pearls

- Manage environmental factors such as thumbsucking and water immersion.
- If nail fold inflammation resolves and proximal nail plate returns to normal, treatment is heading in the correct direction.

Therapy

Reassure parents that recurrent chronic paronychia heals without scarring when infants and toddlers discontinue thumbsucking.

Some have observed that topical steroids such as triamcinolone 0.1% ointment or fluocinonide 0.05% ointment applied twice daily to the involved nail fold alone or with topical antifungal creams decrease inflammation and allow for tissue repair.

Any topical antifungal with activity against *Candida* may be used 2 to 4 times daily. Examples include econazole nitrate cream 1% and nystatin solution (100,000 units/mL).

In severe recalcitrant cases, oral antifungals such as fluconazole p.o. (2 to 3 mg/kg/day) may be effective.

Suggested Readings

Bolognia JL, Jorizzo JL, Rapini RP, eds. *Dermatology*. Vol. 1. 2nd Ed. St Louis, MO: Mosby; 2008:151.

Cohen BA, ed. *Pediatric Dermatology*. 3rd Ed. St Louis, MO: Mosby; 2005:218.

James WD, Berger TG, Elston DM, eds. *Andrews' Diseases of the Skin*. 10th Ed. Philadelphia, PA: WB Saunders; 2006:254–255.

Tosti A, Piraccini BM, Ghetti E, et al. Topical steroids versus systemic antifungals in the treatment of chronic paronychia: An open, randomized double-blind and double dummy study. *J Am Acad Dermatol*. 2002;47(1):73–76.

Diagnosis Synopsis

Balanitis is inflammation of the glans penis. Balanoposthitis refers to inflammation of both the glans and foreskin in uncircumcised males. It is most commonly seen in toilet-trained, uncircumcised boys between the ages of two and five. Most cases are caused by inadequate hygiene of the preputial-glanular sulcus. Exposure to urine, soaps, *Candida*, and bacterial overgrowth exacerbate the dermatitis. Most boys have only one episode.

Abuse affects children of all ages and backgrounds and if suspected needs appropriate referral.

Look For

The glans penis is red, swollen, and tender (Fig. 4-414). Discharge may occasionally be expressed from between the prepuce and glans. The prepuce may also become red and swollen (balanoposthitis). Systemic symptoms, urethral discharge, inflammation of the penile shaft, and inguinal lymphadenopathy are absent. Boys may complain of dysuria.

Diagnostic Pearls

- Urethral discharge is unusual for balanitis and suggests a sexually transmitted disease (*Neisseria gonorrhoeae* or *Chlamydia trachomatis*).
- Inguinal lymph nodes should not be enlarged. Lymphadenopathy suggests an infectious etiology.

?? Differential Diagnosis and Pitfalls

- Group A β-hemolytic streptococcal infection is the most common cause of acute inflammation of the glans penis in prepubescent children. Although it is usually associated with more intense pain, erythema, and discharge than nonspecific balanitis, the diseases may be clinically indistinguishable.
- Other signs that suggest streptococcal balanitis include the presence of perianal streptococcal cellulitis or a preceding throat infection.
- Other diagnoses include the following:

Infections

- Scabies
- Candidiasis
- Syphilis
- Gonorrhea
- Chlamydia
- Herpes

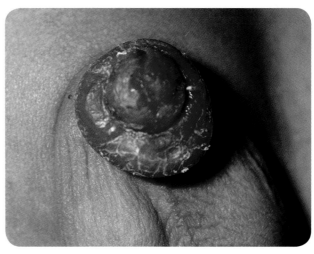

Figure 4-414 Balanoposthitis in infant with erythema, edema, and crusting of the glans and foreskin.

Primary Dermatoses

- Lichen sclerosus (balanitis xerotica obliterans)
- Psoriasis
- Fixed drug eruption
- Plasma cell balanitis (Zoon balanitis)

Contact Dermatoses/Trauma

- Allergic contact dermatitis
- Irritant contact dermatitis
- Sexual abuse

✓ Best Tests

- A rapid streptococcal antigen detection test and/or culture should be performed to rule out streptococcal balanitis.
- If urethral discharge is present and the rapid antigen detection test is negative, the discharge should be evaluated by Gram stain, culture, DNA probes, or other rapid antigen tests for *N. gonorrhoeae* and *C. trachomatis*.
- Consider a biopsy to rule out balanitis xerotica obliterans in recurrent or resistant cases.

Management Pearls

- Patients should follow up within 4 to 6 weeks to ensure inflammation has resolved.
- *Candida* may colonize and exacerbate inflammation of the glans penis but rarely causes primary infection in young boys. Hence, anti-Candida creams are usually unnecessary.

- When abuse is suspected, a thorough history and physical exam should be completed.
- **Reporting:** It is crucial that any recognition or suspicion of abuse or neglect be followed by immediate reporting to appropriate authorities to safeguard the child from further injury. To report suspected abuse, the clinician should contact his/her state or local child protective services agency. The national number, 1-800-4-A-CHILD, is available to help locate the regional department. If unsure whether or not to report, consultation with other health care professionals or Child Protection Services (CPS) is recommended to help determine if the incident is reportable. It is important to remember that the duty to report only requires a reasonable suspicion that abuse has occurred and not certainty.
- In the United States, infections due to invasive group A *Streptococcus* are reportable in all states **except** AL, CO, MS, MT, ND, OR, and UT.
- Per the CDC, infections due to invasive group A *Streptococcus* are nationally notifiable via the National Notifiable Diseases Surveillance System (NNDSS).

Therapy

Nonspecific balanitis usually responds to warm sitz baths, gentle cleansing of the preputial sulcus and glans, and application of a low-potency topical steroid (hydrocortisone 1% ointment twice daily). Boys should be taught to retract the foreskin with each void and to cleanse the prepuce and glans with soap and water twice daily.

Barrier ointments (petrolatum jelly) and topical antibiotics (bacitracin) can also be considered. If local measures are unsuccessful, and in more severe cases with localized cellulitis, an oral second-generation cephalosporin should be added. Circumcision should be considered for recurrent or recalcitrant balanitis. Poor response to therapy should prompt strong consideration for other underlying diagnoses.

Special Considerations in Infants

Phimosis and accumulation of epithelial debris under the infant prepuce is physiologic in uncircumcised males and should be differentiated from inflammatory purulence and scarring that may be associated with balanitis.

Suggested Readings

Escala JM, Rickwood AM. Balanitis. *Br J Urol.* 1989;63(2):196–197.

Krueger H, Osborn L. Effects of hygiene among the uncircumcised. *J Fam Pract.* 1986;22(4):353–355.

Kyriazi NC, Costenbader CL. Group A beta-hemolytic streptococcal balanitis: It may be more common than you think. *Pediatrics.* 1991;88:154–156.

Lafferty PM, MacGregor FB, Scobie WG. Management of foreskin problems. *Arch Dis Child.* 1991;66(6):696–697.

Schwartz RH, Rushton HG. Acute balanoposthitis in young boys. *Pediatr Infect Dis J.* 1996;15(2):176–177.

Diagnosis Synopsis

Candidiasis is a fungal infection caused by the yeast *Candida albicans*. It can be acquired perinatally, in adolescence through intercourse with an infected partner, or occur idiopathically in children of all ages. It frequently occurs in diabetics, in the immunosuppressed, and after treatment with oral antibiotics.

Candida can infect the proximal shaft, scrotum, and crural folds. Candidal balanitis is a fungal infection of the glans penis. It occurs more frequently in the uncircumcised male.

Small erosions and vesicles or pustules present with associated itching and burning. In its mildest form, the condition may be intermittent and transient.

Look For

Look for erythematous to beefy red areas, sometimes with whitish patches or erosions, and surrounding pinpoint papules or pustules (satellite lesions) (Fig. 4-415). There may also be sharply demarcated erythematous plaques

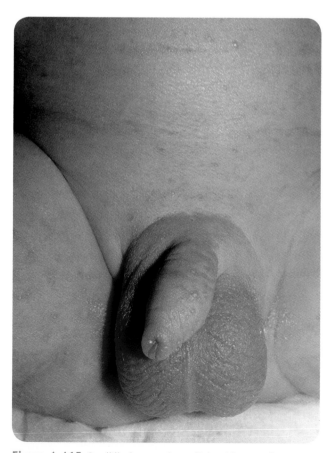

Figure 4-415 Candidiasis on male genitals with extensive scrotum redness and multiple satellite lesions on abdomen and thigh.

with elevated rim and white scale along the periphery on surrounding skin. Rarely, candidiasis can involve the scrotum, presenting with erythema and edema. In rare instances, *Candida* can present as erythema and edema with minimal scale and pustules.

Diagnostic Pearls

Pustules, when seen, are usually subtle and fragile.

Differential Diagnosis and Pitfalls

- Allergic contact dermatitis
- Psoriasis
- Lichen planus
- Irritant dermatitis
- Reactive arthritis (Reiter syndrome)
- Erythroplasia of Queyrat

Best Tests

KOH of whitish spots shows pseudohyphae and budding yeasts.

Management Pearls

If lesion persists despite adequate therapy, consider reinfection from a sexual partner or from a sexual abuser with *Candida* infection or undiagnosed diabetes.

Therapy

- Econazole cream—apply twice daily (15 to 30 gm) for 10 days.
- Miconazole cream—apply twice daily (15 to 30 gm) for 10 days.
- Clotrimazole—apply twice daily (15, 30, or 45 gm) for 10 days.

For teenagers, oral fluconazole (single dose of 100 to 200 mg) can be used for cases that are refractory to topical therapy.

Suggested Readings

Banerjee K, Curtis E, de San Lazaro C, et al. Low prevalence of genital candidiasis in children. *Eur J Clin Microbio Infect Dis.* 2004;23(9):696–698.

Kyle AA, Dahl MV. Topical therapy for fungal infections. *Am J Clin Dermatol.* 2004;5(6):443–451.

Condyloma Acuminatum (Genital Wart)

◼◼ Diagnosis Synopsis

Condyloma acuminatum, or genital warts, is caused by the human papillomavirus (HPV), a DNA virus of which there are over 200 genotypes. While sexual abuse should always be considered, the majority of cases in children aged younger than 4 years represent other modes of transmission, such as autoinoculation from other involved sites or perinatal transmission. The virus can remain latent in skin cells without any visible sign of infection.

Abuse affects children of all ages and backgrounds and if suspected needs appropriate referral.

◉ Look For

Small 1 to 2 mm or larger (sometimes giant cauliflower-like lesions) white, gray, or skin-colored, warty papules on the genitals, crural folds, perineum, or perianal skin (Figs. 4-416–4-419). In incompletely keratinized surfaces, like the vulva or under the foreskin, these papules will have a smoother surface. In males, examine the urethral meatus, frenulum, shaft, scrotum, perineum, and perianal skin carefully.

◉◉ Diagnostic Pearls

- The lesions may show small black dots, which represent thrombosed capillaries.
- Ask parents for history of genital and non-genital warts.
- Ask mothers for history of preceding abnormal PAP smears prior to delivery of child.

?? Differential Diagnosis and Pitfalls

- There are many verrucous-looking lesions of the genitals (e.g., bowenoid papulosis, squamous cell carcinoma, psoriasis, condyloma latum [associated with syphilis], seborrheic keratosis, and lichen nitidus). Other lesions mistaken for warts include normal pearly penile papules, ectopic sebaceous glands (Fordyce spots), lichen planus, molluscum, and the nodules of scabies.
- Patients should be checked for immunodeficiency when there is severe involvement.

✓ Best Tests

The diagnosis of genital warts is made by physical examination and may be confirmed by biopsy, although biopsy is needed only under certain circumstances (e.g., if the diagnosis is uncertain; the lesions do not respond to standard therapy; the disease worsens during therapy; the patient is immunocompromised; or warts are pigmented, indurated, fixed, bleeding, or ulcerated). Presently, there is no evidence for performing HPV DNA typing.

▲▲ Management Pearls

- Wart virus persists and often is present beyond the clinically visible borders of the lesions. This must be considered during destructive therapies. Lesions frequently recur, requiring vigilant surveillance.
- Gardasil (http://www.gardasil.com/) is a quadrivalent vaccine that was approved by the FDA in 2006 for girls

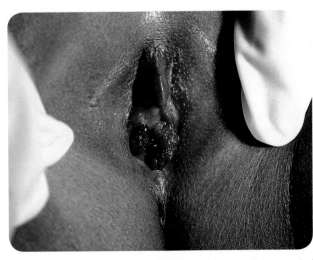

Figure 4-416 Condyloma acuminatum with multiple introital lesions. Sexual abuse must be excluded.

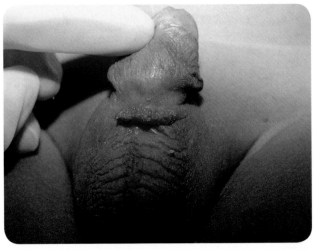

Figure 4-417 Condyloma acuminatum with tightly grouped papules between penile shaft and scrotum. Sexual abuse must be excluded.

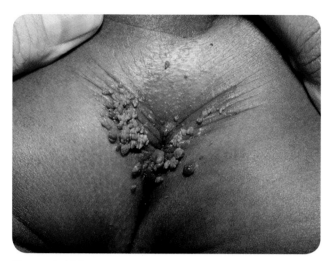

Figure 4-418 Condyloma acuminatum with multiple discrete and grouped lesions. Sexual abuse must be excluded.

aged 9 to 26. It contains virus-like particles of types 16 and 18 (which are responsible for 70% of all cervical cancers) as well as 6 and 11 (which cause 90% of genital warts).

- In the United States, HPV is reportable in the state of Delaware. In Florida, it is reportable in children aged younger than 12.

Therapy

Currently available treatments for visible genital warts include cryotherapy, podophyllin resin, podophyllotoxin, trichloroacetic acid, interferon, carbon dioxide laser, and surgery.

Imiquimod (Aldara) is an immune response mediator for genital warts, which is approved for use in patients aged 12 or older.

Surgical removal—such as tangential scissor excision, tangential shave excision, curettage, or electrosurgery—is yet another provider-administered option. This technique is most useful for larger warts or those causing obstruction (i.e., those involving the urethral meatus).

Condyloma may spontaneously regress, so active surveillance is also an option.

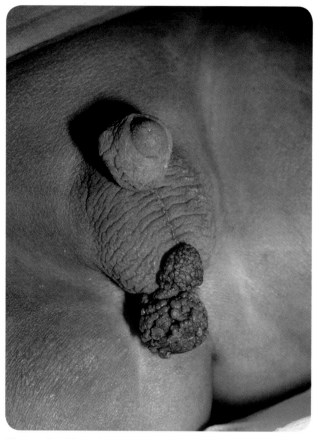

Figure 4-419 Condyloma acuminatum with large cauliflower-like lesions. Sexual abuse must be excluded.

Suggested Readings

Jayasinghe Y, Garland SM. Genital warts in children: What do they mean? *Arch Dis Child.* 2006;91(8):696–700.

Scheinfeld N, Lehman DS. An evidence-based review of medical and surgical treatments of genital warts. *Dermatol Online J.* 2006;12(3):5.

Schöfer H. Evaluation of imiquimod for the therapy of external genital and anal warts in comparison with destructive therapies. *Br J Dermatol.* 2007;157(Suppl. 2):52–55.

Urman CO, Gottlieb AB. New viral vaccines for dermatologic disease. *J Am Acad Dermatol.* 2008;58(3):361–370.

Diagnosis Synopsis

Genital herpes is a sexually transmitted viral infection caused by Herpes simplex virus type 1 (HSV-1) and type 2 (HSV-2), with HSV-2 being the most common cause worldwide. Risk factors for HSV-2 seropositivity are female sex, older age, less education, poverty, increased sexual partners, Mexican-American ethnicity, and African–Americans. The most common patient is a sexually active adolescent. Infection begins within 10 days after direct contact with active lesions on another infected individual; however, asymptomatic viral shedding is another well-established source of infection. Sexual abuse must be considered in all young children with genital herpes. Other sources of infection in young children are autoinoculation from herpetic disease of the fingers (herpetic whitlow), innocent inoculation from a caregiver with herpetic whitlow, and close nonsexual physical contact.

Abuse affects individuals of all ages and backgrounds and if suspected needs appropriate referral.

Look For

Most infections are asymptomatic. If symptomatic, however, one will note grouped vesicles and pustules or grouped erosions or small ulcers on an erythematous base (Fig. 4-420). Vesicles may be umbilicated (Figs. 4-421–4-423). Lesions may be associated with dysuria, vaginal or urethral discharge, constitutional symptoms, and tender inguinal lymphadenopathy. 10% to 15% of patients will have an associated ulcerative pharyngitis.

Diagnostic Pearls

- Vesicles are short-lived when they arise in the genital areas. Thus, grouped erosions are common.
- Lesions, especially erosions or ulcers, may be persistent in immunosuppressed patients.
- Patients may experience a burning sensation before the appearance of lesions. Consider this diagnosis for any recurrent vesicular/erosive eruption.
- It is important to remember that lesions progress from vesicular to pustular, erosive, and crusted stages.
- Painful lymphadenopathy is very characteristic of infectious ulcers (as opposed to noninfectious causes of genital ulcers).

Differential Diagnosis and Pitfalls

- Impetigo
- Molluscum contagiosum
- Fixed drug eruption
- *Candida*
- Aphthous ulcers
- Crohn disease

Best Tests

- Immediate diagnosis to confirm acute herpetic infection—which includes varicella–zoster virus—can be made by demonstrating multinucleated giant cells on Tzanck smear.
- Polymerase chain reaction is the most sensitive and specific test for confirmation.
- Direct fluorescent antibody testing and HSV serologies may also confirm infection.

Management Pearls

- Contact the appropriate authorities if sexual abuse is suspected.
- Symptoms usually resolve spontaneously within 5 to 10 days. However, cutaneous lesions require 2 to 4 weeks to heal. Consider topical 5% lidocaine ointment and oral anti-inflammatories/analgesics for pain management.
- Sexually active adolescents should be instructed that, other than abstinence, there is no way to completely prevent transmission. However, the use of latex condoms and abstinence from sex when lesions or symptoms are present will help reduce the risk of transmission to uninfected partners.
- The sexual partners of patients who have genital herpes can benefit from evaluation and counseling. Symptomatic partners should be evaluated and treated in the same manner as patients who have genital lesions. Asymptomatic partners of patients who have genital herpes should be questioned concerning histories of genital lesions and offered type-specific serologic testing for HSV infection.

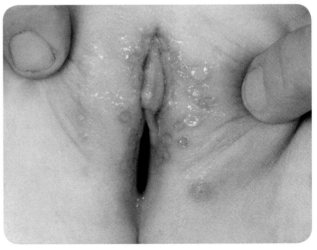

Figure 4-420 Genital HSV with grouped, shallow ulcers on an erythematous base.

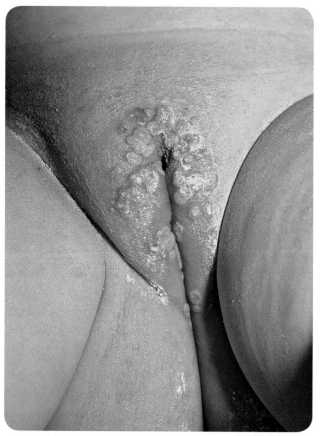

Figure 4-421 Genital HSV with umbilication seen in some of the grouped lesions.

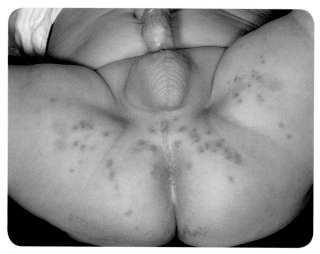

Figure 4-422 Genital HSV with umbilicated vesicles and shallow ulcerations extending to the thighs.

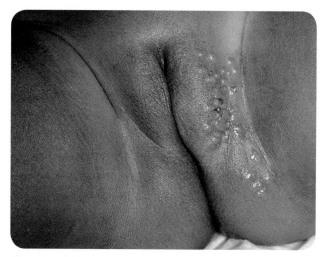

Figure 4-423 Genital HSV with unilateral vesicles suggestive of herpes zoster. PCR is necessary for this differential in a 2 month old.

Therapy

Limited data are available on the use of acyclovir in children aged younger than 2 years. However, no unusual toxicities have been observed in these children in doses up to 80 mg/kg/day. The safety and efficacy of valacyclovir and famciclovir have not been established in children aged up to 18 years.

- First episode of genital HSV (children weighing more than 40 kg): Acyclovir 200 mg p.o. five times daily for 7 to 10 days or 400 mg p.o. three times daily for 7 to 10 days
- Chronic suppression (children weighing more than 40 kg): Acyclovir 400 mg p.o. twice daily

Suggested Readings

Gutierrez KM. Rethinking herpes simplex virus infection in children and adolescents. *J Pediatr.* 2007;151:336–338.

Lafferty WE. The changing epidemiology of HSV-1 and HSV-2 and implications for serological testing. *Herpes.* 2002;9(2):51–55.

Whitley R. Neonatal herpes simplex virus infection. *Curr Opin Infect Dis.* 2004;17(3):243–246.

Xu F, Lee FK, Morrow RA, et al. Seroprevalence of herpes simplex virus type 1 in children in the United States. *J Pediatr.* 2007;151(4):374–377.

Lichen Sclerosus

■■ Diagnosis Synopsis

Lichen sclerosus (lichen sclerosus et atrophicus) is a chronic dermatosis of uncertain etiology affecting individuals of all races. Seventy percent of childhood cases appear in those aged younger than 7 years. Lesions occur mostly on the genitalia, perineum, or perianal skin, but they can appear anywhere. Because of atrophy and hemorrhage, the disease can easily be mistaken for sexual abuse. Lesions can itch, burn, cause dysuria, or cause pain on defecation. Advanced disease may obliterate genital anatomy. Extragenital lesions are rarely symptomatic. In Europe, some cases are thought to be late cutaneous sequelae of *Borrelia afzelii* or *B. garinii* infection. Autoimmune diseases such as vitiligo, alopecia areata, thyroid disease, and pernicious anemia disproportionately affect women with lichen sclerosus. An increased risk of genital squamous cell carcinoma has been observed in adult male and female patients with chronic untreated lichen sclerosus involving the genitals.

Abuse affects children of all ages and backgrounds and, if suspected, needs appropriate referral.

◉ Look For

Extragenital lesions begin as flat-topped, ivory-white papules or macules that coalesce into well-demarcated plaques. Often, there is purpura and widened follicular plugs within the lesions (Fig. 4-424). Over time, the plaques become sclerotic and atrophied with fine wrinkling over the surface (Figs. 4-425 and 4-426). Lesions often prefer sites of trauma.

Female genital lesions often present as atrophic, well-demarcated, white plaques surrounding the vulva and anus (hourglass or figure-eight configuration). Purpura, fissures, and telangiectases are often present.

In boys, lichen sclerosus may present as recurrent erythema, balanitis, and tightening of the foreskins (balanitis xerotica obliterans). Untreated disease can progress to phimosis and urethral stricture (Fig. 4-427).

●● Diagnostic Pearls

- Multiple features of lichen sclerosus (atrophy, purpura, fissures, and telangiectases) are often concentrated at the clitoral hood.
- Epidermal atrophy is often less prominent than in adults.

?? Differential Diagnosis and Pitfalls

- Morphea—indurated, lilac-colored, or hyperpigmented border
- Sexual abuse—disrupted hymen, may have an associated sexually transmitted disease, purpura, and bruising outside of atrophic areas; a diagnosis of lichen sclerosus does not exclude concomitant sexual abuse, and social work should investigate when suspicion is high

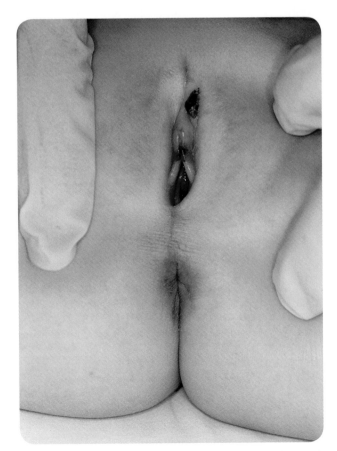

Figure 4-424 Lichen sclerosus hypopigmentation and purpuric lesions. Purpura is part of this condition and is not a sign of abuse.

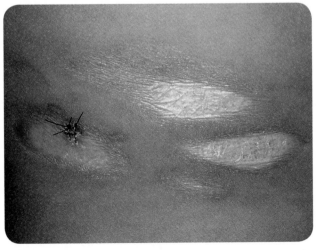

Figure 4-425 Lichen sclerosus may have atrophic plaques on the trunk, sometimes without genital lesions.

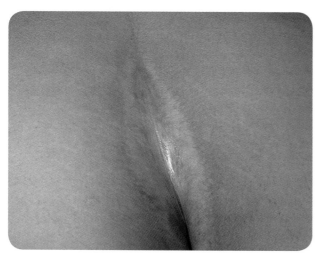

Figure 4-426 Lichen sclerosus with loss of skin markings, a characteristic of atrophy.

- Trauma (straddle injury)—no atrophy, consistent history
- Scars—firm, smooth, indurated plaques
- Vitiligo—well-defined depigmentation, often not in hourglass configuration, lacks signs of atrophy (purpura, telangiectases, fine wrinkling, and fissures)
- Cutaneous candidiasis—may have erosions but no atrophy; erythema and satellite lesions
- Irritant contact dermatitis—may have postinflammatory hypopigmentation, pruritus, erythema, and erosions, but no purpura or telangiectases
- Bacterial vaginosis—vulvar pruritus, but no other specific vulvar cutaneous findings

✓ Best Tests

- Skin biopsy will reveal epidermal atrophy, vacuolization of the dermal–epidermal junction, a hyalinized superficial dermis, and a bandlike infiltrate.

▲▲ Management Pearls

- Despite concerns about potent medicines on genital skin, high-potency topical steroids are universally accepted as the treatment of choice for lichen sclerosus in all patient groups and clinical presentations. Patients should be evaluated frequently and monitored for the correct use of the medication.
- Circumcision may be indicated for boys who fail to respond to topical therapy.
- Lichen sclerosus may resolve after puberty. Patients with lichen sclerosus persisting beyond or developing after puberty should be followed yearly for the development of leukoplakia or carcinoma.

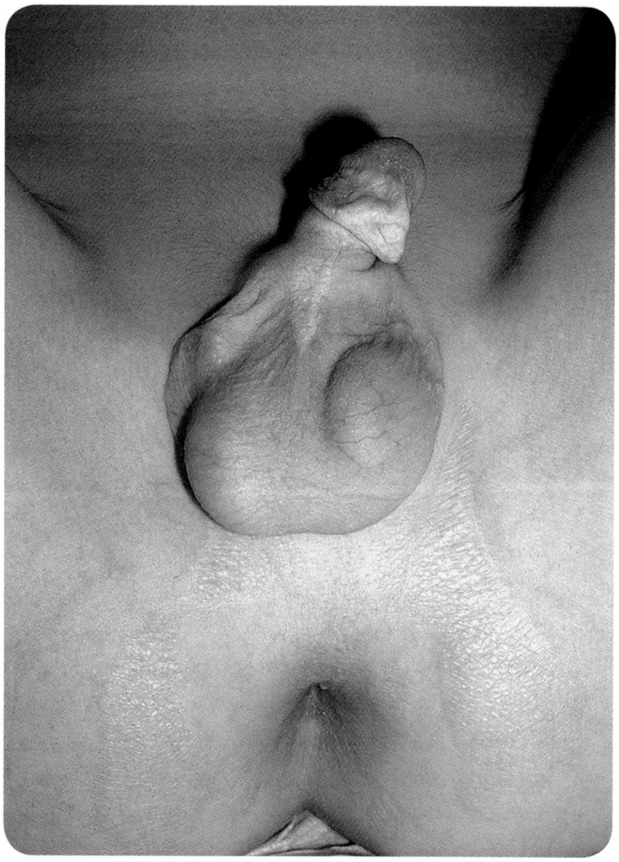

Figure 4-427 Lichen sclerosus with a white penile plaque; more extensive penile lesions may have phimosis.

Therapy

Most patients respond within 6 to 8 weeks to daily application of a class 1 topical steroid such as clobetasol 0.05% ointment. Continued use of these medications may cause atrophy, making close clinical follow-up essential.

Daily application of topical tacrolimus 0.1% ointment has also been shown to be effective in genital lichen sclerosus and is not associated with iatrogenic cutaneous atrophy. However, superpotent topical steroids are considered more effective, and use of tacrolimus should be limited to patients in whom topical steroids are ineffective or not tolerated.

Oral retinoids, topical tretinoin, and topical calcipotriene have also previously been used with varying success in patients who have failed therapy with topical steroids.

Topical testosterone has been shown to be ineffective in this condition and is no longer recommended.

Special Considerations in Infants

Lichen sclerosus is extremely rare in infants.

Suggested Readings

Cohen BA, ed. *Pediatric Dermatology*. 3rd Ed. St Louis, MO: Mosby; 2005:193–194.

Garzon MC, Paller AS. Ultrapotent topical corticosteroid treatment of childhood genital lichen sclerosus. *Arch Dermatol*. 1999;135(5): 525–528.

Poindexter G, Morrell DS. Anogenital pruritus: Lichen sclerosus in children. *Pediatric Ann*. 2007;36(12):785–791.

Powell J, Wojnarowska F. Childhood vulvar lichen sclerosus: An increasingly common problem. *J Am Acad Dermatol*. 2001;44(5):803–806.

Perianal Streptococcal Infection

Diagnosis Synopsis

Perianal streptococcal cellulitis, or perianal streptococcal dermatitis (PSD), is a fairly common, often unrecognized variant of cutaneous streptococcal infection. It may present as chronic diaper dermatitis or, alternatively, as an acute symptomatic cellulitis. Affected children usually range in age from 6 months to 10 years, though cases have been reported in both adolescents and adults. Presenting symptoms include painful defecation, fecal hoarding behavior, or incontinence. Blood-streaked stool and anal fissures may also be noted. Balanitis may occur in male patients. Vulvovaginal involvement has been reported in females but is less commonly reported than balanitis in males. Poststreptococcal glomerulonephritis can occur as a result of untreated perianal streptococcal infection. Guttate psoriasis may be precipitated by PSD. Fever and acral scarlatiniform desquamation have also been reported.

Look For

Perianal erythema and moist superficial erosions with well-defined margins (Figs. 4-428–4-431). Genitalia may be involved. Fissures and scaling plaques may be present.

Diagnostic Pearls

PSD should be within the differential in any patient who presents with well-defined perianal erythema associated with a change in bowel habits.

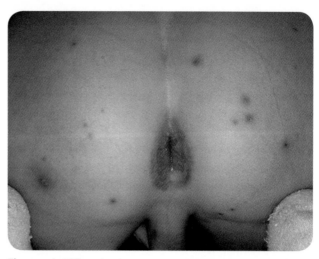

Figure 4-429 Perianal streptococcal infection and associated ecthymatous lesions.

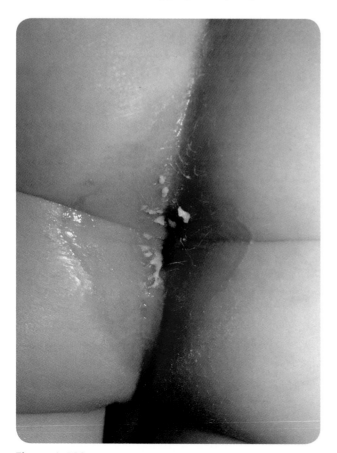

Figure 4-428 Perianal streptococcal infection with a symmetrical bright red lesion.

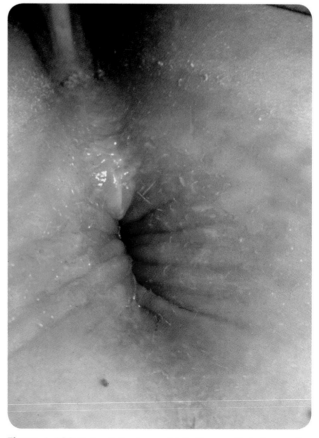

Figure 4-430 Perianal streptococcal infection usually lacks pustules.

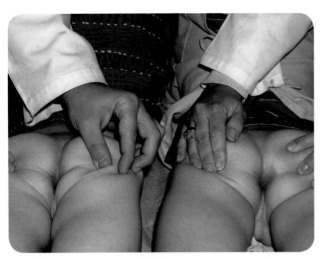

Figure 4-431 Perianal streptococcal infection simultaneously in two brothers.

?? Differential Diagnosis and Pitfalls

- Irritant dermatitis
- Inverse psoriasis
- Candidiasis
- Inflammatory bowel disease

✓ Best Tests

A bacterial culture is necessary to document the presence of group-A β-hemolytic streptococci.

▲▲ Management Pearls

- A post-treatment culture should be sent to confirm complete treatment, as PSD can cause poststreptococcal glomerulonephritis.
- A urinalysis should be obtained around 1 month after treatment is complete.
- Cultures may also be obtained from family members, as they may be carriers.

Therapy

While topical antibiotics may be used as monotherapy for less severe cases, oral antibiotics are recommended as first-line treatment for most patients. Penicillin is the antibiotic of choice. In penicillin-allergic patients, macrolides or clindamycin may be used. The treatment course should last anywhere from 2 to 3 weeks, depending on the clinical response. Topical antibiotics may be used in conjunction with oral antibiotics.

Suggested Readings

Herbst R. Perineal streptococcal dermatitis/disease: Recognition and management. *Am J Clin Dermatol.* 2003;4(8):555–560.

Ulcer, Aphthous

Diagnosis Synopsis

Aphthous ulcers, or aphthae (canker sores), are the most common cause of recurring ulcers of the mucous membranes. They have been reported to occur in 20% of the general population. The etiology remains unknown, but multiple causes have been proposed. These include infection with *Helicobacter pylori*, herpes simplex virus, and rubeola. Other possible etiologies include deficiencies in vitamin B_{12}, folate, or zinc. Crohn disease and food allergies have also been suggested. Aphthous ulcers are divided into three main subtypes: minor, major, and herpetiform.

Minor aphthae (Mikulicz ulcers) represent 80% of all cases and are single or multiple lesions that are 1 cm or less in diameter, mildly painful, and which generally heal within 1 to 2 weeks. They usually develop in childhood or adolescence and continue to occur sporadically throughout life.

Major aphthae (Sutton disease) represent approximately 10% of cases. They are >1 cm in diameter and are usually first seen at the onset of puberty. These lesions are extremely painful, last from 2 to 6 weeks, and generally heal with scarring.

Herpetiform aphthae (10% of cases) are characterized by multiple ulcerations that are 1 to 3 mm in diameter and occur in clusters. Their clinical course is similar to that of minor aphthous ulcers in that they usually heal in <1 month without scarring. They are more common in females and generally do not appear until adulthood.

Look For

Well-defined ulcerations on the nonkeratinized mucosa of the lips, buccal mucosa, or tongue (Figs. 4-432–4-435).

More rarely, they can be seen on the hard palate and gingival mucosa. Ulcers can have a white, gray, or yellow base that is usually surrounded by a slightly elevated erythematous rim.

Diagnostic Pearls

- Aphthous ulcers should remain in the differential in any patient with recurrent oral ulcers.
- It is very unusual to involve any keratinized mucosa (i.e., vermillion of the lips) or any cutaneous surface (other than the scrotum and labia majora).
- Unlike ulcerative sexually transmitted diseases, aphthous ulcers are not associated with lymphadenopathy.

?? Differential Diagnosis and Pitfalls

- Herpes simplex infection
- Crohn disease
- Behçet disease
- Pemphigus

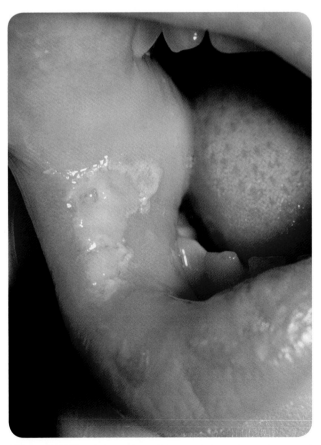

Figure 4-433 Aphthous ulcer with necrotic base, larger than usual, on buccal mucosa near lip.

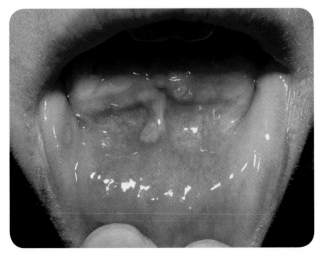

Figure 4-432 Aphthous ulcer on buccal mucosa and side of frenulum.

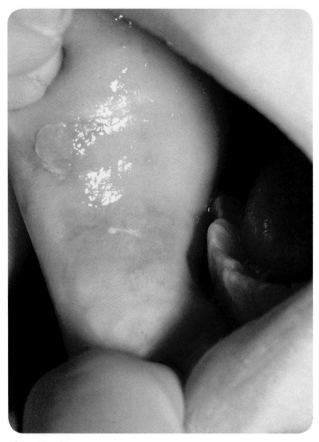

Figure 4-434 Aphthous ulcer in a typical location.

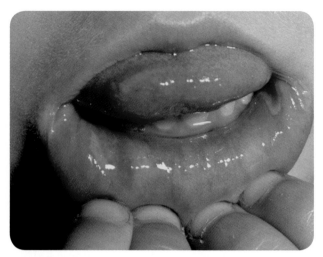

Figure 4-435 Aphthous ulcers on inner lower lip.

- A combination anesthetic mouthwash consisting of aluminum and magnesium hydroxide, lidocaine, and diphenhydramine is sometimes employed.
- Painful urination caused by genital aphthae can be ameliorated by applying a barrier cream or ointment (i.e., Vaseline) immediately before urinating.

Therapy

Treat any underlying diseases and correct any underlying vitamin or mineral deficiencies.

Some clinicians prescribe the use of antimicrobial mouth rinses such as 0.2% chlorhexidine or sucralfate.

High-potency topical steroid gel or ointment (halobetasol or clobetasol) applied four times daily can shorten episodes. These can be applied in combination with an occlusive dressing such as Orabase (carboxymethylcellulose). Intralesional corticosteroids (triamcinolone acetonide, initially 5 to 10 mg/mL) can be used for major aphthae.

Oral tetracycline has been reported to be effective but should not be used in children aged younger than 9 years.

Suggested Readings

Sonis A, Zaragoza S. Dental health for the pediatrician. *Curr Opin Pediatr.* 2001;13(3):289–295.

✓ Best Tests

- This is usually a clinical diagnosis. Biopsies are nonspecific but can help to rule out other causes.
- If pemphigus is suspected, immunofluorescence should be performed.
- Obtain a viral culture or PCR to rule out HSV on initial presentation.
- Consider a CBC; vitamin B_{12}, B_6, B_2, and B_1 levels; serum folate; zinc; iron; and ferritin.

▲▲ Management Pearls

- Symptomatic relief can be provided with topical anesthetics such as lidocaine 2% (one pea-size application up to four times daily), benzocaine 10% to 20% (apply a thin layer up to four times daily), or dyclonine (one lozenge every 2 h).

CHAPTER 5

Dermatological Therapies

Dermatological care in children and adults makes extensive use of topical agents. This chapter emphasizes important practical points for the safe and optimal use of these topical medications. Details of drug use for specific diseases are covered when specific diseases are considered.

Percutaneous Absorption of Topical Medications

The total systemic absorption of topical medicines is related to the concentrations of the drugs in the vehicle, intactness of the epidermis, the maturity of the epidermis, and the percentage of the body to which the medication is applied. Certain characteristics of the vehicle may affect the acceptance of the medication by the child and the parent.

General Considerations

Body Surface Area and Topical Medications

Percent body surface area (BSA) is often used in burn management to predict the severity of burns and is also useful in determining the extent of dermatologic disease and in estimating the amount of topical medication to be prescribed. In contrast to an adult, a child's head makes up a greater proportion of his or her body surface area, whereas legs make up a lesser proportion.

If the BSA of a patient is known, one can utilize percentages found in the Lund–Browder chart (Table 5-1) to calculate the amount of topical medication required for the patient to treat his or her dermatosis. Table 5-2 was created utilizing current NIH values for children in the 50th percentile in height and weight to calculate average total BSA for each age range and assuming that an average patient appropriately applies one thin layer of ointment at $2\,mg/cm^2$.[1] The Lund–Browder chart was then used to fractionate the quantity of ointment required for each anatomical unit. For example, a 5-year-old child requires approximately 1,000 g of ointment to cover his entire body with ointment twice daily for a month, but only requires 3% of 1,000 g (or 30 g) to cover his lower arm for a month.

Vehicle Recommendations

Vehicles, or bases, are major determinants of medication stability, tolerability, absorption, efficacy, ease of application, and patient acceptance. The fundamental ingredients of vehicles are liquids, powders, and lipids. For most conditions in young pediatric patients, vehicles with higher lipid content are preferred (i.e., ointments and oils) due to their increased moisturizing properties, decreased burning on application, and ability to increase percutaneous absorption

TABLE 5-1 Lund–Browder Chart Relative Percentage of BSA as Affected by Growth

Area	Birth–1 year	1–4 years	5–9 years	10–14 years	15 years	Adult
Head (back or front)	9.5	8.5	6.5	5.5	4.5	3.5
Upper leg	5.5	6.5	8	8.5	8.5	9.5
Lower leg	5	5	5.5	6	6.5	7
Trunk (back or front)	13	13	13	13	13	13
Upper arm	4	4	4	4	4	4
Lower arm	3	3	3	3	3	3

TABLE 5-2 Amount of Topical Ointment Required to Cover Each Area Twice Daily for a Month (in Grams)

Area	Birth–1 year	1–4 years	5–9 years	10–14 years	15 years	Adult
Entire body	250	500	1,000	1,250	2,000	2,250
Head (back or front)	25	50	60	75	85	85
Upper leg	15	35	70	115	150	215
Lower leg	15	30	50	70	125	150
Trunk (back or front)	35	75	115	150	250	300
Upper arm	10	20	35	45	80	90
Lower arm	10	15	30	35	60	65

of most medications. As children approach adolescence, vehicles with higher liquid content should be considered (i.e., creams, lotions, gels, and solutions) because older children are less tolerant of the greasy and occlusive film produced by products with high lipid content; prefer the enhanced spreadability of liquid-based products; and are more prone to acne and folliculitis, which may be exacerbated by lipid-based products. Vehicles with powder added (i.e., pastes and shake lotions) are useful in intertriginous areas where they can be used to decrease friction and absorb excess moisture.

Therapeutic Agents

Topical Corticosteroids

Topical corticosteroids are anti-inflammatory and anti-proliferative agents that are used extensively in pediatric dermatology. Multiple assays have been developed to rank the clinical efficacy of topical steroids, and potency ratings may vary slightly depending on the reference utilized. The Stoughton vasoconstriction assay, in which steroids are classed based on their vasoconstrictive activity, is the most commonly used rating system for the potency of steroids. For most topical corticosteroids, clinical efficacy is well correlated with their position on this ladder (Table 5-3). This is an ordinal scale, not a linear ladder, and patients are often confused when they look at the concentration of a steroid and try to correlate that with its potency. Stronger steroids have lower class numbers.

Potential Side Effects of Topical Steroids

The risk for side effects from topical corticosteroids is increased in infants and children due to their thinner skin, increased surface-to-body volume ratio, and decreased ability to metabolize corticosteroids. Suppression of the hypothalamic–pituitary–adrenal axis may result within a week of exposure to small amounts of superpotent topical steroids (Class 1) or extensive and prolonged exposure to medium potency (Classes 3 and 4). Serious adverse effects, however, have been reported after misuse of topical corticosteroid application.[2–4] Local atrophy can occur with repeated exposure of normal skin to superpotent topical corticosteroids.

Therefore, superpotent topical corticosteroids should be used cautiously and appropriately in children aged <12 years; children prescribed medium- to high-strength topical corticosteroids require regular evaluations and education.

Potential systemic adverse effects:

- Suppression of the hypothalamic–pituitary–adrenal axis
- Iatrogenic Cushing syndrome
- Growth retardation

Potential local adverse effects:

- Epidermal atrophy
- Striae
- Purpura
- Hypopigmentation
- Glaucoma and cataracts from absorption around the eyes
- Cataracts
- Hypertrichosis
- Folliculitis
- Perioral dermatitis
- Granuloma gluteale infantum
- Delayed wound healing

Guidelines and tips to the use of topical steroids in pediatric dermatology:

- Familiarize yourself with a small group of generic topical corticosteroid ointments to use as a practical therapeutic ladder (Table 5-4) (Micromedex).[5] Build upon this ladder as you gain experience with topical corticosteroids. One percentage of hydrocortisone is available without a prescription in the United States.
- Utilize the lowest-strength corticosteroid that will clear dermatitis in a short amount of time (fewer than 7 days).
- If long-term, chronic therapy is required (e.g., atopic dermatitis), intermittent therapy is recommended over continuous therapy. An ideal topical corticosteroid will clear the patient's dermatitis within 3 days and maintain clearance for a week without steriod use before requiring more topical corticosteroid.
- Only very mild topical corticosteroids should be used in the diaper area or on eyelids unless under a physician's direction to do otherwise.

TABLE 5-3 Steroid Potency Ladder: From Most Potent (Class 1) to Least Potent (Class 5)

Ointments and Creams

Class 1

Clobetasol propionate 0.05% ointment and cream	12 years
Halobetasol propionate 0.05% ointment and cream	12 years

Class 2

Betamethasone dipropionate 0.05% ointment and cream	13 years
Amcinonide 0.1% ointment	Pediatric approval
Mometasone furoate 0.1% ointment	2 years
Fluocinonide 0.05% ointment and cream	Pediatric approval
Diflorasone diacetate 0.05% ointment and cream	Pediatric approval
Desoximetasone 0.25% ointment and cream	Pediatric approval, 10 years (product information Topicort)
Halcinonide 0.1% cream	Pediatric approval

Class 3

Triamcinolone acetonide 0.1% ointment	Pediatric approval
Triamcinolone acetonide 0.5% cream	Pediatric approval
Betamethasone valerate 0.1% ointment	Safety and efficacy not established
Fluticasone propionate 0.005% ointment	18 years
Halcinonide 0.1% ointment	Pediatric approval
Amcinonide 0.1% cream	Pediatric approval
Desoximetasone 0.05% cream	Pediatric approval

Class 4

Flurandrenolide 0.05% ointment	Pediatric approval
Fluocinolone acetonide 0.025% ointment	2 years
Hydrocortisone valerate 0.2% ointment	Pediatric approval (product information sheet TaroPharma)
Triamcinolone acetonide 0.1% cream	Pediatric approval
Mometasone furoate 0.1% cream	2 years

Class 5

Flurandrenolide 0.025% ointment	Pediatric approval
Prednicarbate 0.1% ointment and cream	1 year
Hydrocortisone butyrate 0.1% ointment and cream	Pediatric approval (Locoid ointment product information sheet and hydrocortisone butyrate 0.1% cream product information sheet TaroPharma)
Betamethasone valerate 0.1% cream	Safety and efficacy not established
Clocortolone pivalate 0.1% cream	Pediatric approval
Flurandrenolide 0.05% cream	Pediatric approval
Fluticasone propionate 0.05% cream	3 months
Fluocinolone acetonide 0.025% cream	2 years
Hydrocortisone probutate 0.1% cream	Safety and efficacy not established (Pandel product information sheet)
Fluocinolone acetonide 0.01% cream	2 years
Hydrocortisone valerate 0.2% cream	Safety and efficacy not established (product information Westcort cream)

Class 6

Alclometasone dipropionate 0.05% ointment and cream	1 year
Desonide 0.05% ointment and cream	Pediatric approval
Triamcinolone acetonide 0.025% cream	Pediatric approval
Flurandrenolide 0.025% cream	Pediatric approval

Class 7

Hydrocortisone 2.5% ointment and cream	Pediatric approval

TABLE 5-4 Suggested Therapeutic Ladder

Potency (Example)	Dermatosis	Skin Thickness	Location	Length of Continuous Use
Superpotent (Clobetasol Propionate 0.05% ointment)	Resistant and chronic	Very thick or lichenified	Avoid face and skin folds Caution on torso	Monitor closely if >2–3 weeks
High (Fluocinonide 0.05% ointment)	Severe and chronic	Very thick or lichenified	Peripheral extremities Avoid face and skin folds Caution on torso	Monitor closely if >2–3 weeks
Intermediate (Triamcinolone Acetonide 0.1% ointment)	Moderate acute or chronic	Moderately thick Mildly lichenified	Torso and extremities Caution on face or skin folds	Monitor closely if >2–3 weeks on face or skin folds or >3 months on body
Low (Desonide 0.05% ointment)	Mild acute	Minimal thickness, no lichenification	Face and skin folds	Monitor regularly if >4 weeks on face or skin folds
Very low (Hydrocortisone 2.5% ointment)	Very mild acute	No thickening, no lichenification	Face, skin folds occluded areas (diaper area)	Monitor regularly if >4 weeks on infants

- Recognize that ointments are usually stronger than other formulations when changing the vehicles (e.g., changing from an ointment to a solution to treat a dermatosis of the scalp).

Systemic Corticosteroids

The use of systemic corticosteroids is limited to specific severe disorders in pediatric dermatology, including lupus erythematosus, autoimmune disease, bullous dermatoses, acute allergic reactions, and complicated hemangiomas. Systemic steroids are very rarely indicated for psoriasis or atopic dermatitis. The most commonly used steroids are prednisone and prednisolone, typically at doses between 0.5 and 2 mg/kg/day (Table 5-5). While on long-term therapy (>2 to 4 weeks), children should be closely monitored for side effects (see below); have their growth and blood pressure followed; and should avoid live vaccines (varicella–zoster, measles, mumps, rubella, and rotavirus).

Potential adverse effects of systemic steroids:

- Suppression of the hypothalamic–pituitary–adrenal axis
- Adrenal crisis
- Hyperglycemia
- Hypertension
- Congestive heart failure
- Hyperlipidemia
- Cushingoid changes
- Growth retardation
- Osteoporosis
- Osteonecrosis
- Peptic ulcer disease
- Bowel perforation
- Cataracts
- Agitation
- Immunosuppression
- Myopathy
- Delayed wound healing
- Pseudotumor cerebri
- Perioral dermatitis
- Steroid acne
- Striae

Antiparasitic Agents

Most cases of lice and scabies are treatable with topical agents and sometimes, systemic agents. Those agents and their usage are listed in Table 5-6.

Topical anesthetics

Topical anesthetics are useful for minor procedures on intact skin (needle or laser procedures). More invasive procedures, such as excisions, require the addition of local anesthetics or general anesthesia. Contraindications to topical anesthetics include allergy to amide anesthetics, nonintact skin, and for EMLA, recent sulfonamide antibiotic use and methemoglobinemia. Dosing and proper application of topical anesthetics are described in Tables 5-7–5-9 (Drugdex [Thomson Micromedex Healthcare Series]).[6,7]

Local Anesthetics

Local anesthetics are required for invasive dermatologic procedures in infants and children (e.g., biopsies and

TABLE 5-5 Systemic Corticosteroids Equivalent Dosing (mg)

Cortisone	25
Hydrocortisone	20
Prednisone	5
Prednisolone	5
Methylprednisolone	4
Triamcinolone	4
Dexamethasone	0.75
Betamethasone	0.75

TABLE 5-6 Common Antiparasitic Agents and Their Uses

Name	Available Formulations	Recommended Age/Weight	Use
Pyrethrins with piperonyl butoxide	0.3% shampoo or lotion 0.18% lotion	>2 years	Pediculosis
Permethrin	1% and 5% cream	>2 months	Pediculosis and scabies
Ivermectin	3 mg tablets	>5 years and >15 kg	Pediculosis and scabies
Lindane	1% shampoo or lotion	>50 kg	Pediculosis and scabies
Crotamiton	10% cream or lotion	N/A[a]	Scabies
Malathion	0.5% lotion	>6 years	Pediculosis
Benzyl benzoate	20%–25% solution	N/A[a]	Scabies
Thiabendazole	500 mg/5 mL suspension 500 mg tablets	>13.6 kg	Cutaneous larva migrans
Precipitated sulfur	6% ointment	N/A[a]	Scabies

[a]Safety and efficacy not established in children.
Source: Micromedex.

TABLE 5-7 Onset of Action for Topical Anesthetics

Brand	Active Ingredients	Onset of Action
EMLA	2.5% lidocaine and 2.5% prilocaine	60–120 min
LMX-4	4% lidocaine	30–60 min
LMX-5	5% lidocaine	30–60 min
Topicaine	4% lidocaine	30–60 min

TABLE 5-8 Maximum Dose of EMLA

Age	Weight (kg)	Maximum Dose (g)	Maximum Application Area (cm²)
1–3 months	<5	1	10
3–12 months	5–10	2	20
1–6 years	10–20	10	100
7–12 years	>20	20	200

Source: *Physicians' Desk Reference: PDR 2003*. 57th Ed. Montvale, NJ: Thomson PDR; 2003.

TABLE 5-9 Maximum Dose of Lidocaine Cream

Weight (kg)	Maximum Application Area (cm²)
<10	100
10–20	200

Source: Drugdex (Thomson Micromedex Healthcare Series).

TABLE 5-10 Maximum Dose for Local Anesthetics in Children and Neonates

Name	Max. Neonatal Dose	Max. Pediatric Dose
Lidocaine	4 mg/kg	5 mg/kg
Lidocaine with epinephrine	5 mg/kg	7 mg/kg
Bupivacaine	2 mg/kg	2.5 mg/kg
Bupivacaine with epinephrine	2 mg/kg	4 mg/kg
Mepivacaine	4 mg/kg	5 mg/kg

excisions).[8,9] Less local anesthetic per body weight can be given to neonates than children and adults, due to decreased metabolic clearance, decreased plasma binding proteins, and harder-to-recognize warning signs of toxic effects. Maximum dosage and onset of action information for local anesthetics can be found in Tables 5-10 and 5-11.

Topical Antifungal Agents

Many topical antifungal agents are available for the treatment of superficial dermatophyte and yeast infections (Table 5-12). They are usually applied once to twice daily, but more frequent application may be required if removed by bathing or perspiration. Several agents, such as clotrimazole, miconazole, and terbinafine are available as over-the-counter medications and are good first-line agents. Undecylenic acid and tolnaftate are usually less effective than prescription medications. It is not recommended to use combination products containing corticosteroids, especially in the diaper area where increased local and systemic absorption occurs.

TABLE 5-11 Onset of Action for Local Anesthetics

Name	Onset of Action	Duration
Lidocaine	<1 min	30–120 min
Lidocaine with epinephrine	<1 min	60–400 min
Bupivacaine	2–10 min	120–240 min
Bupivacaine with epinephrine	2–10 min	240–480 min
Mepivacaine	3–20 min	30–120 min

Acne Medications

The basic principle in treating acne is to utilize the simplest regimen possible that adequately controls the disease. Once a treatment regimen is begun, medications should be titrated regularly to optimize clinical response and minimize irritation.

As retinoids affect all acne lesions, they should be included as first-line agents in every acne regimen. Topical retinoids are ranked by the efficacy of their antiacne action in increasing strength from azelaic acid as the weakest retinoid to adapalene, to tretinoin, and to tazarotene as the strongest agent in the retinoid class (Table 5-13). Irritancy parallels efficacy, such that tazarotene—the strongest retinoid—is also the most irritating. Many physicians start with a topical tretinoin product (e.g., tretinoin 0.05% cream) and titrate up or down the retinoid ladder based on clinical response and level of irritation.

Other medications may be used in addition to topical retinoids to reduce specific acne lesions. Topical antibiotics are most useful in decreasing inflammatory (erythematous or pustular) acne lesions. Oral antibiotics are most useful in decreasing deep acne nodules. Hormonal therapies are especially useful in females who have acne flares with menstrual cycles. Combination products are used to simplify a patient's acne regimen.

Isotretinoin is used when the above regimens fail. Treatment usually lasts approximately 6 months, after which patients are either "cured" of their acne or have residual acne that is much more sensitive to standard therapies. As the use of isotretinoin is highly regulated and requires close monitoring, specialist referral is usually required for its use.

Toxicity from Topical Agents

The literature is replete with cases reports and series of severe systemic toxicity for topical agents (Table 5-14). The key factors are the amount of BSA to which the drug is applied and the decreased barrier properties of the stratum corneum especially in prematurity or in those with extensive blistering or scaling skin diseases.

TABLE 5-12 Topical Antifungal Agents

Name	Spectrum	Formulation	Age of FDA approval
Undecylenic acid	Dermatophytes, *Candida*	Cream, foam, spray, powder ointment	[a]
Tolnaftate	Dermatophytes	Cream, gel, spray, powder	2 years
Ciclopirox	Dermatophytes, yeast	Cream, gel, lotion, solution, nail lacquer	16 years
Clotrimazole	Dermatophytes, yeast	Cream, lotion, spray	Pediatric
Miconazole nitrate	Dermatophytes, yeast	Cream	2 years
Econazole nitrate	Dermatophytes, yeast	Cream	[b]
Sulconazole	Dermatophytes, yeast	Cream, solution	[b]
Ketoconazole	Dermatophytes, *Candida*, *Pityrosporum*	Shampoo / Cream	12 years / [b]
Oxiconazole	Dermatophytes, yeast, *Pityrosporum*	Cream, lotion	Pediatric
Naftifine	Dermatophytes, *Candida*, *Pityrosporum*	Cream, gel	[b]
Terbinafine	Dermatophytes, *Candida*, *Pityrosporum*	Cream, solution, spray	12 years
Butenafine	Dermatophytes, *Candida*, *Pityrosporum*	Cream	12 years
Nystatin	*Candida*	Cream, ointment powder	Pediatric[b]

[a]No specific labeling on safety in children.
[b]Safety and efficacy not established in children.

TABLE 5-13 Dosage of Acne Medications

Class	Name	Dosage/Application
Topical retinoids: Prevent formation of precursor lesions, decrease comedones and inflammatory lesions		
	Tazarotene	0.05%–0.1% gel or cream qhs
	Tretinoin	0.025%–0.1% cream, gel, or solution qhs
	Adapalene	0.3%–0.1% cream, gel, solution, or swab qhs
	Azelaic acid	15%–20% cream or gel qhs
Topical antibiotics: Decrease inflammatory lesions		
	Clindamycin phosphate	1% solution, lotion, pad or gel q.d. to b.i.d.
	Erythromycin	2% ointment, solution, or pad b.i.d.
	Benzoyl peroxide	2.5%–10% cream, gel, lotion, liquid, pad, soap, or solution q.d. to b.i.d.
	Sulfur	1%–10% lotion, ointment, cream, soap q.d.–t.i.d.
	Sodium sulfacetamide	10% lotion, pad, cream, or soap b.i.d.
Combination products: Combined effects two topical therapies in one formulation		
	Benzoyl peroxide/erythromycin	3%/5% cream b.i.d.
	Benzoyl peroxide/clindamycin	1%/5% cream q.d.
	Clindamycin/tretinoin	1.2%/0.025% gel qhs
Systemic antibiotics: Decrease superficial and deep inflammatory lesions		
	Tetracycline	500 mg b.i.d.
	Doxycycline	100 mg b.i.d.
	Minocycline	100 mg b.i.d.
Systemic retinoids: Decrease comedones, superficial, and deep inflammatory lesions		
	Isotretinoin	Up to 2 mg/kg daily or divided b.i.d.
Hormonal therapies: Decreases comedones, superficial, and deep inflammatory lesions in women		
	Spironolactone	50–100 mg b.i.d.
	Estrogens	Various

TABLE 5-14 Potential Toxicities in Children and Infants from Commonly Used Topical Agents

Compound	Use	Toxicity	Risk Factors/Comments
Alcohols	Antiseptic	Hemorrhagic necrosis	Occlusion Preterm infants
Topical corticosteroids	Anti-inflammatory agent	Adrenal suppression	Occlusion (diaper area) Superpotent corticosteroids Use over extensive body surface area
Calcipotriol	Vitamin D analog	Hypercalcemia	Regular monitoring of serum calcium recommended in children and infants
Diphenhydramine	Topical antipruritic	Central anticholinergic Syndrome	Not recommended in infants Apply to affected area not more than 4 times daily
Lidocaine	Topical anesthetic	Petechiae, seizures	Children <2 years Use over recommended amount (see lidocaine dosing chart)
Lindane	Scabicide	Neurotoxicity	Children <50 kg Other skin conditions (atopic dermatitis) Seizure disorder Use over 2 ounces
N,N-Diethyl-m-toluamide (DEET)	Insect repellant	Neurotoxicity	Infants <2 months Use over 30% concentration Reapplication more than recommended by manufacturer
Neomycin	Topical antibiotic	Ototoxicity	Premature infants
Povidone-iodine	Antiseptic	Hypothyroidism	Premature infants
Prilocaine	Topical anesthetic	Methemoglobinemia	Use over recommended amount (see EMLA dosing chart)
Salicylic acid	Keratolytic agent	Salicylism, encephalopathy, metabolic acidosis	Use >20% body surface area
Silver sulfadiazine	Topical antibiotic	Kernicterus, agranulocytosis	Infants <2 months

Source: Micromedex.

Over-the-Counter Medications

Sunscreens

Sunscreens are FDA approved for children aged 6 months and older and should be recommended to all pediatric patients. The American Academy of Dermatology recommends the use of broad spectrum sunscreens that are water resistant, with a sunburn protection factor (SPF) of 15 and above.

Sunscreen Labeling

SPF: Time to produce erythema (redness) on protected skin divided by time to produce erythema on unprotected skin.
Broad spectrum protection: Protection over UVA and UVB spectrum.
Water resistant: Maintains SPF after 40 min of water immersion.
Very water resistant/waterproof: Maintains SPF after 80 min water immersion.

Insect Repellants

Insect repellants are not recommended for children aged <2 months.[10] Products containing *N,N*-diethyl-*m*-toluamide (DEET) or picaridin are formulated for direct use on the skin.[11] Repellants containing permethrin are formulated for use on clothing. DEET is safe in concentrations up to 30% on children. Picaridin is safe in concentrations up to 15% on children.

Systemic Medications Often Used for Children

Commonly Used Oral Antibiotics[12,13]

Some of the common antibiotics used for cutaneous infections are outlined in Table 5-15. The choice of specific antibiotics is discussed in the section for each disease.

H1-antihistamines[14]

Antihistamines can be very useful for pruritus. Age specific dosing is important to prevent side effects (Tables 5-16 and 5-17).

TABLE 5-15 Commonly Used Oral Antibiotics

Name	Formulations	Dose	Max. Dose
Amoxicillin	Drops: 50 mg/mL Suspension: 125, 200, 250, or 400 mg/5 mL Caps: 250, 500 mg Tabs: 500, 875 mg Chewable tabs: 125, 200, 250, 400 mg Tabs for oral suspension: 200, 400, 600 mg	Infant <3 months: 20–30 mg/kg/24 h divided b.i.d.–t.i.d. Child: 25–90 mg/kg/24 h divided b.i.d.–t.i.d. Adult: 250–500 mg/dose t.i.d.	2–3 g/24 h
Amoxicillin–clavulanic acid	Tabs: 250, 500, 875 mg amoxicillin Extended release tabs: 1 g amoxicillin Chewable tabs: 125, 200, 250, 400 mg amoxicillin Suspension 125, 200, 250, 400 mg amoxicillin/5 mL	Infant <3 months: 30 mg/kg/24 h divided b.i.d. Children: 20–90 mg/kg/24 h divided b.i.d.–t.i.d. Adults: 250–500 mg/dose t.i.d.	2–3 g/24 h
Ampicillin	Suspension: 125, 250 mg/5 mL Caps: 250, 500 mg	Infant/child: 50–100 mg/kg/24 h divided q6h Adult: 250–500 mg q6h	2–3 g/24 h
Azithromycin	Tabs: 250, 500, 600 mg Suspension: 100, 200 mg/5 mL	Infant/child >6 months: 5-day regimen: 10 mg/kg on day 1 followed by 5 mg/kg q24h × 4 days 3-day regimen: 10 mg/kg daily × 3 days 1-day regimen: 30 mg/kg once Adults: 500 mg on day 1 followed by 250 mg × 4 days	Multiple day regimens: 500 mg/24 h 1-day regimen: 1,500 mg/24 h
Cefaclor	Caps: 250, 500 mg Suspension: 125, 187, 250, 375 mg/5 mL	Infant/child: 20–40 mg/kg/24 h divided q8h Adult: 250–500 mg/dose q8h	Infant/child: 2 g/24 h Adult: 4 g/24 h
Cephalexin	Tabs: 250, 500 mg Caps: 250, 500 mg Suspension: 125, 250 mg/5 mL	Infant/child: 25–100 mg/kg/24 h divided b.i.d.–q.i.d Adult: 1–4 g/24 h divided b.i.d.–q.i.d	4 g/24 h
Clarithromycin	Film tablets: 250, 500 mg Extended-release tabs: 500 mg Granules for suspension: 125, 250 mg/5 mL	Child: 15 mg/kg/24 h divided b.i.d. Adult: 250–500 mg/dose b.i.d.	1 g/24 h

(Continued)

TABLE 5-15 *(Continued)*

Name	Formulations	Dose	Max. Dose
Ciprofloxacin	Tabs: 100, 250, 500, 750 mg Extended-release tabs: 500, 1,000 mg Suspension: 250, 500 mg/5 mL	Neonate: 10 mg/kg b.i.d. Child: 15–40 mg/kg/24 h divided b.i.d. Adult: 250–750 mg/dose b.i.d.	2 g/24 h
Clindamycin	Caps: 75, 150, 300 mg Oral solution: 75 mg/5 mL	Child: 10–30 mg/kg/24 h divided q6–8h Adult: 150–450 mg/dose q6–8h	1.8 g/24 h
Dicloxacillin sodium	Caps: 250, 500 mg	Child: 12.5–100 mg/kg/24 h divided q6h Adult: 125–500 mg/dose q6h	4 g/24 h
Doxycycline	Caps: 20, 50, 75, 100 mg Tabs: 20, 50, 100 mg Syrup: 50 mg/5 mL Suspension: 25 mg/5 mL	Child: 2–5 mg/kg/24 h divided q.d.–b.i.d. Adult: 100–200 mg/24 h divided q.d.–b.i.d.	200 mg/24 h
Erythromycin	Estolate: Suspension: 125, 250 mg/5 mL Ethyl succinate (EES): Suspension: 200, 400 mg/5 mL Oral drops: 100 mg/2.5 mL Chewable tabs: 200 mg Tabs: 400 mg Base: Tabs: 250, 333, 500 mg	Neonate 0–7 days or <1.2 kg: 20 mg/kg/24 h divided b.i.d. Neonate >7 days and >1.2 kg: 30 mg/kg/24 h divided t.i.d. Child: 30–50 mg/kg/24 h divided q6–8h Adult: 1–4 g/24 h divided q6h	Child: 2 g/24 h Adult: 4 g/24 h
Minocycline	Tabs: 50, 75, 100 mg Caps: 50, 75, 100 mg Caps (pellet filled): 50, 100 mg Oral suspension: 50 mg/5 mL	Child (8–12 years): 2–4 mg/kg/24 h divided q.d.–b.i.d. Adult: 50–100 mg/dose q.d.–t.i.d.	200 mg/24 h
Nafcillin	Caps: 250 mg	Infant/child: 50–100 mg/kg/24 h divided q6h Adult: 250–1,000 mg q4–6h	12 g/24 h
Oxacillin	Oral solution: 250 mg/5 mL	Infant/child: 50–100 mg/kg/24 h divided q6h Adult: 500–1,000 mg/dose q4–6h	12 g/24 h
Penicillin V potassium	Tabs: 250, 500 mg Oral solution: 125, 250 mg/5 mL	Child: 25–50 mg/kg/24 h divided q6–8h Adult: 250–500 mg/dose divided q6–8h	3 g/24 h
Tetracycline	Caps: 250, 500 mg Suspension: 125 mg/5 mL	Child (>8 years): 25–50 mg/kg/24 h divided q6h Adult: 1–2 g/24 h divided q6–12h	3 g/24 h
Trimethoprim-sulfamethox-azole	Tabs (regular strength): 80 mg TMP/400 mg SMX Tabs (double strength): 160 mg TMP/800 mg SMX Suspension: 40 mg TMP/200 mg SMX/5 mL	Child: 6–20 mg TMP/kg/24 h divided b.i.d. Adult: 160 mg TMP/dose b.i.d.	320 mg TMP/24 h

TABLE 5-16 H1-Antihistamines

Name	Antihistamine Effect	Anticholinergic Effect	Sedative Effect
Chlorpheniramine	Moderate	Moderate	Mild
Cyproheptadine	Moderate	Moderate	Mild
Diphenhydramine	Mild	Strong	Strong
Hydroxyzine HCl	Strong	Moderate	Strong
Loratadine	Strong	Weak	Rare
Fexofenadine	Strong	Weak	Rare
Cetirizine HCl	Strong	Weak	Occasional
Promethazine	Very strong	Strong	Strong

TABLE 5-17 Dosing of Commonly Used H1-Antihistamines

First Generation H1-Antihistamines

Diphenhydramine	2–6 years: 6.25 mg q4–6h; maximum 37.5 mg/day
	6–12 years: 12.5–25 mg q4–6h; maximum 150 mg/day
	>12 years: 25–50 mg q4–6h; maximum 300 mg/day
Hydroxyzine	2 mg/kg/24 h divided q6–8h

Second Generation H1-Antihistamines

Cetirizine	0.5–2 years: 2.5 mg q.d.
	2–5 years: 2.5–5 mg q.d.
	>6 years: 10 mg q.d.
Levocetirizine	6–11 years: 2.5 mg q.d.
	>12 years: 5 mg q.d.
Loratadine	2–5 years: 5 mg q.d.
	>6 years: 10 mg q.d.
Desloratadine	0.5–1 year: 1 mg q.d.
	1–5 years: 1.25 mg q.d.
	6–12 years: 2.5 mg q.d.
	>12 years: 5 mg q.d.
Fexofenadine	6–12 years: 30 mg b.i.d.
	>12 years: 60 mg b.i.d. or 180 mg q.d.

Source: Modified from Milgrom H, Leung DY. Allergic rhinitis. In: Kliegman R, Nelson WE, eds. *Nelson Textbook of Pediatrics.* 18th Ed. Philadelphia, PA: WB Saunders; 2007:951 (ref. 15).

TABLE 5-18 Dosage of Commonly Used Immunomodulators

Name	Common Pediatric Dermatologic Indications	Pediatric Dosage Range
Methotrexate	Psoriasis Morphea	5–15 mg/m^2
Azathioprine	Atopic dermatitis Immunobullous disease	0.5–3 mg/m^{2a}
Mycophenolate mofetil	Atopic dermatitis Psoriasis Immunobullous disease	30–50 mg/kg/day
Cyclosporine	Psoriasis Atopic dermatitis	2.5–5 mg/kg/day
Etanercept	Psoriasis	0.8 mg/kg 2×/week
Hydroxy-chloroquine	Lupus erythematosus Porphyria cutanea tarda Polymorphous light eruption	4–6.5 mg/kg/day
Dapsone	Immunobullous disease Pyoderma gangrenosum Pustular psoriasis	0.5–2 mg/kg/day
Etanercept	Psoriasis	0.8 mg/kg/week

^{a}Initial dosing based on TMPT level.

TABLE 5-19 Commonly Used Systemic Retinoids

Name	Indication	Dose
Acitretin	Psoriasis	0.5 mg/kg/day
Isotretinoin	Acne	0.5–2 mg/kg/day

Immunomodulators

Systemic immunomodulators are important agents for patients with significant cutaneous and systemic disorders and should be used by those with experience with these agents and their side effects (Table 5-18).

Systemic Retinoids

Both systemic retinoids have the potential for causing birth defects in females of child-bearing potential and establishing guidelines for their use MUST be followed (Table 5-19).

References

1. Nelson AA, Miller AD, Fleischer AB, et al. How much of a topical agent should be prescribed for children of different sizes? *J Dermatolog Treat.* 2006;17(4):224–228.

2. Katz HI, Prawer SE, Mooney JJ, et al. Preatrophy: Covert sign of thinned skin. *J Am Acad Dermatol.* 1989;20(5 Pt 1):731–735.

3. Gilbertson EO, Spellman MC, Piacquadio DJ, et al. Super potent topical corticosteroid use associated with adrenal suppression: Clinical considerations. *J Am Acad Dermatol.* 1998;38(2 Pt 2):318–321.

4. Warner MR, Camisa C. Topical corticosteroids. In: Wolverton SE, ed. *Comprehensive Dermatologic Drug Therapy.* 2nd Ed. Philadelphia, PA: WB Saunders Elsevier; 2007:595–624.

5. Drake LA, Dinehart SM, Farmer ER, et al. Guidelines of care for the use of topical glucocorticosteroids. American Academy of Dermatology. *J Am Acad Dermatol.* 1996;35(4):615–619.

6. Soriano TT, Lask GP, Dinehart SM. Anesthesia and analgesia. In: Robinson JK, Hanke WC, Sengelmann R, Siegel D, eds. *Surgery of the Skin: Procedural Dermatology.* Philadelphia, PA: Elsevier Mosby; 2005:39–58.

7. *Physicians' Desk Reference: PDR 2008.* 62nd Ed. Montvale, NJ: Thomson PDR; 2008.

8. Berde CB, Sethna NF. Analgesics for the treatment of pain in children. *N Engl J Med.* 2002;347(14):1094–1103.

9. Lubenow TR, Ivankovich AD, Barkin RL. Management of acute postoperative pain. In: Barash PG, Cullen BF, Stoelting RK, eds. *Clinical Anesthesia.* 5th Ed. Philadelphia, PA: Lippincott Williams & Wilkins; 2006:1405–1440.

10. Etzel RA, Balk SJ, eds. Pediatric *Environmental Health.* 2nd Ed. Elk Grove Village, IL: American Academy of Pediatrics; 2003.

11. Katz TM, Miller JH, Herbert AA. Insect repellents: Historical perspectives and new developments. *J Am Acad Dermatol.* 2008;58:865–871.

12. Lee C, Robertson J, Shilkofski N. Drug doses. In: Robertson J, Shilkofski N, eds. *Johns Hopkins: The Harriet Lane Handbook: A Manual for Pediatric House Officers.* 17th Ed. Philadelphia, PA: Elsevier Mosby; 2005, Chapter 27.

13. Schleiss MR. Principles of antibacterial therapy. In: Kliegman RM, Behrman RE, Jenson HB, Stanton BF, eds. *Nelson Textbook of Pediatrics.* 18th Ed. Philadelphia, PA: WB Saunders; 2007:1110–1122.

14. Scheman AJ, Severson DL, eds. *Pocket Guide to Medications Used in Dermatology.* Philadelphia, PA: Lippincott Williams & Wilkins; 2003.

15. Milgrom H, Leung DY. Allergic rhinitis. In: Kliegman R, Nelson WE, eds. *Nelson Textbook of Pediatrics.* 18th Ed. Philadelphia, PA: WB Saunders; 2007:951.

Index

Note: Page numbers followed by "f"/"fs" denote figures and those followed by "t"/"ts" denote tables.